Selective Diagnosis And Causes ofDeath

Dr Benjamin Alli is a Sakellarides Professor of
Medicine and Surgery and the Chancellor of
The Royal College of Physicians and Surgeons
of the United States of America.

Published By: **Elite Exclusivity**
Edited By: **Mugheer Ahmad**
Introduction By: **Dr. Christopher W. Smithmyer**

Elite exclusivity

Dysart Detroit Dallas

Published by Elite Exclusivity LP

Send all Inquiries to: EliteExclusivityPR@gmail.com and
Info@EliteExclusivity.com

ISBN Paperback: 978-1-952651-08-3
ISBN Hardback: 978-1-952651-14-4
ISBN Digital: 978-1-952651-09-0

Printed in the United States of America

Table of Contents

INTRODUCTION

Understanding the development of medicine over the last 40 years requires one to look at what was, what is, and what is coming. While there have been many changes in medicine over the last 40 years, we must always ask, "Are these changes for the better?" Doctors, medical doctors anyway, have an oath to uphold that they do no harm, any time new movements are made in medicine this position needs to be reexamined.

One of the key features that many medical procedures need to review is whether the practice helps the patient or helps the insurance companies. As medicine has become a business, practical methodologies for treating patients have been superseded by profit generating procedures. This takes the patient care out of medicine and creates problems across the board. While the doctors are on the front lines of the treatment process, they are often a patient away from the front lines of the regulatory process. This allows lobbyists from many industries to have a large say in the treatment of patients than the doctors that are actively collaborating with the patients.

Dr. Alli's book is an echo of the medical field of yesteryear, looking at how medicine was conducted before the insurance companies, politicians and lobbyists were involved. Dr. Alli looks at procedures that help patients and look to fulfill the oath of "Do no harm." Too many young doctors are being driven from the field by the "profit now" mentality- hopefully, this text, in some small way will help them realize that the doctors are not the problem- the people setting up regulations for profit are.

What is a Selective Diagnosis book?

This book is a type of medical reference book that might provide healthcare professionals with a comprehensive guide to the diagnosis of medical conditions.

Selective Diagnosis and Causes of Death

In addition to providing information on the diagnosis of medical conditions, this includes information on the differential diagnosis of different conditions, which involves distinguishing one condition from another that may present with similar symptoms.

This book may be a good resource for healthcare professionals, providing examples of information to possibly diagnose and treat a wide range of medical conditions.

Please note that any and all numbers, medicine and more contained in this book are for reference and learning purposes only. Please confirm with healthcare professionals for exact numbers, medicine specific to you and/ or patient needs and more.

Part I: General Principles of Newborn Evaluation and Care

The neonatal period is the first 4 weeks of life. Fetal and neonatal life is a continuum during whichthe growth and development of the human organism are affected by genetic and enviroiienta1 factors (intrauterine and extra uterine). General principles of newborn evaluation and care will include delivery room care where maternal and fetal factors are considered-This care will differ for high-risk and normal infants.

Also, nursery care includes feeding and nutrition, temperature control, and physical examination ofthe neonate.

Intensive care may be needed and includes keeping the airway patent, affording ventilation,and different procedures if needed. Then there are the problems that may arise and must be dealt with, like delivery room care.

The immediate care in the delivery room includes basically clearing the airway, temperature maintenance, and Apgar scoring-Eye care, cord care, and vitamin X administration may be donein the delivery room or on admission to the nursery.

PROCEDURAL METHODOLOGY

Establishing respiratory

The infant should be suspended head downward immediately by holding him with the heels for a few seconds until the mouth, pharynx, and nose are cleared of blood, amniotic fluid, or mucus that has been aspirated during labour by gravity. Blood and mucus are then removed from the mouth, nose, and throat by means of a suction bulb (bulb syringe or soft rubber catheter used.

The mouth should be sucked before the nose, as suctioning of the nose can result in stimulation of gasp and cause aspiration ratio of materials that may be in the oropharynx-Except during resuscitation or the presence of thick meconium, the suction trap should not be used as it may cause cardiac arrhythmia and respiratory arrest due to vasovagal reflex. When respiratory starts, the baby is put on sterile towels on his side, head lower than the rest of the body, to promote drainage from the respiratory tract for 4-8 hours. The reverse position is indicated if there is the possibility of intracranial haemorrhage following a difficult delivery. Ordinarily, gentle body massage, rhythmic flexion of the legs over the abdomen, or gentle dilatation of the rectal sphincter will be sufficient to promote spontaneous breathing within 2- 3 minutes.

APGAR SCORING

Immediate evaluation of new-born at 1 and 5 minutes determines the prognosis and need for closer observation and exceptional care. The infant in the best condition (score 8-10) is vigorous, pink, and crying. A moderately depressed infant (score 5-7) appears cyanotic with slow and irregular respiration but has good muscle tone and reflexes. The severely depressed infant (score four or less) is limp, Pale, or blue, apnoeic, and has a slow heart rate. Taken at 1 minute, it is an index of asphyxia and needs for assisted ventilation; taken at 5 minutes, it is the true index of the likelihood of death and neurological residue (indicates neonatal and long-term prognosis). Asphyxiated babies should (have an Apgar score every 5 minutes till their score is seven or more. In LBW infants, immaturity militates against normal muscle tone; also, their small size predisposes them to more severe shock, so they may have exceptionally low Apgar scores without any prognostic value.

Apgar score taken 1 min and 5 min after complete birth of

infant (after completion of second stage of labour)

	0	1	2
Heart Rate Respiratory Muscle Effort	Absent Limp	Slow (less than 100) Slow, irregular Some flexions of extremities	More than 100 good crying active motion
Response to the catheter in nostril (evaluated after oropharynx is cleared)	No Response	Grimace	Cough or sneezing
Color	Blue or pale	Body pink, extremities blue	Completely pink

CONSERVATION OF BODY TEMPERATURE

Conservation of body temperature is essential because the newborn is prone to subnormal temperatures, and cold stress may result in diminished oxygenation acidosis, excessive weight loss, and increased mortality. Conservation of body temperature is moreimportant in every LBW infant and in the infant severely.

Oxygen consumption in newborns varies with the gradient between skin and environmental temperatures; it is the least when the gradient is less than 1.5 C. Even a slight increase in the body temperature of the infant increase's oxygen consumption. After vaginal delivery and labor, many have mild to moderate metabolic acidosis, which is compensated for by the elimination of 002. This compensation: is more difficult for depressed infants, and progressive metabolic and respiratory acidosis may result from prolonged exposure to usual room temperatures. The body temperature of the newborn must be maintained within a very narrow range of 36.5-37.3 C to minimize the infant's caloric expenditure in response to heat or cold stress. The infant's skin must be dry because the evaporative loss of heat is very large, and it is difficult to support the body temperate if the skin is wet. A radiant heater must be used in the delivery room until the infant is stable and can be taken to the nursery. The infant must be dried immediately and wrapped with blankets to protect him immediately from heat loss. Hypothermia will give rise to hypoglycemia also. In India, the room temperature is usually high. Sometimes, so cooling the roomis needed instead of heating it. Heat loss may be minimized by placing an infant in a Neutral Thermal Environment NTE, which is the thermal condition at which the heat production isminimal, yet the core temperature is within the normal range.

Birth Weight		Incubator temperature for first 24 hours
Kg	Lb.	35
1	2	34.9
	3	34.2
1.5		34.0
	4	33.7

2		
	5	33.5
2.5		33.3
	6	33.2
3		33.1
		33.0

The newborn loses heat readily because of the relatively large surface area in relation to body weight. The heat loss of babies who are wet and exposed to cool air is 5 times that of dried and warmed infants. Body temperature will fall precipitously in a cool environment unless adequate precautions are taken. With a fall in body temperature, the infant becomes cyanotic first in hands and feet, then in the face, and finally over the entire body, and may develop grunting respirations and retractions. A change in cardiac output occurs in hypothermia, and this altered state leads to metabolic acidosis, gradually increasing hypoxia, hypoglycemia, and shock. Examination in the delivery room must be done under a radian warmer.

CARE OF SKIN AND CORD:

To decrease the occurrence of skin and paraumbilical infections, it is important to thoroughly clean the skin and umbilical cord of the newborn. This should be done in the delivery room or upon admission to the nursery using sterile cotton soaked in warm water and a detergent solution. The creases where the cord meets the umbilicus should be cleaned using a cotton-tipped applicator. After rinsing the baby with water at body temperature, they should be thoroughly dried between blankets and covered in a sterilized blanket. In hot and humid climates or unfavorable hygienic conditions, an early bath may be necessary.

To avoid causing any harm to the delicate skin of the newborn, it is important to avoid excessive manipulation. Excess vernix caseosa, particularly in areas like the armpits, neck, folds, and groins, should be gently removed with sterile cotton wool. The bath water temperature should be around 37 degrees Celsius and a mild soap should be used. After drying the flexures, neck folds, axillae, and areas behind the ears, baby powder should be sprinkled on these areas. It is not recommended to use detergent solutions such as 3% hexachlorophene for prolonged periods as it can be neurotoxic. Instead, a single bath with a 3% hexachlorophene solution at 2-4 hours of life, followed by thorough rinsing, can help reduce colonization by S. aureus. Personnel should also use this solution for handwashing.

To prevent bacterial colonization and omphalitis, triple dye or a Bacitracin ointment should be applied to the umbilical cord immediately after birth and daily thereafter. The umbilical area must be kept dry and clean. If there is bleeding from the stump due to a slipped or loose ligature, the cord must be re-tied. Regular inspection of the cord is crucial to detect any possible infection or hemorrhage. In moist areas, dabbing with 70% alcohol is recommended. After the umbilical stump heals, a second bath can be given, but prior to that, only a sponge bath is advised. A daily bath, including washing the scalp, is necessary in tropical regions. The best time for bathing is in the afternoon before feeding.

Promptly change wet or soiled diapers and clean the anal region and buttocks with cotton wool soaked in clean or soapy water. After thorough rinsing, baby powder can be used on these areas, taking care to avoid sprinkling it into the vulva or feet of the infant. If there is diaper rash, mineral or olive oil can be used on irritated areas instead of soap and water. The tender skin of the infant is susceptible to trauma and infection, leading to various skin conditions such as pustules, pemphigus, boils, cellulitis, and exfoliative dermatitis, often caused by staphylococcus and streptococcus bacteria. Strict aseptic precautions are necessary, and attendants must wash their hands every time they touch the infant. Ideally, the care of the newborn should be entrusted to one person, preferably the mother. Infected patients should be isolated from healthy infants and not cared for by the same nurse. If necessary, antibiotics should be administered and infected skin areas should be covered loosely to prevent localized heat or perspiration. The infant should be protected from insect and mosquito bites.

CARE OF THE EYES

Prevention of gonococcus ophthalmic neonatorum is still recommended. One method is to use silver nitrate and instill a 1% solution into both eyes, ensuring that the surface of the conjunctivae is properly bathed in the solution. It is preferable to use single-dose vials for this purpose. After instilling AgNO3, the eyes should not be irrigated with water or saline. However, some believe that promptly irrigating the eyes with isotonic saline solutions can reduce the occurrence of chemical conjunctivitis without affecting the effectiveness of the prophylaxis. Alternatively, some prefer using freshly prepared penicillin solution (2500 units in 1 cc) or bacitracin eye ointment (500 units/gm). It is important to note that conjunctivitis can occur as a result of infection or irritation from improperly prepared AgNO3 solution. Infection usually happens during the birth process due to contact with vaginal organisms, with the most common pathogen being staph. Any neonates with conjunctivitis should be isolated and treated by irrigating the conjunctival sac with normal saline, followed by the instillation of suitable antibiotic ointments (based on culture/sensitivity), which should be repeated frequently until acute symptoms subside.

To prevent hemorrhagic disease of the newborn caused by a greater deficiency of vitamin K-dependent coagulation factors, it is recommended to administer 0.5-1mg of natural vitamin K (KI) to all neonates after birth. This helps to correct any vitamin K-related clotting defects and prevents the usual decrease in plasma Prothrombin level in newborns. It is important to avoid larger amounts of vitamin K as it can increase the risk of hyperbilirubinemia and kernicterus.

Administering vitamin K to the mother during labor is less reliable.

There are several important aspects to consider for the care of the newborn:

1. Mouth care does not require any special treatment, and wiping the palate and pharynx with gauze can cause abrasions and lead to conditions like thrush, pterygoid, ulcers, tooth infections with maxillary osteomyelitis, and retrobulbar abscess formation. Manipulating the mouth in any way can increase the risk of stomatitis and moniliasis.
2. It is important to inspect the nostrils as the presence of mucus can interfere with breathing. If present, it should be removed using a cotton twist.
3. Care of the ears should be limited to cleansing the external ear and external meatus with a cotton twist, preferably after the bath.
4. Identification bands should be placed on either the ankle or wrist of the infant before they are moved from the delivery area.
5. Passing a stomach tube is not a routine procedure, as it can

stimulate the posterior pharynx and esophagus, potentially causing bradycardia and apnea. If necessary, it should be done in the nursery once the infant is stable. However, if the mother has polyhydramnios, a tracheoesophageal fistula (TEF) should be ruled out by passing a soft rubber catheter into the stomach. Additionally, 12-20 ml of clotted cord blood should be collected in two tubes, one for blood typing, Coombs test, serology, and other tests if needed later, and the other tube should be kept in the nursery with the infant in a refrigerator. This tube should be retained.

BIRTH RECOVERY PERIOD

During the recovery period after birth, all newborn infants, except for those who are sick or high-risk, should be admitted to the transitional nursery area. This allows for close observation and detection of any infants needing special care. Within the first few hours of their stay in the transitional nursery, potential issues or risks can be identified. While the normal infant may not tolerate a complete physical examination right away, careful observation can help identify any abnormalities, such as hypotension, pallor, jaundice, respiratory distress, or abnormal birth recovery period. In cases where abnormalities are observed, a complete examination should be conducted.

The birth recovery period can be divided into three stages. In the first stage, which lasts for about half to one hour after delivery, the infant is alert and active, with increased muscle tone and open eyes. The heart and respiratory rates are rapid, and there may be transient murmurs. Bowel sounds are absent, and the infant may drool or vomit mucus. Signs of respiratory distress, such as flaring of the nostrils and retractions of the intercostal muscles, may be present.

The second stage occurs between half to one hour after birth, during which the heart rate and respiratory rate decrease, and the infant becomes less active and falls asleep.

The third stage begins after two hours, during which the infant becomes more alert again. This stage is characterized by an increase in heart rate, vasomotor instability, irregular respiratory patterns with periods of decreased breathing (apnea), the presence of oral mucus, the appearance of bowel sounds, and the passage of meconium. The infant gradually stabilizes, and hunger cues may become evident, such as a loud cry. Any significant deviations from this normal sequence may indicate abnormality. Preterm infants may have a prolonged response.

The use of drugs by the mother, birth trauma, and diseases in the newborn period can affect the events of the birth recovery period. The risk of mortality can be estimated by considering the birth weight and gestational age of the infant. In general, infants with a 10% or greater chance of dying are admitted to the special care nursery. Other factors that are taken into consideration include maternal hypertension, drug therapy, diabetes, Rh sensitization, bleeding, infection, and previous neonatal deaths.

REGULAR NURSERY CARE

Proper hand washing is crucial in preventing infections in the hospital, especially when it comes to caring for the baby. All personnel should wash their hands before and after touching the baby. Bathing the baby with soap and water can be done on a daily basis, but should only be done after the umbilical cord falls off and the umbilicus is dry. It is important to change the baby's clothes daily because the vernix caseosa, a waxy substance, will shed within 2-3 days and can stick to the clothing.

The baby's diaper should be checked before and after feeding and when the baby cries. If it is wet or soiled, it should be promptly changed. When cleaning the baby's buttocks, meconium or feces should be wiped away using sterile cotton moistened with sterile water. It is advised not to retract the foreskin of male infants. It is important to note that hexachlorophene, a substance used to control staphylococcal infections, should only be used sparingly due to its known neurotoxicity, especially in premature infants. The baby's bassinet should be regularly cleaned and it is preferable for it to be made of clear plastic material to ensure easy visibility of the baby. All necessary care, such as physical examination, changing of clothing, temperature taking, and skin cleansing, should be done in the bassinet to limit the risk of infection spreading.

When it comes to clothing and bedding, it is important to keep it minimal for the baby's comfort. Maintaining a constant temperature of 75°F helps simplify clothing choices. The baby's temperature can be taken rectally or in the armpit. During the first 2-3 days, the temperature should be taken every 4 hours, and then every 8 hours thereafter. A normal axillary temperature ranges from 96-99°F. Weighing the baby at birth and on alternate days is sufficient for screening purposes. Infants born in the hospital may undergo screenings for various diseases such as blood group incompatibilities, blood group and direct Coombs test, syphilis serology, phenylketonuria, elevated serum phenylalanine, maple syrup urine disease, leonine (isoleucine valine) alpha ketoacidosis, and homocystinuria.

PHYSICAL EXPLANATION OF THE NEWBORN INFANT:

At no other time than at birth is more information obtained from the genial eve, all visual and auditory appraisal of the naked infant, and less information is obtained from an exhaustive systematic examination. Three categories are of utmost importance, cardiorespiratory status, presence of congenital anomalies, and the effects of the gestation, labor, delivery, anesthesia, andsigns of infection or some other disease. While a fretful infant is quieted by a nipple, the order ofthe examination should be the respiratory system, cardiac status, abdomen, genitalia and rectum, extremities, spine and joints, head, neck and mouth, neurologic examination, and eye. At the time of birth, a rapid examination assessing the heart rate, respiratory, activity, color, and muscle tone and identifying gross abnormalities is done in the delivery room.

The complete physical examination of the infant should be done, ideally in the presence of the parents, within 12-24 hours of the birth and repeated within 24 hours of discharge. The aim of the examination is to note the problems requiring immediate treatment, assess the function of various systems, and rule out any abnormalities. Measurement of the head circumference, weight, and length is made at the time of entry to the nursery. Vital signs are recorded at frequent intervals during the period of stabilization (8-24 hr8). Blood pressure may be obtained from both upper limbs and one lower limb to exclude _ coarctation of the aorta using a noninvasive ultrasonic device if available. If the mother has received no anesthesia or premedication, the 3 distinct stages of reactivity are seen. These are characterized by the alternate reactive(sympathetic and quiet (parasympathetic) periods, the first period of reactivity lasts one and a half hour characterized by increased pulse and respiratory rates, increased motor activity, active mucus secretion from thenose and mouth, and absent bowel sounds are followed by a one and a half hour period of quiet characterized by sleep falling pulse and respiratory rates, decreased secretions, and presence of bowel sounds; again, a 2 hr. period of reactivity, and another period of quiet of 4 hours. The examination of the newborn need's patience, gentleness, and flexibility in the routines of procedures.

GENERAL APPEARANCE:

The general appearance, maturity, nutritional status, presence of abnormal faces or body deformity, and state of well-being are noted. Before the infant is disturbed, observe the resting position, which reflects the position assumed in utero. The normal position is of full flexion ci the limbs, as opposed to the spread-legged, eagled frogs 'leg position of extension in premature or severely ill infants. Physical activity may be absent in sleep relaxation or depression by the drugs given to the mother or by illness. The infant may be lying with motionless limbs when his all energy is conserved for the effort of difficult breathing. Or he may be crying wildly with the accompanying activity of the arms and legs.

Coarse, tremulous (shaky) movements in the ankles or jaw are more common in babies than at any other age, but they are not as significant. These movements typically occur when the baby is active, while convulsive twitching usually happens when the baby is in a calm state. The baby's nutritional status can be determined by their weight, length, and the condition of their body surfaces. If the baby has edema, it may falsely indicate good nutrition, but this edema can either be pitting (leaves an indentation when pressed) or nonpitting. However, the fingers and toes of the baby will lack the normal fine wrinkles over the knuckles when they have fluid retention. Edema in the eyelids can also occur due to irritation from AgNO3. Generalized edema can be associated with prematurity, hypoproteinemia in severe erythroblastosis, congenital nephrosis, Hurler's syndrome, and other conditions. Localized edema may result from a congenital lymphatic system disorder, and if it affects one or more limbs in a female infant, it could suggest Turner's syndrome. The quality of the baby's respiration, color, sleep patterns, muscle tone, mottling, and their response when being picked up are also observed. The baby's breathing may be labored or shallow, and their appearance may resemble that of a baby born to a diabetic mother (cushingoid).

SKIN:

Color and Appearance: The skin becomes erythematous for a few hours after birth and then fadesinto its normal appearance. Vasomotor instability and sluggishness of peripheral circulation are revealed by deep redness or purple lucidity in the crying infant, whose color may darken profoundly with the closure of the glottis preceding a vigorous cry and by harmless cyanosis of the hands and feet when these are cool. Mottling is another example of a general circulatory imbalance.

Persistent central cyanosis or peripheral cyanosis (acrocyanosis) suggests a pathology and maybe due to congenital heart disease, CNS disease, pulmonary disease, abnormal, etc. Significant cyanosis may be masked by pallor in circulatory failure. The relatively high Hemoglobin content of the first few days and the thin skin may combine to give an appearance of cyanosis in the presence of adequate arterial saturation of oxygen-localized cyanosis is differentiated from ecchymosis by the momentary pallor, which follows pressure. This also helps in demonstrating icterus which may pass unnoticed if the skin is suffused with blood-Pallorm may represent anoxia, anemia, shock, or edema. Circulatory failure is evidenced by the pallor of the skin with cyanotic nail beds and lips. The pallor of anemia is characterized by pale skin, pale mucosae, pail nail beds, and tachycardia. Anemia may be due to erythroblastosis, fetal is a rupture of the liver, subdural hemorrhage, fetal-maternal, or intertwined transfusion. Acute blood loss at the time of delivery or gastrointestinal bleeding, or multiple samples of blood from preterm fan May cause anemia leading to pallor. Post-mature infants have whiter skins.

Plethora: plethora suggests polycythemia, which may lead to hyper viscosity syndrome. It occurs in infants of diabetic mothers, SGA infants, Twins who have received a twin-twin transfusion, maternal-to-fetal transfusion, and congenital adrenal hypoplasia. -Petechial and ecchymosis may be normally seen on the face and neck and may be due to a tight nuchal cord. Ecchymosis may be seen on an abnormal presenting pal as foot, leg, buttock, or hand; it is also found in sepsis, hemolytic diseaseof the newborn, thrombocytopenia, chronic intrauterine infection, CID, toxoplasmosis, syphilis, or rubella. -Nevi may be vascular or pigmented. A Mongolian spot is a pigmented nevus, a slate blue, well-demarcated area of pigmentation, seen over buttocks, back, etc., 2-10 cm in size, seen in. 90% of the black, Indian, and Asian infants (mostly in the colored races, but occasionally in the whites also). These disappear within the first year. Capillary haemangiomas are common onthe lower occiput, eyelids, forehead, nares, and lips. These become smaller and fainter as the child grows up. The brown cafe au fait spots are seen as single lesions in 20% of infants; if up to 5 such lesions are present in a baby with no family history of neurofibromatosis, the condition is normal.

Milia, tiny yellowish white papules over the nose and face, arc due to retention of keratin and sebaceous material; occur in 5O of infants. These disappcar within a few weeks. -The skin is usually smooth; dry skin with cracking and peeling of the superficial layers is seen in infants who are poster (more than 40 weeks) or have had intrauterine growth retardation. Normal skin is present underneath; a severe degree of parchment-like skin may suggest ichthyosis congenitally. The skin of the premature infant is thin and delicate and tends to be deep red. In extreme decrees of prematurity, it may be gelatinous. Fine soft immature hair, Lanugo hair covers the translucent skin of the preterm especially in the areas of the scalp and brow and may cover the face. It is roe/aced by villous hair in the term infant. The nails are rudimentary in very premature infants but may protrude beyond the fingertips in infants born post-term. Erythema toxicum may be seen at birth or within 3 days in 30-70% of full-term. infants: these are 1-3 mm white or yellow papules on an erythematous base, which appear anywhere on the body except handed-and palms and soles. They are more corn moons on the trunk. The lesions are seen in different stages. Erythematous macules, papules, or small vesicles containing eosinophilia are less cannon in preterm infants. 3 staphylococcal, or streptococcal infection of the shin in the preterm infant, may resemble erythema toxicum. Diagnosis is made by detection of eosinophil 's on a smear of anaspirated lesion (neutrophils if or lymphocytes in infection), no bacterial growth from a culture ofthe lesion, rapid change in the location-encircle with a ball pen some of the lesions and observing their disappearance within several hours. Vernix caseosa, à whitish, greasy material that covers the body of the fetus, decreases in amount as the term approaches; it is present in the body creases of the term infant but is completely absent from the body of the post-term infant.

Meconium staining OD the umbilical cord, vernix, nails, and skin suggests fetal distress; theseare stained brownish yellow. (Intrauterine anoxia). Head size, shape, symmetry, general appearance of the head and anatomical landmark,

Molding usually resolves itself within a week after birth,

at which time the head circumference that is affected by molding should be premeasured. Caput succedaneum (edema or hemorrhage of the soft tissues of the scalp) is seen on the presenting part. It extends across the suture lines and disappears within a few days.

Cephalhematoma is bleeding into the sub-periosteal space on the surface of a skull bone especially theparietal bone, which is limited by the borders of the individual skull bone. Pamela, there is an underlying fracture. Most resolve within some may persist and calcify. The enclosed hemorrhage is occasionally bilateral: if extensive, it may lead to anemia and hypovolemia, requiring transfusion or hyperbilirubinemia. The size and tension of the fontanelles are determined digitally. Normally the size of the anterior fontanels varies from 1-4 cm at birth in any direction. It is smaller if there is an overriding of the bones. It is soft, pulsates with the infers pulse, and becomes slightly depressed when the infant is upright and quiet. If the fontanels are small at birth, they may increase during the first few months of life. The posterior fontanels are usually less than 1 cm in diameter, while the anterior one is usually less than 5 cm in its greatest diagonal.

It will normally bulge during vigorous crying or in the supine position. Persistent bulging in a resting infant or depressed fontanels (with dehydration or microcephaly) is abnormal. A 3rd fontanel, a bony defect along the sagittal suture in the parietal bones, may be present. The persistence of excessively large anterior and posterior fontanels has been associated with hypothyroidism. Occasionally Sound in the parietal bones at the vertex near the sagittal suture. They are of no consequence. Soft areas in the occipital area suggest the irregular calcification and worming bone formation associated with osteogenesis imperfect, cleidocranial dysostosis, cretinism, and occasionally Downs syndrome. If craniotabes persist, it is abnormal. Craniosynostosis is present as a ridge along the suture and is associated with a cranial deformity- Skull fractures resulting from birth trauma may be linear or depressed and may be associated with a cephalhematoma. Increased ICP in the newborn infant is associated with increasing head circumference and a full anterior fontanelle. Occasionally slight arterial pulsations may be noted; marked pulsations are abnormal. The normal head circumference measured at the most prominent part of the occiput and just above the supraorbital ridges for a healthy full-term infant is 34-37 cm (same or greater than the chest circumference, or the total body length 10 cm). Microcephaly is the abnormality of the size greater than 3 SD belt the mean or 3rd below the3rd percentile macrocephaly is often seen with hydrocephalus. Abnormalities of the shape include anencephaly, encephaloceles (midline defects of the bony and membranous structures), and craniostenosis (premature closure of the sutures).

Trans illumination degree of light transmitted through the head should be determined in any infant suspected of having a neurological disease. A completely darkened room is needed. The circle of light extending beyond the flange of the trans-illumination flashlight should not be more than l5cm in term or up to 2 cm in preterm infants. Excessive light transmission occurs when diminished brain tissue, brain atrophy, hydrocephaly, or porencephaly.

Computerized tomography and ultrasound scans in pre-term infants may reveal sub-ependymal,intra-ventricular, or intra-cerebral hemorrhage during the first 2-7 days of life in the absence of physical signs or symptoms. All newborn infants with a gestational age of less than 35 weeks should have CT or US scans during the first week of life. If hemorrhage into the ventricles has occurred or if the scan was not done, ultrasonography of the brain at 10-21 days of age to rule outprogressive hydrocephalus is indicated. Full-term infants with meningitis or seizure should have CT scanning and ultrasonography for the diagnosis of additional damage to the brain.

FACE

The overall look and balance of the face are examined. The face may appear uneven due to the fetal position. If the head is positioned on its side and the shoulder pushes against the jaw, it can cause a noticeable dent. The jawbone may noticeably shift away from the center. However, these irregularities typically resolve within a few weeks or months. Abnormal facial features are often seen in conjunction with specific syndromes. Swelling, bruising, or differences in movement can occur due to pressure during birth or the use of forceps. When the infant cries, facial nerve paralysis can be observed. The unaffected side of the mouth typically moves, resulting in a distorted sound.

NOSE

The nose should be evaluated for both its shape and function. Some deviation and deformity may be present, which can be attributed to the positioning in the womb. In cases where birth trauma is suspected, it is important to rule out fractures or dislocations of the nasal septum. A bony fracture can be diagnosed through an x-ray, while a septal dislocation (found in 1-7% of newborns) can be identified by observing the displaced septum in either nostril, either by compressing the nose or by determining the angle of the septum in relation to the floor of the nasal cavity using an applicator. These deformities can be caused by the positioning in the womb or by congenital syndromes.

Newborns primarily breathe through their nose, except when they are crying. Confirming the openness of the nostrils can be done by passing a catheter and listening to the sounds of breathing while keeping the mouth closed. Premature babies may have more audible sounds due to narrower air passages. Secretions from the nose can occur for a few hours after birth. If the mother has taken reserpine for congenital syphilis, the nasal secretions may become purulent or bloody. An examination with a speculum is conducted to ensure normal anatomy and the integrity of the nasal system, as well as to rule out choanal atresia, rare tumors, and encephaloceles. Symptoms such as nasal discharge, noisy breathing, or complete obstruction may indicate choanal atresia. In cases of obstruction, the infant may experience cyanosis or apnea since they are reliant on nasal breathing. Nasal obstruction from mucus discharge can occur in infants with upper respiratory tract infections acquired as viral infections in the womb. Flaring of the nasal alae is observed in cases of respiratory distress or cold stress.

Abnormal nose shapes are observed in various syndromes, such as beaked, aperts, croutons, Hallerman-strife, Teacher-Collins syndrome, upturned, achondroplasitidiiopathic, hyperkalemia, Downs, Conradi's syndrome, and flat nose, often in conjunction with cleft palate.

EYES

Precautions must be taken before administering Ag No 3 prophylaxis to newborns to prevent potential side effects such as periorbital edema and conjunctivitis. The eye examination should include an evaluation of the periorbital structures, nerve function, interior orbital structures, and light reflex. In premature infants, the remnant of the pupillary membrane can also be used to determine the gestational age.

Newborns typically have their eyes open and are alert for the first 30 minutes, after which they close their eyes during sleep for a few hours. When awake, the baby will open their eyes, especially when picked up in a semi-dark room. The eyes can be further examined by gently tipping the infant forward and backward or by lifting them from a supine to an upright position.

During the examination, the size, shape, and position of the eyes, as well as the presence of epicanthal folds, should be noted. Swelling of the eyelids and conjunctival discharge may occur within the first day after the use of silver nitrate, but this is not always indicative of effectiveness. Observing eyelid movement is important, as normal eyelids should function independently.

Some newborns may exhibit setting sun signs, where the lower borders of the irises are partially below the level of the lower lid. This is normal in some premature and full-term babies, but if it persists, it may indicate underlying conditions such as hydrocephalus, kernicterus, or brainstem irritation.

Occasional uncoordinated eye movements are common in newborns, but persistent irregular movements like nystagmus deviation are abnormal. Epicanthal folds may obscure the medial corner of the eyes, giving the appearance of strabismus (pseudo strabismus). This can be confirmed by directing a light at the eyes and ensuring its reflection appears in the center of each pupil.

Evaluation of eye movements can be done by rotating the baby while holding them upright. Doll's eye movements, where the eyes lag behind the turning of the head from side to side, are usually observed during the first 10 days and should not be present at 2-3 months of age when the baby can fixate well.

Newborns are sensitive to light from birth, and while initially only capable of monocular fixation, binocular convergence develops during the second month. The pupillary reflex may be sluggish at birth but becomes more apparent in a few days. A simple flashlight can be used to observe corneal or lens opacities and pupil size. Eliciting the red reflex can help evaluate the presence of tumors or cataracts. Focus and equality of the pupils usually develop a few weeks after birth. The blink reflex, triggered by bright light, loud noise, or touching of the eyelashes or cornea, is already present.

The presence and color of the iris should be noted, as the absence of the iris may be familial autosomal dominant or sporadic and associated with Wilms tumor. The color of the iris will continue to change as the infant grows older, and the final color may not be determined until they are 6 to 12 months old. The presence of Brushfield spots (salt and pepper speckling) may be normal but can also be associated with Down syndrome. Colobomata may also be present. The pupils, which are normally constricted for the first few weeks, should be evaluated for their response to light.

In all newborns, an ophthalmoscopic examination for the red reflex should be conducted. A white reflex may indicate retinoblastoma, while cataracts can appear as black spots. If necessary, an ophthalmoscopic examination through dilated pupils can be performed to assess for glaucoma or interior chamber hemorrhage. Dilating eye drops, such as 0.2% cyclopentolate or 1% phenylephrine, may be used, but they can have side effects such as vagal slowing of the heart and cold stress.

Anterior chamber hemorrhage may occur following birth trauma but may not be noticeable for several hours. Congenital glaucoma may be present if the cornea is cloudy due to edema and measures more than 11 mm. Photophobia is common, and the enlargement of the entire eye is a late finding. Chorioretinitis can be caused by infections, while a greyish yellow or absent light reflection, dilated pupil, or strabismus may indicate retinoblastoma. Conjunctivitis may occur after the use of AgNO3 or due to infections like gonococcus or chlamydia trachomatis. Ptosis, drooping of the eyelid, may be secondary to birth trauma, a hazy cornea, or an enlarged eye due to trisomy 13 or 18. Retinal hemorrhages can be associated with trauma, hypoxia, or subdural hematoma. Excessive tearing or epiphora that occurs several weeks after birth and the obstruction of the lacrimal duct (dacryocystitis) should also be considered.

EARS

The external ear should be examined for size, shape, and position. The size of the ear in relation to the head should be noted. Large protruding ears when bilateral main Be normally inherited. IfUnilateral other ear anomalies are also present normal shape of the ear can include the lop ear floppy or bent over pinna resulting from the absence of antihelix. Premature babies may have an incompletely developed helix because of the deficiency of cartilage. Occasionally a nodule of Darwin's tubercle along the posterior segment of the outer Rim of the ear helix may be present on one or both ears.

Deformities of the pinna are seen occasionally. Low-set or rotated ears are often associated withother deformities and anomalies in the urinary tract anomalies, including renal agenesis (potters' disease) because the two organs develop at the same time embryologically. Other syndromes associated with low-set ears include chromosome abnormalities and acrocephalosyndactyly (Apert's syndrome).

Unilateral or bilateral preauricular papilloma's skin tags frequently occur, maybe often as a familiar trait. Fleshy skin tags on the line drawn between the tragus and the corner of the mouthaccompanied by a small low set ear

and stenosis or atresia of the external meatus in Goldenhar's syndrome(Facio-auricula vertebral dysplasia). When pedunculated can be tightly ligated at the base when they undergo dry gangrene and slough away, the amount of cartilage in the pinnas is related to maturity. The tympanic membrane can be visualized easily on otoscopy through the short straight external meatus, which is slightly directed upwards. It is usually dull and directed horizontally (vertically in an older child); fluid may be present behind the drum for the first few hours.
The insertion of the superior part of the ear is normally at or above a line drawn between and extended from the medial canthal of the eyes. This is more accurate than using the medial andLateral canthal of the eyes since an upward or downward slant of the eyes could be misleading. Otitis media occurs fairly frequently in neonates, especially, in preterm infants, in thosewith deformities of the palate, or in those who have been intubated for long periods of time, particularly with nasotracheal intubation. Otitis media may be due to usual bacteria or may be dueto syphilis.

Gross hearing must be evaluated for both ears. The newborn can hear a loud noise, not avibration that can be felt, which should be associated with a blink in a newborn.

MOUTH

Observing the lips and mucous membranes for pallor and cyanosis. In a normal hydrated infant, the membranes are moist. The mouth should be examined when the baby is crying to confirm that the movement is symmetrical. Asymmetry may be normal or due to facial paralysis.

Circumoral pallor is seen in shock cyanosis may be present. Abnormal shape of the mouth maybe associated with various syndromes, broad mouth, idiopathic hypercalcemia, fish-like mouth, Treacher Collins, Praguer Willi, and silvers syndrome, open mouth, downs, and apert syndrome and myotonic dystrophy, small, Schwartz jampel and Hallerman-Streiff syndromes, craniocarpotarsal dystrophy.

Natal teeth precocious teeth are rarely present, maybe soft in scissors in the lower Incisor position oraberrantly placed. These are shed before the deciduous teeth erupt; sometimes, these need to be removed to avoid aspiration.

If true deciduous teeth have erupted (incidence 1:2000 births), the normal root is present in X-ray these are left as such. Predacious teeth (1:4000) are always loose with non-roots and should be removed to prevent aspiration. Epithelial pearls (Epstein pearls) are retention cysts of keratin, multiple, small firm, grayish white nodules seen on the alveolar mucosa over the gums and on the half palate and at the junction of the hard and soft palate on either side of the median raphe. These are temporary accumulations of epithelial cells. These are present in 85% of newborns and are shed spontaneously within a few weeks of birth. Congenital epulis, a smooth-surfaced tumor occurring mostly in females (10:1), is usually associated with the alveolar mucous membrane by a pedicle and can be excised. Clusters of small white or yellow follicles or ulcers on an erythematous base may be found on the interior tonsillar pillars, most frequently on the third dayof life. They clear without treatment within 2 to 4 days. The high-arched palate may be normal or abnormal with abnormal facies.

There may be a cleft lip and cleft palate. Most new bones have asmall mandible, but if it is very small (Pierre Robin Syndrome), difficulty in breathing may occurwhen the tongue blocks the airways as it falls back against the pharynx. Tonsils and adenoids are quite small in newborns. Some drooling of the mouth is normal in the first few hours, but excessive drooling suggests esophageal atresia. The tongue appears relatively large the frenulum may be short. Occasionally the sublingual mucous membrane forms a prominent fold. A lymphangioma or hemangioma may be seen on the tongue as a local area of macroglossia.

Unnecessary cutting of the triangular in the ankyloglossia may lead to infection and uncontrolled bleeding. A tongue tie usually does not interfere with function, therefore, should not be cut. A retention cyst of the sublingual salivary gland ranula may normally be seen on the floorof the mouth filled with clear or yellow contents. Ankyloglossia superior fusion of the tongue to the hard palate and gums may occur. Macroglossia at birth may be seen in down's syndrome, beck with the syndrome, or hurlers syndrome. After birth, it is associated with the hormonal disease as hypothyroidism or hyper pituitaries, infection, mechanical trauma, and neoplasm. The palate must be visualized and palpated to ensure that the soft and hard palates are intact. Jaundice may be noted on the palate. A high-arched palate with no other abnormal findings may be normal, but it is frequently seen in chromosomal abnormalities or arachnodactyly. The cheeks have fullness on both sides, Buccal as well as external, due to the accumulation of fat, which makes up the sucking pads. Sucking calluses and dry cornified epithelium are normally seen in the central part of the lips. Both sucking pads and the labial tubercle on the upper lip disappear when the suckling days areover. The throat of the newborn is difficult to see because of the Arch of the palate. There may be clefts of the posterior palate or uvula.

Mucous retention cysts (mucoceles) are elevated translucent bluish compressible. Lesions found onthe tongue and lips usually but may be seen in any area containing salivary glands, not on the interior half of the hard palate. These may Rupture and collapse and re-appear for months. Are Ling uvula may be a cause of frequent gagging. Excess Secretions on the bearings may be due to TEF. Oral moniliasis, a thrashed localized oral infection by candida Albicans may appear as elevated gray-white or white patches that resemble the appearance of crowded milk or keratin-containing cysts and do not come off when scrapped with a tongue blade. If they are scrapped off, the underlying area is raw and occasionally bleeding.

Micrognathia is seen in Pierre-Robin, Treacher Collins, and Hallermann-Strieff syndrome and may cause respiratory distress secondary to pharyngeal obstruction by the tongue. Prognathismprotruding jaw may be seen in Crouzons disease, Apert syndrome, and cerebral gigantism.

Redundant skin or webbing in a female suggests turner's syndrome. Webbing is also seen in an isolated finding l. in Downs syndrome, Noonas Syndrome, and trisomy 18. The abnormally short neck may be seen in Noonas syndrome, Turners syndrome Klippel Fiel Syndrome, Spondo-epiphyseal dysplasia, or trisomy 13. Congenital torticollis may be due to cervical spine abnormality, sternomastoid muscle mass, or from the position in utero. Opisthotonos may be caused by kernicterus, cerebral palsy, or rarely meningitis. Cystic hygroma will cause edema. A thyroglossal duct that is high in the midline and moveable should be identified. A persistent tonicneck reflex assumed spontaneously and maintained by the infant may be caused by brain damage.

THE CHEST

The thorax must be examined for shape, symmetry, position, nipples and breast tissue, respiratorypattern, and the character of respiratory, including rate, rhythm, and depth. The anteroposterior and lateral diameters of the chest are normally equal. The fullness of the thorax due to. Increased anteroposterior diameter leads to the barrel-shaped chest, which is due to the overexpansion of lungs as severe meconium aspiration or congenital emphysema. The short wide thorax is seen in Morquios disease, and the small but immobile thorax with short hypoplastic ribs is seen in thoracic asphyxia dystrophy of the newborn as part of the generalized chondrodystrophy. Pectus excavatum may be an isolated deformity or is associated with Margfans or Pierre Robin syndrome. Pigeon-shaped chest (protruding sternum) is less commonly occurring as an isolated finding and not due to rickets or osteoporosis as in older children. Separation of the sternum or sternal clefts are rarely seen. Note asymmetry in the expansion of 2 sides or retractions during inspiration in the sub-costal, intercostal xiphoid, and suprasternal areas. These indicate pulmonarydisease, airway obstruction, or airway leaks. Asymmetry of chest movements during respiratory suggests pneumothorax, phrenic nerve palsy secondary to birth trauma, diaphragmatic hernia, congenital emphysema, or pulmonary agenesis.

Absent clavicles permit unusual anterior movement of the shoulders. Clavicular fracture is detected by tenderness and crepitus at the fracture site, and limited movements of that the arms must be noted when the Moro is elicited. After a few days callus willbe formed, and the deformity can be easily visualized and felt.

LUNGS:

Almost as much can be learned about lungs by observation of breathing as by auscultation and percussion. Evaluation of respiratory status includes color, presence of acrocyanosis, respiratory rate, and presence of apnea. The rate of respiratory varies from 20-100/min in normal infatuate, depending on physical activity and state of wakefulness or presence of crying. The usual at rest is 40-60, with the rhythm somewhat irregular. Counting of the rate should be done during sleep for one full minute since fluctuations are rapid. For premature infants, rates are higher and more fluctuant. Rates that are consistently higher than 60/min during periods of regular breathing usually indicate cardiac or pulmonary insufficiency. Bradypnea (rate less than 30) and apnea (defined in the premature infant as cessation of respiratory longer than 20 seconds and possibly associated bradycardia or cyanosis may be due to CNS diseases, drug infection, or acid-base imbalance. The premature infant normally breathes with Cheyne stokes rhythm (periodic respiratory or with complete irregularity. Periodic respiratory is rare in the first 24 hours of irregular gasping, sometimes accompanied by spasmodic movements of the mouth and chin, strongly indicating serious impairment of respiratory centers.

Expiratory grunting occurs with respiratory distress due to many causes, but deep RDS. Inspiratory stridor is associated with partialobstruction of the upper airway during inspiration as it occurs with the soft, collapsible tray, and cheal structures of the congenital strider. A high-pitched cry suggests brain damage. A hoarse cryresults from inflammation or edema of the larynx or vocal cord paralysis. A whining cat's cry occurs with partial deletion of the short arm of chromosome 5. A weal cry may be due to illness. A delay in vocalizing the cry after the infant appears to be crying is congenital hypothyroidism. The breathing of the newborns. It is almost entirely diaphragmatic so that the soft front of the thoraxis commonly drawn in during inspiration, and the abdomen gets protruded. If the baby is quiet, relaxed, and of good: color, this paradoxical movement may not be evidence of insufficient ventilation. Labored respiratory is a sign of abnormal pulmonary ventilation, pneumonia, or other mechanical dist branches of the lungs; often, the mechanical difficulty is too much or too little air in the lungs, and the intercostal tissues are drawn in during respiratory.

Group I include infants who, while quiet, breathe approximately 40/min from birth on without fluctuation greater than 1/in-group II infants with respiratory rates being high, usually over 60/min, during the first hour, who showed no significant increase after the first hour and subsequently decrease to normal levels. Within 48 hours. After birth. In these two groups, there is no associated mortality. In group II, infants whose respiratory rates show a significant increase, 15/min or more over the mean for the first hour, during the first 48 hours. In this group, there is a 25% mortality, more so if birth weight is less. Retraction scoring with respiratory rate and cyanosis is a gauge of respiration difficulty in newborns. It is applicable 1-2 hours after birth, unlike Apgar that is. Used to evaluate the infant in the first 1-5 minutes after birth,

	Grade 0	Grad2 1	Grade2
Upper Chest	Synchronize d	Lag on Inspire	Seesaw
Lower Chest	No Retracts	Just Visible	Marke d
Xiphoid Reduction	None	Just Visible	Marke d
Nares Dilata	None	Minima l	Marke d
Expirator	None	Steth	Naked

y Grunting		Only	Ear

These are the criteria of respiratory distress ; grade 0 for each criterion indicates no respiratory distress , and grade 2 indicates severe respiratory distress Percussion may be more informative than auscultation because of the small total area of the lungs. Breath sounds from an adjoining region may be heard as though directly under the stethoscope. Auscultation Normal breath sounds are Broncho vesicular (or bronchial). There may be incomplete, deceased, or absent breath sounds.6uspicion of the decreased breath sounds should be verified by inducing deeper breathingand, if a local area is suspected, by altering the position of the infant. Fine riles are heard normally for the first some hours, but persistent Tales suggest pneumonia, atelectasis, or rarely pulmonary edema. The fine crackling riles of early pneumonia may be heard only at the end of a deep inspiration induced by crying. When there is pneumothorax or pneumomediastinum, the breath sounds, and heart sounds may be distant.

Percussion: Normal resonance should be present; hyperresonance suggests free air: in the thoraxfrom a pneumothorax, pneumomediastinum, or emphysema. The diaphragmatic hernia may be associated with either hyper-resonance or hypo resonance, depending on the amount of gas in the herniated intestine. Hyperresonance suggests fluid or atelectasis. Grunting heard with or without a stethoscope may be due to pulmonary, cardiac, or CIS disease or with infection, anemia, or coldstress. The presence of bowel sounds in the chest, and the left hemi thorax, suggests diaphragmatic hernias, but these may be transmitted from the abdomen. A cheat X-ray must be taken since the physical findings alone are of limited lit use in diagnosis. The location of the nipples and pigmentation of the areola should be noted (hyper-pigmentation suggests congenitaladrenal hyperplasia). Breast and nipple size are normally related to gestational age. In full-term infants of either sex, milk may be present. And may persist for 1-2 months. Any redness or heat of tenderness suggests mastitis. If the infant is otherwise well, riles and questionable breath sounds are usually: insignificant.

HEART:

The heart is examined primarily by auscultation for rate, rhythm, quality of sounds, size, and told position. Percussion is of no value in estimating heart size, but palpation of the ape beat is helpfulin detecting cardiomegaly. Evaluation of cardiac status should include perfusion of skin, the strength of the pulses, the position of the maximal cardiac impulse, palpation of the femoral and brachial pulse, and auscultation of the heart for rate, rhythm, presence of murmurs, etc. Because of rapid alterations inthe systemic and pulmonary pressures, murmurs do not always reflect the presence of significant heart disease. Murmurs may be transitory or intermittently present. There is only a 1:12 chance that a murmur heard at birth: represents congenital heart disease. Innocent murmurs and murmurs of a transient PDA can be heard in the normal neonate. 80-90% of murmurs present during the first week disappear in 1 year; in most cases, they will disappear after 3 months. Murmurs existing beyond the first or second day should be suspected as evidence of cardiac abnormality. The absence of a murmur can ‘t always means a normal sign.

Otherwise, the arrhythmias are most frequently observed during drowsiness or deep sleep. Many are accompanied by a startle Response . Immaturity of the ANS has been postulated as a possible cause of arrhythmias. Tachycardia (rate greater than 170 beats/min) may be due to fever, hyperthyroid sm, hyperactivity, drug toxicity, or cardiac abnormalities such as atrial tachycardia Bradycardia (less than 90/min in full term, 70 in premature) is commonly due to heart block, digitalis toxicity, hyperkalemia increased CSF pressure or acute myocarditis. Pulses altering withalternate strong and weak peripheral pulses are associated with left heart failure or primary myocardial disease. The point of maximal impulse is barely palpable in the normal full-term infant Femoral, brachial, and radial pulses. It should be palpated, and the pulses should be of equal quality bilaterally. On auscultation, the heart sounds are normally of equal intensity and appear distant. The sounds are best heard over the value areas. In the newborn, the first sound is normally not split in contrast to the second sound, which is a split sound that normally widens to inspiration.

ABDOMEN:

The abdomen is examined for asymmetry, including musculature, masses, and fullness. Palpation with gentle pressure from the lower to the upper quadrant is most useful. The abdomen is primarily examined by observation and palpation. The abdomen is slightly scaphoid at birth but becomes more prominent as the bowel fills with air when the abdomen becomes convex. The umbilical cord normally has 3 vessels and two contracted arteries. And one large thin-walled vein. There is nobulging aril and the umbilicus or inguinal area, which may represent a hernia. Occasionally diastasis recti are seen in the midline. In the premature baby, bowel patterns normally may be seen on the abdomen. Visible gastric or bowel-patterned full-term infant suggests the presence ofobstruction. A pacifier or flexing the knees and hips will frequently calm an agitated baby to permit palpation. The abdominal organs are most easily palpated before the bowel becomes distended with air.

A scaphoid abdomen (with respiratory distress) is neonate

will suggest a diaphragmatic hernia. It isgenerally on the left side. Visible dilatation of veins on the anterior abdominal wall (caput medusa) is present with venous obstruction. Distention of the abdomen, which can be quantitated by serial measurement of the abdomen al circumference, may be due to air, within or outside the bowel fluid, clear or chorus blood, or Pusan enlarged viscus or a tumor cystic, solid but commonly renal in origin. Palpation should be done for both kidneys. The lower poles of both kidneys can frequently be palpated, especially. before the abdomen fills with gas in the deep flank. The liver edge isnormally distinct, and maybe 2 am below the right costal margin (usually less than 2 cm, below the- costal margin in the right midclavicular line and may remain palpable up to 1.5 am throughout childhood. At birth, the liver is relatively larger and weighs. 1/18th of the birth weight as compared to 1/50th of the body weight in adults. Abdominal musculature may be absent prune belly syndrome), there may be gastroschisis, omphalocele, which at times is so small that it is incorporated into cord clamp, and exstrophy of the bladder.

Umbilical hernias are common. Prune belly syndrome may occur in association with severe urinary tract abnormalities-Spleen is usually not palpable but may be felt just above or below: the left costa/ margin. The approximatesize or location of the kidney can be determined by deep palpation. Unusual masses should be immediately investigated by flat film, cross-lateral table film of the abdomen, followed by IVP, if needed, exploratory laparotomy. The commonest masses encountered are urinary tract anomalies, renal embryos, ovarian cysts, and intestinal duplications. Abdominal distension at or shortly after birth suggests perforation of GIT, which often is due to meconium ileus; later, it is due to lower bowel obstruction or peritonitis. Abdominal distension may occur with paralytic ileus in sepsis also.

The outline of the distended bladder may be seen above the syphilis pubis and may be felt as a ballotable mass in the lower abdomen. Palpation may lead to the contraction of bladder muscles with voiding.

The umbilical cord begins drying within hours after birth, becomes loose from the underlying in by 4-5 days, and falls off by 7-10 days. Occasionally a granulating stump remains that heals faster if treated with AgNO3 cauterization. The umbilicus may show signs of infection (redness,foul odor, and presence of pus), bleeding, polyp, granuloma, or an abnormal communication with the abdominal viscera (urine from a patient urachus or bowel contents from a patent omphalomesenteric.

Anatomy and muscle tone of the anus must be observed. Imperforate and is not always: visible, and if meconium has not been passed, gentle insertion of the little finger or a soft rubber cathetershould be passed, not a rigid object as a rectal thermometer. Irritation or fissures may occur after the immediate neonatal period. The dimple or the irregularity of the skin often fold normally presentin the sacrococcygeal midline and may be mistaken for an actual or potential pile-nidal sinus.

Perianal fistula is abnormal, and the associated imperforate anus should be sought. The examination should include the passing of a soft catheter into both nares and the stomach. The presence of thecatheter tip in the stomach is confirmed by palpation and auscultation of the bubbling of 1-3 ml of air infused through the catheter. The stomach is then aspirated, and the contents (normal clear gastric fluid versus bloodstained or meconium-stained fluid) and quantity are recorded. Clear gastric fluid more than 25 ml suggests a proximal bowel obstruction. The presence of blood suggests ingestion of maternal blood or neonatal bleeding, a test that can differentiate maternal from fetal hemoglobin. Meconium most frequently is evidence of fetal distress. Or breech delivery.The catheter is then passed per vaginum to assure patency and per rectum to exclude anal ages: A firm meconium plug may be present. Meconium plug syndrome may occur in the newborn infant with hard meconium producing total intestinal obstruction. These infants appear well with marked abdominal distension. Once the plug is passed, the distension is rapidly relieved and doesnot recur. Abnormal meconium occurs in cystic fibrosis and leads to meconium plug syndrome.

GENITALIA:

The genitalia and mammary glands normally respond to trans placentally obtained maternal hormones. Male and female genitalia show findings characteristic of gestational age. In most term male infants, the scrotum is relatively 14rge. Its size may be increased by the trauma of the breech delivery. And a transit rye hydrocele. A large scrotum must be Trans illuminated to differentiate a fluid-filled hydrocele from a bowel-containing hernia. However, the bowel will also occasionally transilluminate. The scrotum is pendulous, with reggae completely covering the scrotum should be examined for size, presence of testes, and the quality of the skin (thickness, presence of rugae, and pigmentation). In the full-term infant, the testes. They are present in the scrotum (completely descended), but sometimes they are retractile. In premature infants, they may not be completely descended and may be palpated in the inguinal canal. -When found in this area, and they may be drawn down into the scrotum by gently stripping the skin of the inguinal area Proximal to the soft mass of the testes. If the mass can be pushed into the scrotum, it is normally descended into the testis and will descend spontaneously in several weeks. The black male infant usuallyhas dark pigmentation of the scrotum before the rest of the skin assumes its permanent color.

The normal penis measures 2-3 cm from the pubis. A small phallus is normal if the. The urethral meatus is at the tip of the glans, and both the testes are descended. Erection of the penis normally occurs and is common. The prepuce of the newborn is normally tight and adherent. Non retractable foreskin is normal for the first 2-3 months after birth. Small phallus, hypospadias, epispadias, or cryptorchidism is suspicious of abnormality of the sex chromosome, or the infant is a masculinized female with an enlarged clitoris. Apparent hypospadias or epispadias may be the first evidence of adrenogenital syndrome. End pigmentation of the scrotum in males, and the labia major in females may normally be present in dark-skinned people. It is less prevalent in a premature baby. Labia majors should be separate and not fused and, at term, completely cover the labia minor and the clitoris. Both the labia major and theclitoris are normally large in newborns. A hymnal ring may be seen as a protruding tab of tissue. During the first few days after birth, a white mucous discharge may contain blood issues from the vagina. Occasionally a thin septum produced by the fusion of the labia minor covers the vagina, the fusion. It is easily disrupted by a blunt probe. The vaginal and urethral orifices should be seen. The urethral meatus is located just posterior to the clitoris. If the external genitalia are ambiguous, e.g., showing thickening corrugation or abnormal pigmentation of the labia major or fusion of the labia major, which can be an isolated congenital abnormality. If the stool is present in urine, the rectovaginal fistula should be suspected. Urine is passed usually during or immediately after the birth, and then a period of no urine follows normally, which may even extend to 24 hours. The urinary stream should be seen by the examiner. The stream is usually continuous.

Normally the extremities of the full-term baby are held in partial flexion. The lower extremities are normally bowed with separation of the knees when the ankles are held together, and the legs fully extended. The hand, if closed, may normally assume the cortical-thumb position (fingers flexed with the thumb inside). Femoral torsion (longitudinal twisting of the femur, the most common cause of toeing out in children) may be a normal finding, diagnosed by rotating the femur while the baby is- in the supine position. The normal range of femoral rotation is 30 degrees inward to 60 degrees outward. With inward femoral torsion, the patellae may even face each other (90-degree rotation) when the femurs are rotating Medical. Abnormal tibial torsion may be present. In the normal extended leg, a line drawn from the anterosuperior iliac spine across thecenter of the patellae should project to the second toe. If excessive tibial torsion is present, the line projects lateral or medial to the second toe in internal (the commonest cause of the toeing in) or excessive torsion, respeciallyectively. It may also be detected by extending the legs with the patella and tibial tubercles facing forward.

Tibdal torsion is present if a line drawn through all 4 malleoli is not parallel to the table and the normal foot, the forefoot, and the hindfoot lie in a projected straightline. Inward and outward deviation of the toes may be due to deviations of the foot. These deviations may be positional abnormalities (from the in-utero position) or structural (bony) deformities. The mild positional abnormalities will correct spontaneously or maybe 1 helped by passive exercises. This can be assessed by determining if the foot straightens out by stroking the inner and outer/sides of the foot or by passive manipulation without force. The foot of the newborn is normally flat because of a fat pad around the arch. The arch is not normally present until the child has walked for 1-2 years (is 2-3 years old. The extremities should be equal bilaterally. Spontaneous and passive movement of the extremities should be noted for all joints. Spontaneous movements are usually symmetrical. Passive movements ensure the full range of motionof all joints and assess muscle tone as well. Examination of the hip; Examined by 2 signs and 3 maneuvers.

The skin creases in the inguinal area (in the supine - position) and on the buttocks and thighs (in the prone position) are most often symmetrical on full extension of the legs, though asymmetrical folds may be seen sometimes. The 2nd sign, length from the hip to the knee, shouldbe checked with the knees and hips is flexion. In this position, the knees normally should be at t esame level of full extension, and the total length should be the same. The 3 maneuvers test. Abduction, rotation, and mobility. In abduction of the hips, the knees are flexed to 90 degrees and grasped by the examiner's hands, with the thumb resting on the medial aspect of the thigh and the index finger on the. Lateral aspect (the fingertip on the greater trochanter, the thighs are then abducted. Normally the thighs abduct to about 180 degrees, with the lateral aspects of the knees touching the examination table. Limitation of tightness may be evidence of dislocation. While in the position of abduction, the thighs should be gently pushed laterally by the thumbs and up by the index fingers to test for subluxation of the hip joint do click should be. Felt during any of these maneuvers, the: presence of a click is. Evidence of subluxation (Ortolanis click). Rotation assesses the ability of the femoral head to remain in the. The acetabulum confirms that the jointis not dislocated. It is performed by holding the knees in flexion and thighs partially abducted.

The femur is then rotated externally and internally normally, full range of rotational movement is -present and smooth without any resistance or spasm to determine the mobility of the hip joint in the supine position. One hand is placed on the area of the iliac crest, the other around thethigh. The two are gently pulled apart. Normally less than a centimeter of separation is possible. Polydactyl (presence of supernumerary digits) is frequently seen in normal babies, inherited. as a dominant trait, or maybe a manifestation of Laurence-Noon Bied or Ellis-van Creveld syndrome. Often these are simple skin tags, usually of the hand, which may be ligated or excised. Fleshy or born di fits may require surgical excision. Syndactyly (fusion of the bones or webbing) most often involves the third and 4th fingers or the second and third toes. It may be normal or be a part of acro-cephalo-syndactyly. Muscle tone and development must be assessed. Babies atbirth are frequently limp with good tone after the 1st or 2nd breath. Persistent poor tone after birth may be due to narcotics or depressants administered to the mother at the time of delivery. The spine should be aligned but flexible.

The arms and legs should be relatively symmetric in anatomy and function. Obviously, major abnormalities of the extremities include the absence of a bone, clubfoot, fusion or webbing of digits,or missing parts. Hip dislocation is suspected when there is a limitation of abduction of hips or when there is a click that can be felt when the femur is pressed downwards and then abducted.

The length may be unequal in length, and extra folds in the thighs are seen (skin folds). Palsies are seen in the extremities and recognized by limited movements of the extremities especially. if only one is involved. Fractures may be present, swelling and crepitation are felt, and limited movementof the extremities in the spontaneous movements or stimulated activity. Viable deformities or discontinuity found on palpation of the limbs ma: he due to a fracture from trauma at birth or bone disease as ontogenesisimperfecta. Circumferential constrictions or amputations on an extremity may be due (to constricting bands in utero. Talipes equinovarus(clubfoot), talipes calcaneovalgtu, and metatarsus adducts may be present. Abnormally short limbs may be real, as seen in Amelia or phocomelia, with the absence of a distal or proximal segment of a limb or may beapparent, as seen with a fracture of a long bone or congenital dislocation of the hips. Short and broad extremities are seen in Downs syndrome, gargoylism, and achondroplasia. Short thumb and 4th and 5th fingers are seen in pseudo-hypoplasia euthyroidism-Abnormally long limbs may be seen with lymphangiomas, large hengi-omas, arteriovenous fistulas, neurofibromatosis, hemihypertrophy, or lymphedema (Milroy 's disease or Turners syndrome), Long and thin extremities are found in arachnid dactyly.

Abnormalities of movement include diseases of bones, joints, muscles, the nervous system, and metabolic diseases. Arthrogryposis multiplex congenital is characterized by multiple dislocations and severe contractures. The excess motion of joints may be an isolated finding due to fetal position (genu redurvatum or hyperextension of the knee) or a manifestation of disease such as Down syndrome, Ehlers-Danlos syndrome, or amyotonia congenital). Lack of spontaneous movement may be due to paralysis from nerve damage during a traumatic birth, such as brachial nerve palsies, or fracture CNS abnormality such as myelomeningocele. Pseudoparalysis seen in congenital syphilis is due to pain in the motion of theextremities from periostitis. Fractures may be detected by deformity, decreased movement, diminished range of motion, excess motion in a bone associated with pain or crepitation, swelling, or absence of a pulse distal the fracture. Bones most often fractured at birth are the clavicle and homers. And femur. Increased muscle spasms may result from tetanus, kernicterus (early stage), seizures, hypocalcemia, and neonatal narcotic withdrawal. Poor tone or weakness may be associated with metabolic diseases (hypokalemia, hypoglycemiahypoxia, and asphyxia), drugs such as narcotics and sedatives, CNS diseases such as myasthenia gravis, cerebral edema, C hemorrhage, LMN disease, cerebellar lesions, cerebral palsy, endocrinopathy lee as hypothyroidism, hypoadrenalism, hypopituitarism, Downs syndrome, muscle cyst trophies. Hypotonia may be due to any other severe illness.

NEUROLOGICAL EXAMINATION:

It has been discussed in detail in the chapter on the neurologic examination of children and neonates. The neurological examination is performed partly while observing the patient during the physical examination. The activity, movements, state of consciousness, and position of the baby are noted. During a period of activity or hunger, a baby will be more responsive or even irritable compared to a baby who is in a postprandial state, at rest, or depressed from maternal drug administration. Although many reflexes can be elicited in the neonate, Moro and grasp reflexes are the most valuable in the clinical evaluation of the neonate. Moro should be symmetrical. The grasp reflex is useful as a test of strength since wealthy full-term infants should be able to partially support their weight while acing lifted from the supine to the sitting position. The degree of headlag dines lifting the baby assesses the baby's general tone. Placing and stooping Response s test the strength of the legs of the deep tendon reflexes; knee jerk is present at birth, followed shortly afterbirth by the Achilles and brachial reflexes. Chvosteks sign may normally be present, and upgoing, Babinski's sign is normal.

Transitory ankle clonus for several beats may be normal. An excellent method of evaluating the general tone of a baby is by suspending him ventrally in the palm of the hand. The healthy, alert baby will dorsiflexion the back and elevate the head to be in line with the back or even in slight extension while the legs are partially flexed. A baby with a poor tone willdroop. Vertical suspension holding the baby by the trunk under the arms tests the tone and strength of the shoulder girdle. A normal baby can be easily held in this way, but a baby with a poor tone will slip through the examiner's hands. High frequency, Low Amplitude movements of the extremities, a hyperactive Koro reflex is associated with hypocalcemia, tetanus, CNS infection, or cerebraldamage. A reverse-Loro reflex (extension and external rotation of t arms followed by rigidity) may be seen in babies more than 5 days old with base ganglion disease as kernicterus. Hyperactive deep tendon reflexes are seen with hyperthyroidism, hypocalcemia, hypomagnesemia, or lesion. Hypoactive reflexes may be from flaccid paralysis, Downs syndrome, malnutrition, brain injury a myotonic muscular.

Dystrophy, myasthenia gravis, hypomagnesemia, when the mother is eaten with mag sulfate, or LMN disease. The physical examination of the newborn child should be appropriate for its age (The first examination performed immediately after birth is aimed at identifying any life-threatening abnormalities that may need immediate attention and evaluating the infant 's ability to adjust to extrauterine life. A complete examination can 't be done at this time. The second examination may be done in the transition period when the pt. is observed but not disturbed except for weight, height, and to be classified by birth weight and gestational age. The complete examination should be ideally performed 12-24 hours after birth. The final evaluation should be done at the time of discharge.

FEEDING:

More mistakes are made by feeding too much than too little. Customarily feedings are startedafter the infant stabilizes in glad condition, sleep, then wake up hungry and start crying.
Usually, 6 hours after delivery, gradually feeding the infant. Adequate nutrition is achieved if theinfant is no longer losing weight by the 7th day and is gaining by the 14th. Some delay occurs in the establishment of breastfeeding. Scheduling is not important. Four hourly feedings are sufficient. It is better that infants Are given 5% dextrose for first feeds since regurgitation of this will not lead to significant irritation of the respiratory tract in case aspiration occurs. Till two weeks of age, no vitamins are added. Glucose rater also causes some pneumonitis. It is better to give sterilewater first. On the first day, it is best to limit. Sucking to 5 min at each feeding, 10 min the 2nd day, and 15 min the 3rd day. Breastfeeding should be done whenever the baby is hungry, at least 2-4 hours. Immediate sucking after birth will enhance the appearance of colostrum. Dextrose water should be given after nursing as fluid-supple meat until milk volume is sufficient.

During hot water, sterile water should be given to prevent dehydration and fever. Demand feeding allows the infant to eat when awake and hungry and leads to optimal attar intake and the eventual establishment of a suitable schedule. The first feeding of sterile water should be offered as the birth recovery reward is ending and the infant appears hungry, which is normally at 3-6 hours of age. The most important criteria to be considered in starting feeding are the infant should appear actively hungry, should have normal bowel sounds, and should have no abdominal distension. When these conditions are met, the first feeding of sterile water is given. If it is tolerated full, strength milk formula (20 kcal/oz.) or breast feedings can be given by the 3rd day, and the infant must receiveat least 100ml/kg/day, which may increase to more than 180ml/kg/day, allowing for hunger satisfaction. About the 4th or 5th day, the infant becomes hungrier, but this lasts for one to two days only, and the infant will return to a less frequent schedule soon after.

Schedule for Special Care for the High-Risk Infant is in Appendix III

The occurrence of chromosomal anomalies, congenital anomalies, inborn errors of metabolism, mental retardation, or any familial disease in blood relatives increases the risk of the same condition in the infant. The lowest neonatal mortality, 2%, occurs in infants of mothers 20- 30 years. of age; it is doubled if the mother 40-45 years and quadrupled if she happens to be morethan 45 years. The mother is less than 15 years. of age, the neonatal mortality is high-Maternal illness incites the risk. Infants born to mothers with infections or with a h/o any illness during pregnancy, with premature rupture of membranes, toxemia, diabetes, or any other metabolic disease, with a h/o a severe social problem, such as teenage marriage, drug addiction, absence of the mate, absent or delayed prenatal care, with minimal weight gain during pregnancy, prolonged infertility, with 4 or more pregnancies, who are 35 years. or more of age, or who have taken any teratogenicitydrug during pregnancy, are all high-risk neonates. A gestation beginning within 3 months of a previous pregnancy is also included. Infants born to mothers who had stressful events lent during gestation, such as severe emotional problems, hyperemesis gravidarum, serious accidents, or generalized anesthesia.

Polyhydramnios is present in 80% of cases of trisomy 18. The conditions associated with polyhydramnios include anencephaly (205 meningoceles, encephalocele, esophageal or duodenal atresia, pyloric stenosis KlippiFell syndrome, cleft palate, harelip, achondroplasia, diaphragmatic defects, multiple anomalies-Atresia of the upper intestinal tract interfere with the reabsorption into the circulation of swallowed amniotic fluid; faulty fetal formation or release of ADH is involved in fetuses with anomalies of the CNS. Oligohydramnios is associated with renal agenesis, ureteral dysplasia, urethral atresia, pulmonary hypoplasia, or amnion nodosum. Congenital aplasia of the fetal kidneys is often accompanied by a reduced amount of amniotic fluid because fetal urine is not formed.

Iighydramnios before the last few weeks of pregnancy may result in mechanically induced abnormalities such as genu reeurvatum. Intrauterine amputations may be due to local constriction during fetal growth caused by amniotic bands or fibrous strings (formed because of rupture of fetal membranes early in gestation). Pregnancy is an elevated risk if the uterus is inappropriately largeor small. A uterus that is large for estimated stages of gestation suggests. Multiple fetuses, hydramnios, or excessively large infants and appropriately small one indicates retardation of intrauterine growth. Rupture of membranes earlier than 24 hours. Before delivery carries a risk of infection of intrauterine contents and increased perinatal mortality. Prolonged and difficult laborincreases the risk of mechanical and hypoxic damage. The risk of neonatal death in uncomplicated labor lasting less than 24 hours is 0.3%, and it increases 6-fold in labor lasting over 24 hours. and 20-fold (6%) in those over 30 hours. A precipitate delivery with short labor increases the risk of intracranial hemorrhage. Cesarean infants have problems that necessitate surgery and the effects of prolonged maternal anesthesia. In the absence of these factors also, delivery through the abdomen carries a greater risk than through the birth canal. Some of them may die, while a small number have some degree of respiratorydifficulty for a day or two after birth, and idiopathic respiratorysyndrome may have the most unfavorable outcome. Infants born before 37 or after 42 weeks of gestation are also elevated risk. Most high-risk infants are either born prematurely born or have a low weight for gestational age. For any given duration of gestation, the lower the birth, the higher the mortality. For any given weight, the shorter the duration of gestation, the higher the neonatal mortality. The highest risk of neonatal mortality is among infants who weigh less than 1000 gm. at birth and whose gestation was. Less than 30 weeks, the lowest risk is in infants with birth weights of 3000-4000 gm. and whose gestational age was 38-42 weeks.

MULTIPLE BIRTHS (TWINS)

Twining occurs in 1:90 cases on average, but the incidence is high in blacks and low in east Asian races (1:150-300). Twins may develop from single ovum, money gothic, constituting1/3rd of twins in all races. About 1/3rd of these monovular twins have a double placenta (amnion and chorion). Twins may develop from two ova, dizygotic. The incidence of females arises with the number of fetal products of multiple pregnancies. The occurrence of monovular twins appears to be independent of genetic or environmental factors. Polyovular pregnancies are more frequent beyond the second pregnancy in older women and in families with a history of polyvular twins. They may result from the simultaneous maturation of multiple ovarian follicles.

Conjoined twins (Siamese twins) and the presence of two embryos in one amniotic see are the results of late monovular twining. Twins who are of opposite sexes are dizygotic. When both are of the same sex, zygosity can be determined by examination of the placenta at birth or later through comparison of physical characteristics, detailed blood typing, or trial of tissue transplant from twin to twin. A careful examination of the placenta is. The best way of differentiating monovular and polyvular twins. If the placentas are separate, they are dichromic, but the twins are not necessarily dizygotic. Twins of the same sex, if not monochromic, should be reevaluated between the ages of 2 and 4 years. At this time, physical characters for the identification of monovular twine become most valid. If there are important physical differences by this age, dichromic twins may be presumed to be dizygotic. If the partition between the twins consists of 2 layers of transparent amnic without an intervening chorionic, monozygotic twining is diagnosed. The fetal growth pattern is different than in a single fetus pregnancy. Intrauterine growth retardation occurs at a given total weight of all fetuses regardless of the number. The greater the number of fetuses, the earlier pregnancy labor will occur. Therefore, the fetuses in multiple pregnancies are more likely to suffer from preterm delivery and intrauterine growth retardation than singletons.

Discordant twins whose birth weights differ by 20% or more are often associated with twin-to-twin transfusion syndrome and are more common when there is a single chorionic, as in monozygotictwins. Thus, twins of widely discrepant sizes are usually monochorionic. Vascular anastomosisin monochromic placentas may be artery to artery, vein to vein, or artery to vein. Usually, they are well-balanced, so neither twin suffers. In rare cases, one umbilical cord may arise from the other after leaving the placenta when the twin attached to the secondary cord is usually malformed or dies in the uterine. Uncompensated placental arteriovenous shunts the monochromic twins on the arterial side are oligohydramnios, small premature, who are malnourished, pale, anemic, hypovolemicila in shock, and microcoria, while as those on the venous side it is. Polyhydramnios, large premature well nourished, plethoric, polycythemia, and hypovolemic, and suffers cardiac failure and cardiac hypertrophy. Maternal hydramnios in a twin pregnancy suggest fetal transfusion syndrome.

When a donor twin may need a transfusion and the recipient twin is bleeding, the additional cardiac load, as evidenced by arteriolar hypertrophy in a distressed recipient twin, suggests digitalization of the infant. Death of the donor twin in the uterus may lead to generalized fibrin thrombi in the smaller arterioles of the recipient due to transfusion of thromboplastin-rich blood from the macerating donor fetus. Postnatal identification: Physical criteria for determining the monovulartwins –

Both must be of the same sex –

Their features, including ears and teeth, must be obviously alike –

Their hair must be identical in color, texture, natural curl,

and distribution –

Their eyes must be of the same shade and color –

Their skin must be of the same texture and color –

Their hands and feet must be of the same conformation and of equivalent size –

Their anthropometric values must agree closely.

Dermatoglyphics is of limited use in the diagnosis of zygosity. Prints of monozygotic twins mayhave a similar pattern; they are not identical. Detailed blood typing can offer absolute proof only that twins are dizygotic, and if no blood group discrepancy can be demonstrated between twins, homozygosity can be presumed.

Complications of multiple births:

Most twins are born prematurely; pregnancy is usually several weeks shorter.

Maternal complications of pregnancy are more common.

Polyhydramnios is 10 times more common, placenta previa from the increased placental mass is more frequent, and abruption placentae may occur with the second twin placenta due to a reduction in the size of the uterus following delivery of the first twin. Breech and other abnormal presentations are more common. There is an increased risk of velamentous insertion of the umbilical cord, with a higher incidence of bleeding during labor. Uterine contractions after delivery may be poor, with subsequent bleeding. Prolapse of the cord is 7 times more frequent because of the abnormal presentation and rupture of the second twins' membranes when engaged. Monoamniotic twins have an increased likelihood of entangling theircords, leading to asphyxia. If one of the fetuses is macerated, the live twin is usually delivered first. The 2nd twin is more subject to anoxia than the first because the placenta may separate after the birth of the first twin and before the birth of the 2nd. Differences in size at the birth of the monovular twins usually disappear by 6 months.

LOW BIRTH WEIGHT (LBW) AND PREMATURITY.

All over the world, birth weight is recognized as the single most significant factor which influences perinatal survival and the incidence of disorders and deals in the early weeks of life. Birthweight is important because many physiologic and metabolic processes, such as temperature regulation and the need for environmental temperature support, are a function of size and are relatively independent of the infant 's gestational age. Relative surface area increases as weight decreases.
LBW:

Infants who weigh 2500 gm. or less at birth are LBW infants. They may be so due to a less-than-expected rate of intrauterine growth or a shortened gestational period, or both.

PREMATURITY:

Live-born infants delivered before 37 weeks of gestation (from the first day of the LMP) have shortened gestation and are thus called premature. Prematurity and LBW are usually concomitant.2/3rd of LBW infants are prematurely born, while 8% of infants, more than 2500, are premature. Prematurity is especially seen in those weighing less than 1500 gm. (i.e., infants ofexceptionally low birth weight}. Their problems of w metabolism, thermal regulations, and water and electrolyte balance are exceedingly complex regardless of their gestational at Gestational age is calculated based on LMP, uterine size, the time when fetal heart sounds and movements were first noted, other tests as serial ultrasound examinations to determine the parietal diameter andits rate of growth, amniotic fluid examination, for creating concentration assessment of lecithin/sphingomyelin ratios. After delivery, clinical estimation of gestational age is based on physical examination and neurologic assessment, both of which change with increasing gestational age. Inmany parts of India, the average birth weight is less than 2500gm. In the USA, 7.2%-of whites and 14% of blacks are LBW. Based on the 2500 gm criterion, 34.7% of Indian infants are LBW, and if less than 2500 and is taken as the standard Weight, 19 of the institutional births are LBW.The mortality in the very LBW is 50%.

CAUSES OF LBW AND PREMATURITY.

Birth weight is influenced by biological pathological, and social factors. Length of gestation is the most important single factor. In developed countries, 2/3rds of LBW are born too soon, i.e., before 37 weeks. The incidence of pre-term birth is slightly higher in Asian countries than in developed. World, but the incidence of LBW among babies born at 37 weeks. or later is much higher. Thus, the most crucial factor of LBW in the developed world is the length of gestation, but in developing countries, a higher incidence of maternal pathology and inadequate maternal care are mostly respeciallyonsible. Boys weigh more than girls at all fetal ages after 37 weeks and average 100-200 gms at 4.0 weeks, up to the 28th wk. The growth of twins is slightly less than the singleton fetus, but subsequently, the velocity of growth decreases so that after 35 weeks, there is slight further weight gain, and a loss may occur after 38 weeks. Mothers who had themselves LBW have a higher incidence of LBW infants. Short maternal height also correlates. Disorders that shorten gestation or which interfere with placental blood supply, such as pre-ecliptic toxemia, hypertension, antepartum hemorrhageotaternal anemia, due to undernutrition and infection. The fetus may be small because of gross congenital anomalies, chromosomal anomalies, or because of the growth retarding influence of the fetal infection.

Toxoplasmosis and other torch infections, and many other fetal viral infections, may cause generalized fetal disease, often with meningoencephalitis leading to microcephaly and hepatitis, and thus retard fetal growth, particularly of the brain and skull. -Life at high altitudes may reduce birth weight. High flying in. the last 6 weeks. May precipitate labor and thus lead to LBW. Low socioeconomic status correlates both with short gestation and LBW. Excessive physical work during pregnancy may lower the birth weight. The incidence of LBW is high in illegitimate pregnancies. Early marriage and short- spacing between pregnancies may lead to LBW. Illiteracy, cultural patterns, and indigenous customs controlling nutrition, etc., all affect the birth weight of the baby. Cigarette smoking, even in moderate amounts, will lower birth weight may be due to a steady rise of CO in smoking pregnant women towards the term. In general, premature birth is associated with conditions in which there is an inability of the uterus to retain the fetus through artificial interference.

LBW infants are divided d into two groups; one is preterm, i.e., LBW infants born before 37 weeks of gestation, whose pattern of growth has been normal and there has been no fetal growth retardation, infants suffering intrauterine growth retardation (the infant may be preterm, term, or post-term) when the birth weight is less than 2 SD below the mean for the gestational age. The intrauterine growth rate of an infant is affected by the mother's general health, the health of the fetus, and the condition of the placenta.

PRETERM INFANTS WITH NO FETAL GROWTH RETARDATION

The clinical state of these babies depends entirely on gestational age; the most striking changeswith increasing maturity are seen in the body proportions. –

At 28-31 weeks, the head appears relatively large with an average circumference of 25 cm, which increases up to 32-33 cm by 37 weeks. Skull is soft and shows little molding; fontanels and sutures are wide open, and thin. Skin through which the veins and venules are easily seen is covered with fine, downy hair. The circumference of the head is 4-5 cm greater than the thorax, and this difference reduces to less than 3 cm at term. The face is small in comparison to the vault of the skull, with the absence of the sucking pads and very shallow orbits so that the eyeballs protrude. Eyebrows are just defined and eyelashes scanty, the chin is pointed, and the nose and mouth are exceedingly small. The pinna of the external ear is almost flat of skin with little or no incurving of the upper edge and fold over as the chili lies on them. Advancing maturity is shown by increasing firmness and development of cartilage extending towards the periphery. The upper part of the pinnae develops well-defined incurving. At 32-36 wk. The skull molds markedly during labor, the increase in the subcutaneous. Fat diminishes the angularity of the face, and as the orbits deepen, the exophthalmic appearance is lost. Lanugo hair is abundant on the face and back arms from 30-35 weeks.

THORAX.

At 28 weeks thorax is cone-shaped and short, about 1/4th of the total trunk length. This ratio increases to 245 at term. The lower ribs lie almost horizontal, and the intercostal muscles are poorly developed. Inspiration often causes marked retraction of the lower end of the sternum. The abdominal wall has poor musculature and facial development; visible peristalsis in the stomach and intestine is always seen, and distension occurs readily. The umbilicus lies well below the mid-line of the abdomen and is closest to the symphysis pubis in the three most immature infants. The liver and kidney are easily palpable. Limbs are very thin with little muscular development. Skin is fine and transparent and has a dark red color although pigment begins to appear in the deeper layer, sit rarely shows through in the preterm infant. Lanugo hair is soft hair that is abundant but decreases on the back and arms after 36 weeks. –

EDEMA.

Almost invariably present to some degree on the first 2 days giving the skin a stretched and shinyappearance. Subsequently, it hangs in loose folds. Vernix caseosa is scanty and gradually increasing in an amount up to term. Nails are incredibly soft, and the toenails particularly don ‘t reach the end of the phalanges.

ASSESSMENT OF THE GESTATIONAL AGE:

To assess the quality of intrauterine growth, gestational age must be known. The most useful external characteristic of the clinical estimation of the gestational age is skin color and texture, edema, lanugo hair, skull hardness, ear form and firmness, external genitalia, breast size and nipple formation, and plantar creases. These physical signs distinguish infants under 2500 gm who are of appropriate weight for their gestational age from those with retarded growth. Infants of either group lack sc fat, but infant with retarded growth is likely to be shorter than expectedfor gestational age and appears to have a disproportionately larger head for their body size than a premature infant of the appropriate weight-brain growth is generally less affected than the linear growth or growth of other organs by factors that adversely affect the intrauterine growth (excepting in the chronic fetal nonbacterial infections and chromosomal anomalies). Functional development of the fetal nervous system correlates with gestational age. Development of the external genitalia provides one of the most reliable indications of gestational age. In the male, by the 32 wk, the testes have not descended but are just palpable in the inguinal canals. By the 36 wk, the testes are not usually completely descended, and the scrotal rugae arefew and limited to it.

SIZE OF THE BREAST NODULE

Two finely pigmented brown areas of 1-2 cm diameter, with a tiny depression in the center, represent the primitive mammary glands at 28 weeks. It is usually not palpable at 33-34 weeks. At 36-37 weeks, the primitive nipple rises above the surface, and the breast nodule becomes palpable, but at this stage, it is not more than 3 mm in diameter; in term infants, the areola is wellraised above the surface and is 4-10mm in diameter. Extraordinarily little colostrum is produced in the immature infant so that physiological mastitis is only seen in term infants. –

PLANTAR SKIN CREASE

No plantar skin creases are present at 28 weeks, and then

faint remarks develop over the interior part of the sole; by 36 weeks. There are only one to two creases seen on the interior of the sole of the foot. By 38 weeks, more creases have appeared, and by term, areas other than the anterior part of the sole (i.e., the whole o the sole) are seen to have deep indentations of the crisis cross creases covering the whole ofthe sole. Scalp hair: tends to be short and fuzzy up to 37 weeks by 40 weeks, coarse and silky strands are seen individually standing. -The cartilaginous development of the ear lope, which makes the folds of the helix and antihelix stand out, occurs chiefly between the 36 and 40 weeks of gestation. -Radiological markers; Ossification centers at the knee joint; that for the lower end of the femur usually appears at 34 weeks, and the upper end of the tibia appears at 39 weeks. The center for the cuboid appears at term. The size of the center is important in the assessment of infants believed to be born at term or post-term.

ASSESSMENT OF NEUROLOGIC DEVELOPMENT:

The immature infant is characterized by hypotonia. The infant is observed for posture in quiet and in a supine position. A froglike posture may be adapted initially; an asymmetrical posture with extended limbs is soon assumed, and there is little or no flexion in Response to muscle stretching. The head can 't be lifted in the prone posture and lags in the sitting position till 39weeks. Heal angle, with the infant supine and the pelvis flat on tie examining coach, and the thigh is held in the knee-chest position by the examiner's left index finger with the thumb supporting the knee. The leg is then extended by gentle pressure from the examiner's right index finger behind the ankle, and the popliteal angle is measured. The popliteal angle steadily reduces from 150 degrees at 28 weeks to 100 at 34 weeks and to 80 at L0 weeks.

Ankle dorsiflexion the foot is dorsiflexed onto the anterior aspect of the leg with the examiner's thumb on the sole of the foot and other fingers behind the leg; enough pressure is applied to getas full flexion as possible, and the angle of the dorsum of the foot and anterior aspect of the leg is measured. Maximum dorsiflexion of the foot is only achieved by 36 weeks when the dorsum of the foot touches the skin of the leg.

Leg recoil: with the infant supine, the hips and knees are fully flexed for 5 sec, then extended bytraction on the feet, then released maximal Response is one of full flexion of the hips and knees. -Free movements of the limbs are continually active at 28-32 weeks and then gradually decrease until, at term, the infant remains relatively still. The traction Response is present at 33-36 weeks.

Square window: the hand is flexed, and the forearm is between the thumb and index finger of the examiner. Enough pressure is applied to get as full flexion as possible, and the angle between the hypothenar eminence and the ventral aspect of the forearm is measured and graded. Care is taken not to rotate the infant 's wrist while doing this maneuver.

Heel-to-ear maneuver with the baby supine, the baby 's foot is drawn as near to the head as it will gowithout forcing it. The distance between the foot and the head and the degree of extension at the knee are observed. The knee is left free, and I draw down alongside the abdomen.

Scarf sign with baby supine, the infant's hand is taken and tried to put around the neck as far posteriorly as possible around the opposite shoulder. The maneuver is assisted by lifting the elbow across the body. Ventral suspension: the infant is suspended in the prone position withthe exam inners hand under the infant's chest. The degree of extension of the back and the amount of flexion of the arms and legs are noted. Relation of the head to the trunk is also noted.

Please See Dubowitz Scoring of Neurological Signs in Appendix 1.

A discrepancy in maturation between the physical and neuromuscular characteristic: often indicatea problem in intrauterine growth. Evaluation of physical character is done within 24 hours of age and neurological examination after 413 bras of age. Intrauterine growth retardation due to undernutrition(rather than due to fetal malformation)alters the physical growth more than the neurological characteristics so that there is diminished growth or absence of breast tissue and in the female, relatively small labia major, loss of vernix and desquamation of the skin prior to term, meconium staining 06 the skin and nails due to fetal distress with bower evacuation, weight is affected first followed by decreased growth in length, and in severe undernutrition, head circumference, while the neurologic examination is lest affected and is usually appropriate for the actual gestational age.

REFLEXES in the assessment of the gestational age; -

Sucking and swallowing reflexes which are essential to survival, are present weekly from 32 weeks but usually are inadequate and insufficiently coordinated to allow the sufficient intake of food by sucking until 36 weeks. The sucking reflex is absent before 31wk, and its presence shows more than 33 weeks. The rooting reflex is also similarly timed. Moro grasp and trunk curving reflexes are present but weak at 28 weeks.

The development of patterns can also give useful confirmatory evidence of the stages of fetal brain maturation. 29-32 weeks high amplitude slow waves with occipital evidence, at 33-36 weeksmoderate amplitude faster waves with no localization, and at 37-39 weeks low amplitude waveswith a frequency of either cycles/second or indeterminate and no special dominance.

PATHOLOGY IN LBW INFANTS:

Neonatal deaths among premature and term infants of low birth weights, and thus low birth weight for gestational age, result from the same general group of t the pathology. Prematurity is not a cause of death, and the principal causes of death in both premature and term infantsare anoxia, cerebral birth injury, malformations, RDS, bronchopneumonia, septicemia, and other infections. Hyaline membrane diseases associated with desorption atelectasis are found in 50% of LBW infants, dying 1 hour to 4 days after birth. Hemorrhage associated with traumaranoxia, infection, and defect in the clotting mechanism is frequent and severe.SC ecchymosis, bleeding into the choroid plexus, subependymal or intraventricular, is frequent in premature infants with LBW and is due to increased capillary fragility. Sudden shock and collapse during the first few days of life are often due to intraventricular hemorrhage. Fatal hemorrhage into the lungs may also occur. Retrolental fibroplasia occurs in premature infants treated with oxygenat concentrations above ambient air levels. Kernicterus associated with hyperbolic binomial is seen in 2-20% of autopsies on premature infants. Immaturity of anatomy, physiologic, and biochemical functions is an index of the relative inability of the preterm and LB infant to survive.

Deficiencies in these functions affect infant's ability to withstand demands that do exist within the uterus, such as temperature control, pulmonary function, nutrition, disposal of metabolic waste, immunologic function, detoxification, and excretion of toxic substances. The developmentof each tissue and function is variable with gestational age. Cuboidal epithelium of lung alveoli prevents gaseous exchange prior to 28 weeks but disappears by 31 weeks. The immature infants' respiratoryfunction is limited by the under-ventilation of perfused alveoli, decreased surface for gas exchange, and insufficient surface-active lipid surfactant to prevent the collapse of alveoli. Underdeveloped airways and lung tissue and the persistence of fluid in the lung results in increased resistance to airflow. The ability to minimize heat loss in Response to cold stress is proportional to body size, and there is a decreased capacity for non-shivering thermogenesis.

There are decreased stores of hepatic and myocardial glycogen, which compromise the infant's ability to withstand asphyxia-The nephrogenic zone of the kidney is used as a dependable guide to gestational age since it disappears by 35-36 weeks. Renal blood flow, glomerular functions, and tubular functions are decreased. The liver shows a progressive reduction in mesenchyme tissue and amount of erythropoiesis by 35 weeks, except in fetal hemolytic disease and the in rant of the poorly controlled diabetic mother, where erythropoietin tissue can be present till 38 weeks. Cardiopulmonary circulation is transitional between that of a fetus and an adult; increased shunting through ducts arteriosus and foramen ovale may occur in Response to stress and result in circulatory insufficiency or under perfusion of vital organs. The shorter the period of gestation, the more unprepared the infant to meet the extrauterine life. Based on pathologic changes, infants of low birth weight for gestational age are divided into two groups; one group has anatomic changes like those found in infants with postnatal alimentary malnutrition, as diminished sc fat decreased alas of and organs the adrenal liver spleen and thymus the small size of orphans due to a subnormal amount of cytoplasm in individual cells rather than to a diminished number of calls. These infants with fetal malnutrition include infants of toxemic mothers, multiple pregnancies and prolonged pregnancies, or placental abnormalities which interfere with nutrition-The other group has a reduced number of cells in various body organs butwith a normal amount of cytoplasm /cell. This hypo-plastic group of infants includes infants with chromosomal abnormalities and congenital heart disease except for TGA, congenital rubella, and CID.

PROBLEMS OF PREMATURITY:

Problems of prematurity are due to anatomic and functional immaturity of the various organs. Atterm, the ability to suck and swallow is already developed, and failure to do this may be due. To immaturity, damage to mental brain deficiency (but nasal obstruction, thrush, anomalies of the mouth such as cleft palate may be respeciallyonsible). Weak suckling, swallowing, gagging, and cough reflexes lead to difficulty of aspiration. Pulmonary immaturity and a pliable thorax led to hypoventilation and hypoxia, which leads to respiratoryand metabolic acidosis.

Problems of major clinical significance associated with prematurity or infants of LBW include respiratory distress (hyaline membrane diseases, Pulmonary hemorrhage, aspiration syndrome, congenital pneumonia pneumothorax), recurrent apnea, hypoglycemia, hypocalcemia, hyperbilirubinemia, anemia, edema, neurologic signs related to cerebral anoxia, circulatory instability, hypothermia, bacterial sepsis, In infection syndromes withcongenital anomalies, persistent viremia with organ localization, and disseminated intravascular coagulopathy. Infants who are small for gestational age suffer fetal distress, CNS depression, meconium aspiration, hypoglycemia, chronic IU infection, pulmonary hemorrhage polycythemia, or congenital anomalies. Preterm infants whose weight is appropriate for their gestational age have a higher incidence of hyaline membrane disease, nonhemolytic hyperbilirubinemia, neonatal bacterial infections, thermal instability, poor feeding, prolonged failure to gain weight, apnea, cardiac arrhythmia, anemia, bleeding intraventricular hemorrhage in infants less than 1200gm, and late metabolic acidosis.

CARE OF THE PRETERM AND LBW INFANTS (ORDINARY AND SPECIAL)

The preterm infant may need only ordinarily care or may need exceptional care both a birth (in the delivery room) as well as in the nursery. Infants born at 36-38 weeks may need only a routine nursery, stabilizing uneventfully after birth. But the more premature infant will need exceptional care in a specialized nursery. The aim is to provide exceptional care to these babies who have a reduced chance of surviving without such care by counteracting their various handicaps. If the principles of routine neonatal care are more effectively applied to LBW infants. The survival rate improves considerably with quite simple methods and without incubation (or sophisticated equipment. At birth, the same measures for clearing the airway, initiation and maintenance of breathing, and care of the cord and eyes are required as for normal-weight babies. Simple care can be affected at homeor in a hospital, and this is all that is needed for most babies weighing 2000gm or more and even m any weighing 1750 gm. perinatal hypoxia and apnea should be anticipated and treated. Fluid overload (should be avoided as FDA is common in premature. Blood components, packed cells: Plasma platelets may be needed for anemia, hypovolemia, or bleeding. Hyperbilirubirubinemia, hypoglycemia, hypokalemia, hypernatremia, temperature control problems, and special nutritional needs must be anticipated.

Indications for hospitalization:

- All mothers with pregnancy complications or in premature

labor (before 37 completed weeks ofgestation) should be delivered in the hospital.

- After birth, the absolute indications for Hospitalization are -

- The extremely low birth weight, i.e., less than 1600gm, or short gestation, i.e., less than 36 weeks. -respiratory distress needing continuous oxygen therapy.
- Evidence of cerebral irritation, apneic spells, and convulsions, -Development of early jaundice requiring investigation, Inability to bottle feed
- Inability to maintain body temperature
- Development of neonatal diseases such as congenital malformations, severe infection, hemolyticdisease, etc.

If possible, infants less than 30 wk gestation should be delivered in e hospital that has an intensive care nursery since the need for transport adds to morbidity and mortality. Preterm infants at 35-36 weeks gestation often thrive with the simple care provided for term LM if they have escapedthe special hazards of stress in labor, the difficulty of delivery, and asphyxia. The survival of preterm infants with truly short gestation of those with severe neonatal problems depends mainly on specialized care, and with limited facilities and overload, the selection at birth is needed according tothe prospect of survival.

- Prevention of infection is especially important for preterm and LBW babies. Scrupulous attention to hand washing by personnel before and after handling each baby or any equipment tobe used for it. Organisms multiply more actively on the body of the neonate's umbilical cord stump, groins, perineum, and nose than elsewhere and are carried on the hands and clothing of personnel in contact with babies to each new baby admitted to the ward.

Chemical disinfection isunsatisfactory, and scissors, cord dressings, mucus catheters, etc., should be heat sterilized to prevent infection during and after birth.

- Loss of body heat is poorly tolerated, so the body should be quickly wrapped in a cloth and placed in a warm cot or by the mother 's body while awaiting transport. Tight wrappings should be avoided as these impede respiratorymovements. Blankets can do the same. Extra heatis provided by hot water bottles in the cot on bags arranged around the cot, protecting the baby from direct contact. Poor maintenance of temperature is a critical factor in improved survival and prevention of morbidity. Infants with extremely low are most vulnerable to cold stress. They have limited capacity to produce heat because of decreased brown fat and diminished muscle mass, and therefore less no shivering thermogenesis. They suffer greater heat loss because of a larger surface-to-volume ratio, the extension of the extremities (the normal position of premature infants), increased peripheral circulation, and decreased insulation due to diminished ac fat (less than 2% of body weight in a 1000g infant versus 16% in a 3000g infant). Cold stress can be prevented by warming the delivery room, drying the baby immediately after birth, and placing the baby under the radiant warmer. In the nursery, the baby should be maintained in a thermal-neutral environment (the temperature at which a resting infant maintains normal body temperature alongwith a minimal rate of oxygen consumption) under radiant heaters or in standard incubators the sickest infants who need continuous accessibility should be cared for under the radiant heaters. A thermo-neutral temperature can always be achieved in these infants if the abdominal skin temperature is maintained at 36.3-36.5C by means of a thermistor probated to the right upper quadrant of the anterior abdominal wall, which controls the heat output of the radiant heater or incubator. Preferably small, preterm, or growth retarded infants should be cared for in incubators set to maintain skin temperature at 36-37C with an air temperature of 32-36 C. Modern incubatorsconserve body heat through the provision of a warm atmospheric environment and standard conditions of humidity provide a regulated oxygen supply, reduce atmospheric contamination, and thereby minimize risks of infection and prevent excessive evaporative water loss. The air temperature of the incubator will depend on the size and maturity of the infant; infants of 1000g or less usually need a temperature in the upper ranges. Relative humidity should be maintained at 50% (40-60%), which reduces the heat loss at lower temperatures and prevents the drying and irritation of the lining of the respiratorypassages, especially. during the administration of oxygen and during endotracheal or nasotracheal incubation, and in thinning viscid secretions and reducing insensible water as from the lungs. If the humidity is lower, the temperature should be higher thanthat 14 the table. Incubators and radiant heaters must be kept away from coolers, air conditioners, cold windows, and cold walls double-walled incubator may be used, preferably. High humidity is undesirable as it encourages the growth of the hydrophilic organisms, pseudomonas, on the inner surfaces of the incubator. The administration of oxygen to reduce the risk of hypoxia and circulatory insufficiency must be balanced against the risks of hyperopia for the eyes and lungs. If there is cyanosis, dyspnea, and apnea, these are definite clinical indications for oxygen therapy. If an incubator is not available, the general conditions of temperature and humidity control can be attained by the intelligent use of blankets, heating lamps, heating pads, and warm water bottles and by control of the temperature and humidity of the room. If oxygen is needed, it can bedone by a face mask or through an intubation tube.

Umbilical cord infection, tetanus, is a real hazard, and a sterile dressing should be applied atonce, and the use of hexachlorophene 33% in a sterilized dusting powder is recommended strongly to keep down colonization with ale eve organisms on the umbilicus, groins, and perineum, and buttocks. There should be no attempatient to clean the baby's skin, as this involves chilling and increases liability to infection. Before removal from the delivery room, the baby should be examined for clinical characteristics, which determine the type of care according to gestation and birth weight and classified as preterm and of appropriate weight for gestation, or term or preterm large for dates or small for dates. The advantage of involving the mother in the child 's care is that the risk of cross-infection is reduced, and the mother can keep continuous observation of her own child, reducing the risk of regurgitation and inhalation of gastric contents in an unattended baby's tendency for hard-pressed nursing personnel to hurry to overfeed or resort unnecessary gavage feeding is avoided.

Role of the special care baby units. These can be set up in association with the delivery room and lying in the wards. Staff must change their shoes before entry to the unit and may even wear face masks. In hot, dusty climates, wet mopping of the floor may be needed. Cots on the star should be suitably placedspaced in the rooms, 50 sq ft allocated for each cot and 30 sqft for each incubator. Linen and equipment must be kept in cupboards. Each room should have simple equipment for respiratoryemergencies. The apparatus that has direct contact with babies should be heat sterilized. The incubator can be a source of danger from infection if not cleaned thoroughly with water and soap and sterilized with formalin vapor after each baby's stay. Admission to such nursery is restricted to babies of very short gestation, who are unable to maintain body temperature without incubators or heated cots, or who require gavage feeding or treatment of special problems such as RDS, hyperbiliriinernia, etc. If possible, the room must be air-conditioned and equipped with oxygen, a mechanical sucker, a resuscitation trolley with a laryngoscope, tubes for intubating, a pressure gauge, and masks for oxygen therapy. The room must be under the continuous supervision of a trained nun to see who is flied gavage feeding and has no duties in connection with follow-up clinic or any potentially infected mother or baby. Infected babies must be removed from a nursery immediately. The essence the specialized care is constant observation of the behavior and appearance of the child, which is accurately recorded with temperature, pulse, and respiratory rates at regular, frequent intervals, i.e., 2, 3, 4 hourlies according to the condition of the baby throughout 24 hr. period, and immediately attended if there is change it his condition as cyanosisor apnea, etc. The survival of small or frail infants often depends entirely on the skill of the nurse as it is easy to cause regurgitation and inhalation pneumonia if food is administered inexpertly and the baby is not watched subsequently. Sophisticated equipment for artificial ventilation and condition monitoring depends on regular electric supply, is of very limited value, and makes great demands on staff, and its users can ‘t be recommended in the existing circumstances of most tropical countries. A single mattress type of apnea monitor is useful for alerting the nurse when apneic attacks occur and is easy to use and clean.

Note- The premature infant who is swaddled and able to maintain body temperature without added environmental heat is 'placed in an open bassinet; this can be done when the infant is reached 1800-2000g; in order to monitor growth, hydration, nutrition of preterm infants, standard postnatal growth curves can be used in conjunction with the infants own growth cure Each clay the infant's weight total water intake, (milked) and total caloric intake (kcal/kg/day) are plotted on thegraph. The advent of noninvasive techniques for physiologic monitoring of infants reduces manipulation of the infant, as doppler technics for measuring arterial BP and transcutaneous electrodes fur measuring continuous arterial PO2.h

Transport of the baby; a premature baby may have to be transported from the place of birth to a hospital for simple or special care. During transport, the baby must be kept warm, and respiratory maintained adequately. In tropical countries with cool nights, the same type of portable incubator is needed, in which the child can be easily observed, and oxygen can be administered if respiratorydifficulty occurs. If not possible, a wooden or basket-work cot, made draught proof with blankets and heated with hot water battles. An oxygen cylinder, mash, a simple mucus extractor, simple cotton wrapper is to be kept handy for instant use. The baby should not bebathed or fed before transport, about the umbilicus must be dressed as described earlier.

FEEDING THE PREMATURE BABY:

It is important to avoid fatigue and aspiration of food during feeding or by regurgitation. Therefore, the person using any of the methods of feeding must be well-trained. Ural feedings should not be instituted or should be discontinued in infants with respiratory distress , hypoxia, circulatory insufficiency, excessive secretions, gagging, sepsis, or signs of serious illness. These infants will require intravenous alimentation. Large premature infants can often be fed by bottle or at the breast. Breastfeeding is least likely to be successful since the sucking effort is the limiting factor. In bottle feeding, the effort can be reduced by using special soft nipples with largeholes. Infants as small as 3 lb. at birth are occasionally vigorous enough for bottle feeding.

Human milk is. Preferable, if possible, should be obtained by manual expression at 3-4 hourly interval in the hospital units, it is possible to collect milk from several mother's pool strain it into sterilized glass jars, and pasteurize at 75C for several minutes, followed by rapid cooling with cold water of high standard of purity preferably boiled. The milk is then stored in the refrigeratorand used.

Human milk is. Preferable, if possible, should be obtained by manual expression at 3-4 hourly intervals in the hospital units; it is possible to collect milk from several mother's pools, strain it into sterilized glass jars, and pasteurize at 75C for several minutes, followed by rapid cooling with cold water of high standard of purity preferably boiled. The milk is then stored in the refrigerator and used.

The danger of abdominal distension, regurgitation, and aspiration Gavage feeding has the same risk as nipple feeding. A soft polyethylene tube of No 5 F external and 0.05 cm internal diameter, with a rounded atraumatic tip and 2 holes on the alternate sides, is preferable. The tube is passed via nose through the esophageal-bas Riu junction until 1 inch of the lower end is at least in the stomach. The free end of the tube is then placed under water. If bubbles appear with each expiration, the catheter is in the trachea and must be withdrawn and reinserted. The free end has an adapter into which the tip of a glass syringe is fitted, and a measured amp of feeding is allowed to flow in slowly by gravity. These tubes can be left for 3-7 days (average 4 days) if rinsed with a few drops of boiled water at the end of each feed. The milk is. Pour into the barrel of the syringe raised about 10-15 cm above the infant's face and given slowly with the infant lying inclined to the right side. Only polyethylene tubes should be used as indwelling catheters. If only rubber catheters are available, interrupting feeding should be used organically since the rubber has an irritating effect on the nasal and pharyngeal mucosa. In the dwelling or gastric polyethylene, tubes can also be used. The location of the end of the tube must be checked for each feeding. Nasogastric tubes tend to obstruct breathing, especially in preterm infants who are obligate nasal breathers, and they constitute a FB in the nasopharynx and thus can give rise to otitis media and blockage of the auditory tube. An occasional preterm infant of fewer than 32 weeks.

Gestation can 't tolerates gastric feeds and should be given duodenal or naso Sejunal tube feeding. The use of these tubes is associated with bill° reflux or perforation of the viscous with rupture and infection into the perioral cavity, the renal pelvis, or the retroperitoneal space. Therefore, these tubes must be taped with the clear markings of the proper location, must be changed every 4-5 days, and must never be advanced after initial placement is established. When replaced, it should be done through the alternate nostril. The tubes though single, can be cleaned, sterilized, and reused. Those infants who show considerable local irritation from an indwelling tube with excess secretions gathering around it in the nasopharynx, or there may be gagging; in these cases, a sterile 1OF rubber cats' titer is used orally. Sometimes gastrostomy is needed, and the main indications are in surgical conditions such as TEF and chest surgery. Certain types of bowel surgery in the preop and opstocare, and for some children with severe CNS dysfunction. The main principle in the feeding of premature is to proceed gradually. Comparatively, activity, low heat production, and larger body water content all reduce the immediate need for calories, water, and electrolyte; careful early feeding of glucose or saline solutions tends to reduce the incidence of hypoglycemia and hyperbilirubinemia without any risk of aspiration. As soon as the infant has recovered from the stress of delivery and appears active and in no distress, oral feedings may be instituted. This may be only 1 hr. after (birth, usually given 6-12 hours of age or earlier if the child becomes restless. Early feedings are preferable over a period of prolonged starvation and dehydration. If the infant is in distress or is sick, he may have to be given active feedings for some days before giving oral feeds. Most infants below 1500g and many larger ones need initial tube feeding. Start by giving sterile water, and if tolerated, give l ml of 5% dextrose solution for the infant under 1000 g, 2-4 ml for those between 1000-1500g, and 5-10 ml for infants over 1500g by a rubber-tipped medicine dropper. If the starting amount is 1 ml, feeding may be given hourly for the 1st 8 hours. Increasing the amount by l.ml at every other feeding. Feedings may then be given every 2 hours. With a more rent of 2 ml at every other feeding until 12 ml is reached. Then 12 ml is continued every 2-3 hours for 24-48 hours, at which time a mixture of 8 ml of 5% dextrose + 4ml of a half-skimmed milk formula (containing 0.67 Cal/ml or 20 Cal/oz.) It may be substituted for 2 feedings; then 4 ml of 5% dextrose and 8ml of formula for 2 feedings; then full-strength formula is used. Then the amount of for mule is gradually increased so that the intake is about 150 ml/kg/day. If the infant still seems hungry or fails to gain weight, the amount should be further increased. Some infants with small gastric capacities fail to gain on tolerated amounts of the formula containing 0.67 Cal/ml, when more frequent feedings may be given to increase the total daily intake, or the calorie intake may be increased to as high as 1 Cal/m1 (=30 Cal/one). To infants of 1000-150 0g, the glucose and water feedings may be given every 2-3 hours, with 4 ml increments at every other feeding until feedings of 16 ml are reached, at which point formula may be substituted gradually.

When tube feeding is used, the contents of the stomach should be aspirated before each feeding. If only air or small amounts of mucus are obtained, the feeding is given as planned; if any of the previous feedings is obtained, the amount of feeding must be reduced and gradually increased thereafter, 3 hourly regime is suitable given a day, and night, but in smallest of babies, less 2 hourlies may be needed. Nipple feeding can be substituted for gavage feeding at 24 wk gestation, and the infant begins to suck on the gavage tube. As the infant tires easily with the nipple, the transition is made gradually. Feeding is satisfactory when optimal neigh gain occurs but gain in. weight may not be achieved for 10-12 days, and more than 120 Cal/kg and 180 ml/kg per 24 hours may be needed. Gastrostomy is contraindicated in premature infants for risks of increased mortality, except as an adjunct to the surgical management of specific gastrointestinal conditions. IV fluids are always needed in preterm, VLBW, and critically ill infants. The fluids are given primarily to ensure adequate hydration and electrolyte intake. A multivitamin preparation should be added by the 5th day if feedings have not b started yet. Water and electrolyte intake must be adjusted to the needs of each infant, based on a record of intake and output that is reviewed every 12 hours; the amount given should maintain normal plasma Na concentration, a plasma osmolality near 280 kg of water, and a urine flow rate between 150-250 kg of wale and a urine flow rate between 1-3 ml/kg/generally the amount of water given 1O5 glucose should be 80-150 ml/kg/day and sodium gate at intake between 1.5-3 mEq/day. After the infant has begun to urinate, potassium 2 mEq/kg/day should be added to the iv fluids, In the absence of metabolic acidosis, sodium is given as NaNCO3 or NaCl and potassium as KC1, and in the presence of acidosis, both are given as NaHCO3 and Potassium acetate (metabolizable anions). Total parenteral nutrition is not a substitute for oral or gavage feedings in premature infants' routine feeding. But when oral feeding is impossible for prolonged periods of time, TPN may provide sufficient fluids, calories, electrolytes, and vitamins to sustain growth. Especially those neonates who are benefitted tight and have gastrointestinal abnormalities that donut allow adequate oral feeding or infants with associated severe malabsorption.

IV fluids are discontinued gradually to avoid reactive hypoglycemia and to provide supplemental fluids until oral intake is satisfactory; then, several oral feeds are retained, and the infusion is discontinued. The digestive enzyme systems of premature infants are mature enough to permit efficient absorption of protein and carbohydrates. The premature infant will require an IV infusion of 10% glucose at a rate sufficient to provide 7 mg/kg/min. The rate may be adjusted to maintain a blood sugar of over 40 mg/dl but under 120 m7 /dl/ When milk feedings are given, these will provide additional sugar in the form of lactose, which is rapidly taken by the infant's liver and converted into glucose. Occasional hypolactasia may cause diarrhea from lactose intolerance and failure to gain weight. Glucose is the preferred sugar for addition if it is necessary to dilute the milk on account of fat or lactose intolerance, and after 2-3 weeks c cane sugar is usually tolerated satisfactorily. Protein may be given as amino acids in TPE (Proteinhydrolysates) but preferably as protein contained in milk. The infant can tolerate larger content of protein, but an intake of 2g/kg/day is sufficient (some smaller infants may need 3-4 and Human breast milk or modified cow ‘s milk with a high whey/curd ratio are preferred feedings in VLBW. The usual substitutes for human milk are half-skimmed milk (dried or evaporated). Premature have a poor tolerance for fat for several weeks, and fat ingestion appears to be important in establishing normal postnatal liver and gastrointestinal function. Unsaturated fats and fats in human milk are absorbed better than that in cow ‘s milk. Formulas with medium-chain triglycerides and complex fats should be used. Then the introduction of milk feedings is markedly delayed. In neonates, essential fatty acids must be given in other forms. Some believe that better weight gain can be achieved with formulas made with half-skimmed milk than with human milk, which has a higher fat content and lowers protein and mineral content; high protein and mineral content of cow's milk formulas of high-calorie content constitute a large solute load for the kidneys. There is an incensed need for vitamins C and D and calcium. Metabolism of phenylamine and tyrosine depends in part on vitamin C, and loss of focal fat involves loss of fat-soluble vitamins, also, and calcium. Vitamina is added at 7-10 days of life as in the artificially fed. 50 mg of C and 1000 in D daily is sufficient. Vitamin D intake from all sources should not exceed 1500 daily. Then mother 's diet is polished rice adequate. B1 should be added. If acute deficiency develops in the neonate, and signs of heart failure occur, 5-10 mg of BI is given or followed by oral treatment for some weeks. Infants with birth weights of less than 1830g need supplemental iron since their iron stores are limited and there is increased growth with an increase in red cell mass during the first years. of life. Both these factors exaggerate physiological anemia in premature owing to postnatal suppression of erythrocytes poiesis. The anemia develops earlier and reaches a lower ultimate level. Fetal or neonatal blood loss will accentuate this problem in premature dietary iron is never adequate to supply the iron needed by him because of the rapid growth.

Therefore, iron supplementation is needed; 6 mg/kg/day of iron orally started at 8 weeks of age. The iron supplementation should not be done up to at least 38 wk gestation in VLBW since iron causes hemolysis in them. Zinc and copper deficiency may occur in prematurely. Small babies are especially prone to die from malnutrition and infection later in the neonatal period. They should be retained in the hospital or receive trained nursing supervision at home until birth weight has been regained and feeding is well established. The properly fed - premature may have 1-6 stools of semisolid consistency daily; a sudden increase in number or a change to a watery consistency should be of concern. More than 1 and a half of preterm Lag infants pass their first stool within 12 his and 80 % 'by 24 hours. The child, on leaving the hospital, should be free from infection and other medical disorders, with breast or bottle feeding well established, and should be above the BW and at least 2000-2500g.

The infant follow-up should take place as near as possible, and the baby must be reassessed at 3 months of age. 10-20% of surviving infants whose birth wt is less than 1500g later had physical problems, neurologic difficulties, visual impairment, deafness, learning and perceptual problems, or mental retardation, The mortality rate of LBW infants who survived (to be discharged from the hospital is 3 times that of term infants, during the first 2 years of life many of these deaths being due to infection. There is an increased incidence of SID syndrome; defects in the regulation of the cardiorespiratory system secondary to immaturity and high environmental risk factors secondary to socio-economic factors also play their part.

INTRAUTERINE GROWTH RETARDATION

The IU growth rate is affected by multiple factors, including the mother 's health, the health of the fetus,and the condition of the placenta. Any organ system disease can affect the growth of the child inutero, temporarily or permanently-The weight of the infant reflects the total genetic and environmental status. Maternal toxemia may lead to small-for-gestational-age (SGA) infants. The longer the toxemia, the more pronounced the degree of growth retardation-Congenital viral infection, chronic ingestion of alcohol, nicotine, or heroin, multiple births, chromosomal aberrations, and birth defects produce some degree of retardation. All the infants who have IU growth retardation, irrespective of the cause, will suffer fetal distress during labor and delivery and are high-risk infants.SGA infants are at increased risk of birth asphyxia, meconium aspiration, renal injury leading to oliguria, hyperviscosity syndrome, hypoglycemia, and hypocalcemia. Conversely infants of diabetic mothers are large for gestational age (LGA); excessive size in infants is associated with increased incidence of trauma, especially during vaginal delivery. In a vertex delivery, there may be injuries to the head and neck, including stretching or tearing of cervical or brachial plexus leading to peripheral nerve injuries as Erb's palsy or phrenic nerve palsy-They are also at increased risk of having congenital anomalies, cardiomyopathy, hypervisoosity syndrome, hypercoagulability, hyperbilirubinemia, hypooalcemia, and hypoglycemia. Many newborn infants whopresent with 1U growth retardation in weight show relatively less deviation from normal in length and head circumference. Length and head growth appear to be protected to some extent during IU undernutrition. But in severe and prolonged IU undernutrition (as occurs in discordant twins) all body proportions may be affected. Weight-length ratio increases with fetal age (the infant becomes heavier in relation to his length as he approaches term). In IU growth retardation, the W-L ratio decreases since the rate of growth in weight is affected more than length. IU growth retardation dysmaturity is an erogenous group containing infants that vary diversely.

SMALL FOR GESTATIONAL AGE (SGA, IGR, LFD, SFD)

Small for dates or small for gestational age are infants whose birth weight is below the 10th percentile for gestational age, irrespective of other clinical features. They constitute 1/3-2/3rd of all LBW babies. The conditions associated with SGA are advanced maternal age, multiparty, race, previous spontaneous abortions, unwed mothers, drug abusers as alcohol and heroin addicts and smokers, maternal vascular diseases as cardiac renal diabetes, toxemia, hypoxia due to high altitude or sickle cell anemia, multiple fetuses, abnormal placentation or placental lesions, congenital anomalies chromosomal abnormalities, chronic Ill infection, single umbilical artery, drugs, and radiation. They tolerate the stress of labor poorly and frequently suffer perinatal asphyxia and meconium aspiration. These babies show a general reduction in size, showing that growth stimulation has been inadequate for a much longer period-They have grown very slowly for a long time; therefore, their general appearance is undersized as well as under-weight, and they resemble infants of the same birth weight horn preterm, but their behavior is more appropriate to the length of gestation. There is an increased incidence of congenital anomalies, vascular ones as detected by a single umbilical artery, chromosomal anomalies, and other anomalies handicapping life. Bird-headed dwarfs fall into this category, and the chronic twin transfusion may cause a gross discrepancy between the sizes of the 2 fetuses. Maturation of the organs proceeds normally btthere are differences in size from babies of normal weight for gestation. The lungs, liver, and thymus are considerably reduced. The kidneys and adrenals are not significantly affected; there is a slight increase in the size of the heart, spleen; the brain is much larger, and the weight ratio of brain tolive may be increased to as much as 6-7:1 as compared to 3:1 in the normal full-term infant.

Biochemically, Hemoglobin is high at birthmother is often metabolic acidosis and raises blood NPN; neonatal hypoglycemia is a problem of the first 3 days for all babies whose birth weight is low for gestation on-esterified fatty acids which may have a glucose-sparing action may be failed to rise adequately in some of the severely growth retarded babies. These features are not seen in preterm with typical features of an SGA infant are exceptionally awake wide-awake hungry appearance; if given sufficient food, there is no weight loss in the first week and usually a gain inweight above BW by 7th day. These infants start gaining weight soon after birth in contrast to the wt loss of the first few days after birth, which is characteristic of the normal newborn. Lack of SC far and brown adipose tissue makes the maintenance of body temperature in a cool environment difficult, and cold injury occurs if chilling occurs when there is a fall in environmental temperature at night in the tropics. There is an increased incidence of cerebral edema in the first 3 days; because of the frequency of fetal distress, asphyxia, and metabolic acidosis, they are at high risk for hypoglycemia because of diminished hepatic glycogen stores in high brain-to-liver weight ratio and decreased SC fat. In infants who are SGA, the overall incidence of transient neonatal hypoglycemia is 20%, but at least 40% of such infants who are born prematurely have blood-glucose levels below 20 mg%. The highest incidence, more than 70, has been reported in smaller of the discordant twins when the smaller twin weighs less than 2000g and the larger more than 2700g. HyPerviscosity syndrome, polycythemia, frequently occurs because of lU hypoxemiasney are particularly prone to develop massive pulmonary hemorrhage,which causes death on 3rd clay and other hemorrhagic manifestations such as hematemesis and melena. During pregnancy, fetal well-being must be monitored by urinary measurements and ultrasonography. At delivery, fetal distress, meconium aspiration, hypoxia, and heat loss must be anticipated. After the infant is born, to identify existing conge vital anomalies, do serial screening for hypoglycemia up to 72 hours. If perinatal asphyxia is present for hypocalcemia, also monitor for polycythemia. Examination of the placenta and umbilical artery is helpful. Once the cause is unknown in the majority of cases, I level and serum antibody titers for chronic torch infections should be done. The light for dates is those whose weight is disproportionately low relative to other measurements such as head circumference and body length, which are within the range of normal for the gestation, estimated for the menstrual history, antenatal observation of the pregnant uterus, and for the clinical characteristics of the infant. A relatively short period of growth retardation, probably less than tires late in gestation, may reduce weight out of proportion to skeletal growth. The appearance of the infant often suggests that not only has therebeen a lack of it.

Skin is relatively hairless, often paler than normal, with meconium staining and lack of Vx cases umblical cord may be thin and yellow. Lack of SC fat in the face gives the childa wizened appearance. Most of them are of 3 or more weeks of Gestation, and other clinical features, ildg neurological signs and one maturation pattern coincide with expected maturity. Theincidence of hyperbilirubinemia coincides 'with the gestational age and not birth weight.

CARE OF SGA INFANT (LFD AND SFD)

They need to remain in the hospital longer but are more likely to have a problem; in the first 3 days. the easiest approach is to set aside a room or part of a ward where the mothers and babies can be nursed together. The mother should do most of the nursing, and other relatives shouldn ‘t beallowed to handle the tilt. Baby and the cots may have to be moved for supervision to nurses ‘rooms during visit hours. Infection is minimized cap if the mother does as much as possible of the routine care of the baby. Hand washing should be. A routine, water at is available preferably running watt from the tap. The mothers must be taught to do Han thrashing at the correct time. An adequate supply of soap and clean towels must be available. Unless the mother ‘s outer clothing is washed daily, a gown must be given to her to wear before handling the baby. All the procedures are done by the nurses, including feeding and cleaning of the babies, must be done in the cot and not on a table or nurse's lap, as far as possible. Each baby must be barrier-nursed with his own equipment for the toilet, such as cotton swabs, thermometer in antiseptic solution, etc, kept on a tray or a small locker attached to the cot. A gown should be kept on or by the cot and worn while carrying out any procedure which involves contact of the baby of its cot linen with her uniform. Medical personnelshould wear gowns for examinations or procedures where contact with the infant is unavoidable. Room temperature must be recorded morning and evening, and extra heat must be used if it falls below 25C. The optimum temperature is 26-30C. Each baby must have its own sill pie draught-proof cot on astand raised off the floor. The cot should have a cotton lining with pockets at the sides and foot, into which hot water bottles or substitute containers containing hot water enclosed in cotton bags may be placed to provide extra warmth. Body temperature, preferably rectal, must be recorded twice daily, using a min low-reading thermometer, and must hey maintained by adequate environmental heat so that it records at least 350 in the first 12 hours and subsequently 36-57, skin temperature is recorded; it should be taken in the carefully dried groin or axilla for at least 2 min.

If a low reading thermometer is not available, a temperature of 350 should be regarded as too low and extra heat provided. In very hot weather, if the baby becomes restless. And pyrexia, the cot should allow a free flow of air, but the direct draught of a fan is undesirable as it cools the skin excessively. Tepid sponging with boiled water and sterile swabs s should alsobe employed with careful aseptic precautions to avoid skin infection Clothes may only be neededat night but should be loose, changed whenever soiled and made from a material that lauders easily and does not chafe the skin. Swaddling should not be allowed, but quilted bags may be helpful in a cool environment. Fly-proof netting fitted to windows and mosquito netting for individual cots may be provided. Blinds for shade from sunlight may be needed, and if it is not possible to provide these facilities for mothers as well as babies, it is necessary to equip a smallerroom for the babies only, which should be very close to the ward where the mothers are nursed, so that they can give all the routine care during the day. A whole-time nurse must be provided forthe babies during the night since they require supervision. And 3 hourly feeding at night at least for the 1st week. Regular charting of all fluid taken at the time of each feed and the baby's reactionsas vomiting, regurgitation, food refusal, and cyanotic attack, should be done; also, each passage of urine, meconium, faeces, etc. must be recorded by a nurse. Breastfeeding is even more importantthan for the larger infants and must be put to the breast at one hr after birth or even sooner, and subsequently 3 hourly or more often if demanded. If the child is lethargic or sucking inadequate nasogastric polyethylene tube must be passed with 10% dextrose water, 15 ml 3 hourly, till the baby can feed on the breast without tiring. Small dates with short gestation have double problem fetalmalnutrition with all the perinatal hazards and the handicaps of preterm infants. Their care is determined by their gestation and is like other pre-term babies with additional problems.

The greatest risk of this complication is seen when the ratio of head circumference to body weight is 6-7:1. Regardless of the cause of the intrauterine growth retardation. These infants are atincreased risk of hypoglycemia. Symptomatic hypoglycemia may occur in more than 6% of small for gestational-age infants, and the risk continues for the first 3 days. Hyperexcitability, jitteriness, or apathy, Are usually present, and it is likely that underlying brain damage is responsible for the increased demands for glucose and has precipitated the failure in blood sugar.

PREVENTION OF HYPOGLYCEMIA IN SGA INFANT

Very early feeding, within the first hour after birth, with subsequent sufficient calories in the first 3 days to cover the basic metabolic requirements. Feeding is started in the first hour with 15-20 ml of 10% dextrose in water, and the say is given every 3 hourlies. Milk, half diluted with 5% dextrose, is instituted at 6 hours. The strength and amount of milk mixture are increased rapidly so that at 4 days of age, the intake is 150 ml of undiluted milk/kg/day. Blood sugar determination isadvised. Others believe that all SGA infants must receive 100 ml/kg/day of 10% dextrose infusion to maintain blood glucose concentration at more than 40 mg monitored continuously with dextrostix or any other means. Some infants will develop hypoglycemia ditethis therapywhen the glucose concentration or the flow rate must be increased proportionately.

Vomiting, cyanotic attacks, or abdominal distension are indications of smaller especially. but more frequent feedings by nasogastric tube or continuous intragastric milk drip, or iv 10 dextrose for not longer than 24 hours, for the risk of venous thrombosis or infection. Rarely SGA infants may develop marked hyperglycemia and a transient diabetes mellitus-like syndrome. Insulin therapy, if needed, rarely is not required beyond the first week. The GSA infant with hypoglycemia and a very high hematocrit, capillary hematocrit of more than 75, is likely to show the most severe clinical signs of hypoglycemia, reflecting a reduction in cerebral blood flow. A small exchange transfusion with plasma should be given to reduce the hematocrit and to correct the hypoglycemia. For symptomatic hypoglycemia with cerebral signs, initial slow iv transfusion of 50% glucose, lgm/kg followed by

20% fructose + 5% dextrose at the rate of 75mg/kg/24 h.rs.Fructose has a glucose-sparing action and is less irritable to the veins than glucose, but it passes so quickly into the tissue and the brain that it fails to elevate the blood sugar if It is not available, 105 glucose should use. If the clinical condition allows, oral feeding mustbe continued carefully 5 units of ACT may be given to elevate blood glucose, which is useful foremergency use while waiting to start iv therapy or to reinforce it. Glucagon is of no proven benefit.

POST-TERM INFANTS:

Infants born after 42 weeks of gestation are post-term. About 25% of all pregnancies end on or after the 287th day, 12% on or after the 294th day, and 5% on or after the 370th day. The cause is unknown, but is associated with anencephaly, trisomy 18, and sickles dwarfism-Clinically they may be indistinguishable from term infants, but some resemble an infant of 1-3 weeks again, appearance and behavior, called post mature. The infants are characterized by the absence of lanugo hair, decreased or absent vernix caseosa, long nails, abundant scalp hair, white skin, parchment-like ordesquamating akin, and increased alertness. Some of these features may be seen in term or preterm infants. Then delivery is delayed 3 or more weeks beyond the term, and mortality may be increased 3 times. During pregnancy, they need a careful estimation of gestational age from LNP, ultrasounds, and monitoring of fetal wellbeing. Delivery must be elective depending on the lung maturity or fetal distress since primigravida, and more than 25 years of age increase the mortality rate further. Caesarean is performed on elderly primigravida who go beyond a wk or two beyond the term, especially if there is evidence of fetal distress. Their problems include intrapartum asphyxia, meconium aspiration, neonatal hypoglycemia, and polycythemia.

LARGE FOR GESTATIONAL AGE (LGA)

Birth weight of more than the 90th percentile for gestational age. The LGA infant may be constitutionally large (familial infants of diabetic mothers the primary association is with material diabetes since 1/3rd of them is LGA post-term infants, those with transposition of great vessels erythroblastosis fetalis.

Infants who are very large have an a-higher incidence of birth injuries such as cervical and brachial plexus injuries, phrenic nerve damage with paralysis of the diaphragm, fractured clavicles, cephalhematomas, and ecchymosis of the head and face. The incidence of congenital anomalies is also higher than in term infants of normal weight-Polycythemia and hypoglycemia may be present. There is significant evidence for intellectual and developmental retardation in high birth weight term and preterm infants at school age. The primary association of LGA infants is with maternal diabetes (since 1/3rd of them is LGA)-About 1 of live-born infants are productsof diabetic pregnancies 0% are associated with frank maternal diabetes class A, B, C, and 60% with the fiesta. Tonal diabetes. In severe diabetes, class D, E, F, many of infants are appropriate for gestational age (ACA), and about 10 are SGA, due to maternal vascular complications that affect the placental circulation-Compared to normal infants) wants to have 3 times the incidence of congenital anomalies, esio cardiac and spinal (particularly spinal agenesis).

Neonatal problems include hypoglycemia, hypocalcemia, polycythemia nerviscosity syndrome renal vein thrombosis), laundice, and RDSreven in pregnancies at term. Hypoglycemia may occur in 50% of infants of diabetic mothers. Of the babies born to insulin-dependent mot,) ers,10% are symptomatic, and 50-75% have blood glucose values below 30mg/dl, but only 2 of infants of mothers with gestational diabetes are symptomatic, but 20-30% have abnormally low blood glucose without symptoms. Serial screening for blood glucose tab and her autocrat (maximum value is reached at 3-4 hours after birth), serum calcium at 24-C hours after birth, and bilirubin. Also, observe for respiratory distress , hypoglycEutia, and hypocalcaemia. If maternal blood glucose levels are well controlled during pregnancy, labor, and delivery, the incidence of large size for gestational age and its associated morbidity is like that of a normal population, but these infants have an increased incidence (10%) of diabetes mellitus later.

PLACENTAL DYSFUNCTION SYNDROME.

12% of all births show some clinically recognizable or placental dysfunction, such as abnormal fetal heart pattern retarded intrauterine growth, low maternal levels of estriol, contamination of the amniotic fluid by meconium, etc. Incidence of the clearly recognizable form of the syndrome. (With yellow staining of the Vx and skin) is 1.2% of all births. The majority of the affected are term or pretax' especially SGA infants of toxemic mothers, elderly primigravida, and women with reproductive Live Inefficiency. About 20% are postaierm, the placentas are small or poorly attached, and the syndrome is thought to be due to degenerative changes in the placenta resultingin progressive reduction in oxygen and nutrition supply to the fetus. The infant may become thus be born at term, preterm or post-term. Some are premature SGA, but those who are born post-term may have any of the 3 stagesStage 1; they are infants with usual signs of post maturity (desquamation, long nails, abundant hair, white skin, alert facies, loose skin especially around the thighs and buttocks, giving the appearanceof the recent loss of weight sage 1- These have increased mortality that is due to prolonged gestation but not war left due to the syndrome itself 1/3 of them show some evidence of respiratory distress or CNS irritation.

Stage II; in addition to the signs of post maturity as above, they have meconium stared amniotic fluid, skin, vernix caseosa, umbilical cord, and placental membranes due to fetal anoxia. Since they are born at the height of DJ anoxia or after a moderate to severe hypoxic episode, 2/3 of them have severe respiratory distress apparently resulting from aspiration of meconium-stained amniotic fluid; some of them have signs of anoxic cerebral damage; the overall mortality is 35%.

Stage III; they have the same signs, and in addition, their nails and skin are stained a bright yellow, and the umbilical. Cord yellow green. The live-born infant in this stage have survived the severe acute anoxic sage-e4-phase of stage II trey and have the same problems, but their morbidity is low,and mortality is 15%. The treatment of placental dysfunction syndrome lies in the prevention of the conditions that cause the condition, treating episodes of fetal distress during labor and aspiration pneumonia, and cerebral anoxia after birth,

DELIVERY ROOM CARE OF THE HIGH-RISK INFANT

(Pediatric emergencies in the delivery room)

The commonest and most important emergencies in the immediate neonatal period are failure toinitiate respiratory and to maintain satisfactory respiratorys. Less frequent are shocked, severe anemia, plethora, and convulsions.

If respiratory distress movements are made with the mouth closed, but the infant fails to move air in and out of the lungs, bilateral canal atresia or other obstruction of the upper Respiratory tract should be suspected. The mouth should be opened, and the mouth and posterior- pharynx clearedof secretions by gentle suction. Nasal obstruction or hypoplasia of the mandible can be identifiedand relieved by pulling the tongue forward to allow air exchange. Or pharyngeal airway should beinserted, and the source of the obstruction should be sought immediately; effective respiratoryflow is notproduced by opening the infant's mouth and clearing the airway. Laryngoscopy is indicated. With obstructive malformations of the epiglottis larynx, or trachea, an endotracheal tube should be insertedand; prolonged nasotracheal intubation of tracheotomy may robe needed. Respiratory failure from depression or injury to CMS may require continuous artificial ventilation with a facemask and bag or through an endotracheal or nasotracheal tube. Hypoplasia of the mandible with posterior displacement of the tongue may result in symptoms like those of canal atresia; they may be temporarily relieved by pulling the tongue forward. A scaphoid abdomen suggests hernia or eventuation of the diaphragm, as does the asymmetry of the contour of movement of the chest, or shift of the apical impulse of the heart (latter manifestations are also compatible with tension pneumothorax classification of respiratory distress and failure in neonates:

1. CNS failure manifests as apnea, slow irregular gasping respiratoryefforts (seen in narcosis,prenatal or perinatal anoxia, IC hemorrhage or trauma, CNS anomalies)

2. Peripheral respiratorydifficulty manifests as rapid respiratoryrate, or increased respiratoryrate, chest large intercostal subcostal and xiphoid retractions, chin tug, expiratory grunt, and frothing atlips) (seen in primary atelectasis, congestive pulmonary failure, RDS, aspiration of amniotic fluid containing formed elements, pneumonia, diaphragmatic hernia, lung cysts, lobar emphysemai pneumothorax, aspiration of food or mucus).

FAILURE TO INITIATE OR SUSTAIN RESPIRATORY

Failure to initiate or sustain respiratory originates in the CNS (immaturity is seldom a causative factor) -Narcosis, resulting from heavy doses of morphine, pethidine, barbiturates, reserpine, or tranquilizers administered to the mother shortly before delivery, or from maternal anesthesia, especially if prolonged, during delivery. The infant is cyanotic at birth and slow to cry or breathe; if respiratory is established, it is extremely slowed Treatment consists of physical stimulants such as frequent snapping of the soles of the feet to stimulate crying and deeper breathing or insertion of a catheter through the nostril into the nasopharynx to produce reflex irritation and breathing. The efficacy of stimulants of the CNS in the initiation of respiratory effort has not been established. If narcosis is due to morphine or its derivatives, naloxone hydrochloride, 0.01mg/kg should be injected IV. Oxygen should be administered if cyanosis is present; some form of artificial respiratory is necessary until a regular and adequate respiratory pattern is established. Prenatal or perinatal anoxia, if sufficiently severe, will produce a central nervous system type of respiratory failure (irrespective of the cause of anoxia), secondary apnea, which does not respond to sensory stimulation. Death is due to apnea and may be resuscitation. External cardiac massage, correction of acidosis, and circulatory support may beimportant ad junctures to ventilation. Hypotnemia as a means of temporarily reducing the metabolic needs of the infant for oxygen during the period of oxygen shortage is not proven and is contraindicated. -Intracranial hemorrhage and trauma and CNS anomalies may be the cause of respiratory failure in the neonate.

DELIVERY ROOM CARE OF THE HIGH-RISK INFANTS

Be aware of the maternal and fetal historya) Maternal

factors-

1. Prior obstetric history: abortions, premature births, congenital anomalies, infants dying shortlyafter birth –

- Maternal diseases: chronic disorders such as renal diseases and diabetes may require premature birth,cause delayed maturation, or may dispose to malnutrition o infants.
- Maternal infections: syphilis, gonorrhea, TB torch infections –
- Medications: fetal depression, narcotic addiction, fetal alcohol smoking, teratogenicity
- Perinatal maternal factors: toxemia, abruption placenta, placenta previa, prolonged labor,multiple births, prolonged rupture of membranes.

2. Fetal factors—

- Gestational age: relates to the timing of elective surgery, therapy for jaundice, temperature, feeding,and postnatal growth rate –
- Pulmonary maturation: Amniotic fluid lecithin/sphingomyelin ratio, an Indic form of pulmonary maturation. –
- Oxytocin challenge test fetal distress following oxytocin-induced uterine contraction gives arelative index of fetal risks. –
- Metal monitoring during labor will predict asphyxia. Immediate care after delivery the high-risk infant: -
- Place Cue infant on a warming table. Auction the flares

and mouth with a bunion bulb. Gastric suction and deep suctioning in the first 5 minutes of life may produce bradycardia. And shouldnot be done routinely. If thick meconium is present, suction the oropharynx and trachea before the onset of breathing. Dry the infant. –

- Evaluate by the Apgar score; 7f heart rate is below 100, clear the airway and ventilate with a bag and mask with pressures of 20-25 cm of water at 30 breathes /Min the score is 0-2;(baby blue andlimp, heart rate less than100)
- Suction oropharynx; stimulate and give oxygen by mask; if the heart rate is less than 60, cardiac massage is done; bag and mask may be inadequate, in which case intubation is done and oxygengiven by endotracheal tube; umbilical vein catheter is introduced for medication; If there is no improvement; see if the mother has received a narcotic drug.

NO -

NaHCO3 iv 2mg/kg (o.5mEq/ml) if no improvement/Epinephrine iv (0.5-1ml of 1:10000 solution) if no improvement/Calcium gluconate,10% iv, 2ml slowly/if no improvement/Volumeexpanders iv, as whole blood 10ml/kg or 5% albumin 10 ml/kg or NaCl 10ml/kg/if there is still no improvement Epinephrine, intracardiac 0.5-1ml(1:10,000)

If there is improvement, observer and monitor the baby.

YES - give naloxone, 0.2mg/ml(premature ml, full-term 2ml). Be sure that the bag delivers 100% oxygen endotracheal tube in the trachea, 02 connections are secure, pressure is adequate to ventilate, and cardiac massage is adequate. All infants should have a brief general examination foranomalies. If the mother is awake and the infant appears well, permit her to hold the infant as soon as she wishes.

APGAR SCORE

(Infant is scored at 1 minute and 5 minutes)

Signs	0	1	2
Heart Rate	Absent	Slow, less than 100	100 or more
Respirator y Effort	Absent	Weak, cry, and hypoventilation	Crying
Muscle Tone	Flaccid	Some flexion extremities	Well flexed
Reflex irritability	No Respons e	Some motion	Cry
Color	Blue Pale	Blue Hands and feet	Entirely Pink

RESUSCITATION OF THE NEWBORN

Resuscitation may be needed in the delivery room in the nursery. The principles of resuscitationinclude maintaining patency of the airway and assisting ventilation.

The upper and central airway should be cleared of the foreign material as adequately as possibleby removal of accumulated liquid contents (meconium, vomitus); resuscitation should lie start with some method of simple, gentle physical stimulation such as snapping of the feet soles with afinger or repeatedly passing a nasal catheter. If this is unsuccessful in initiating satisfactory respiratory upper airway should again be suctioned, and patency of the airway should be established by using a par oral airway (a size 00-1 plastic or metal airway inserted to lift the tongue off the posterior pharyngeal wall. The infant can be adequately ventilated with a bag and mask until preparations are made for intubation. The need for resuscitation is determined by the baby 's condition at birth and Lakiotis

Apgar score.

Normal infants with Apgar scores of 7-10. Require no treatment. Moderately asphyxiated babies whan Apgar score of 4-6, should be ventilated by providing up to 100% oxygen by mask. If there is no Response , IPPV should be used at less than 40 cm of water pressure. If there is no improvement, intubation should be carried out immediately. Babies with severe asphyxia apgarscore of 0-3, and heart rate less than 100 •Some method of artificial respiratory or pulmonary inflation should be employed; he should immediately be intubated with the rapid aspiration of the secretions via the endotracheal tube and given IPPV with up to 100% oxygen.

INTUBATION:

IN the delivery room and in an emergency, oral intubation is quiches and easiestwith sizes 14, 16, and 18. For term, and 10, and 12 for premature infants. If in doubt, the correct size of French endotracheal tube, care be estimated from the diameter of the child and 5th finger. When the infant's condition is stabilized, Cole tubes are changed to a soft, cuffless tracheal tote (a Ported tube) for chon intubation.

Size for infant weighing	Portex Tube Size (Internal diameter in mm)
less than 1250	2.5 mm
1250-2000g	3.0
More than 2000g	3.5

Method of intubation:

Suction the mouth and the upper airway. If the intubation is elective, empty the stomach and attach a cardiac monitor. For endotracheal intubation, measure proper tube length prior to intubation (can be done by charts showing a relation of naris-carina and nares-glottis (vocal cord) distance to the birth weight. The baby should be ventilated with a bag and mask just prior to intubation. The infant's head should be in a neutral position, avoiding excessive extension of the neck. The laryngoscope is held between the thumb and first finger of the left hand, with the fingers holding the chin and stabilizing the head. Pushing down on the larynx with the 5th finger of the left hand (or having an assistant do it) and keeping the infants head straight may help to visualize the vocal cords (tracheal. The laryngoscope is passed into the right side of the mouth and then to the midline, swinging the tongue out of the way. The endotracheal tube is held between the right hand and inserted between the vocal cords to about 2 cm below the glottis.

During nasotracheal intubation, Magill forceps can be used to guide the tube between the vocalcords. If the 5th finger is pressing on the trachea, the tube can be felt as it slips into place. Check the tube position by auscultation to ensure equal aeration of both lungs. If air entry is poorover the left chest, pull back the tube until aeration improves. During the procedure, one person should continually observe the infant and monitor the heat rate. The infant should be allowed to become hypoxic or have bradycardia during the intubation. If bradycardia occurs, stop the procedure, and ventilate the fare with a bag and mask. Attaching an anesthetic bag on one side to 1040 oxygen and on the other side to the intubation tube adapter will deliver 100% oxygen to ti pharynx during the intubation procedure. An inline pop-off valve should be pleasant so that pressures don 't exceeds 25 cm of water. Intubation in the delivery room is usually temporary, and the tube can is held in the place by hand. If prolonged ventilation is required, the tube should be secured by paper tape and obtained to check its position. –

VENTILATION:

a) In the delivery room: Artificial ventilation is used to oxygenate the infant and, if necessary, to initiate spontaneous ventilation. Usually, the airway is cleared, and ventilation is established witha mask and an anesthetic bag capable of delivering a Fi02 of 1. A maximal pressure of 25 cm with a rate of 30 breaths/min is usually adequate. Pressure should be measured by an inline manometer. Pressure should be increased if the chest wall is not moving ditea tightly fitting face mask. A good Response will be shown by a rise in heart rate.

Indications of CDAP are RDS, when a Fi02 of more than 0.4-0.6 is required to keep aet444e4e4- arterial F02 (PaC2) at 50-70 torr or when apnea does not respond to otter therapy. Itincreases arterial P02 allowing the reduction of Fi02. Contraindications to CDAP without eve pressure are increasing PaCO2, persistent acidosis, and diseases not associated with decreasedpulmonary compliance. *

Intermittent positive pressure ventilation (IPPV) is indicated in PDS (when Pa02 is less than 50 torr, F102 is more than 60, and CDAP is 10 cm- water), when PCO2 is more than 70-80 from anycause, in persistent respiratoryacidosis, and when apnea dot snot responds to other therapy, The actual levels of arterial P028, PCO2 selected for intervention depend on the disease course. Respiratorysupport is adjusted so that Pa02 is 50-10 torr, PaCO2 is 35-50 torr, and pl is 700-7.40. These values are optimal and differ for a certain disease.

If there is no Response to the above measures (no spontaneous respiratory, persistent flaccidity, or bradycardia) within 1-3 minutes, chemical resuscitation should begin. An umbilical catheter should be inserted with sterile precautions (venous placement is easier and quicker during resuscitation blood for pH and measurement of P02, and PCO2 should be obtained. Blood gas samples: can be obtained a via med heel in a heparinized tube by heel stick or by direct puncture of the radial, temporal or posterior tibial arteries. If his condition is unstable, annulation of the umbilical, radial, posterior tibial, or temporal arteries may be needed. Brachial and femoral artypunctures should be avoided.

Maintenance of circulation is an important adjunct to artificial respiratory in infants in circulatory collapse with slow, weak heartbeats ad the heart is absent, or bradycardia prestartexternal cardiac massage should begin immediately. In the newborn, this is done by Ly depressing the midstream area about, i.e., 5/4 in at a rate of 100-120 times /min using the thumbs while holding the back with the rest of the hand. The ratio of closed heart massage should be synchrony: zed the ventilation0:1 ratio), Interrupatient the cardiac massage every 5s for one to two insufflations of the lungs.

Laryngoscopy, intubation, and cardiac massage should be carried out by experienced personnel negative intrathoracic pressures of 20-50 cm of water have been recorded during the firstfew breaths positive pressure much below 20cm is unlikely to introduce oxygen into the lungs.

Pressures of 25 cm may rupture the lung if only a small area is being expanded. On the other hand, a positive pressure of 40cm has been safely applied by using a resuscitation apparatus that automatically limits the inspiratory phase to 0, 1 second and provides an expiratory phaseof 5.9 seconds. Mouth-to-mouth breathing may be helpful in some and harmful for others by introducing infection or alveolar rupture from uncontrolled pressures. If the infant is making feeble but spontaneous respiratorymovements, the. Effectiveness will be increased by raising the partial pressures of oxygen at the nose and mouth, even without any change in atmospheric pressure.

Supplementary oxygen (up to 100*) should be used during resuscitation to abolish cyanosis and provide adequate oxygenation. Monitoring of arterial blood gases is imperative during oxygen administration. Oxygen administration, especially in the premature, should be at the lowest effective concentration while monitoring arterial blood gases. Levels. As the baby improves, oxygen concentration should be decreased gradually (decrements of 10-20%) while monitoring the blood oxygen level. Oxygen should be discontinued as soon as the baby can get along without it.

After the infant's airway has been cleared and adequate ventilation provided, severely asphyxiated,and acidotic infants often require the below (ml/min) administration of NaHCO5 (5-4mEq/kg) through an umbilical catheter to correct the associate metabolic acidosis; a solution containing 0.5-1mEq Al of NaHCO3. It may also be a necessity to administer epinephrine (0.1m1ikg of a 1:1.0,000 solution) via a catheter or intracardiac injection. While infusing sodium bicarbonate during resuscitation, assisted ventilation may be needed to wash out the excess CO2 producedby the bicarbonate. No drug advocated as a respiratoryStimulant has proven of value, and mostof them are convulsants, in doses slightly greater than those supposed to stimulate breathing.

Drugs used in resuscitation:

Sodium bicarbonate 44mEq/50ml (mix 1:2-1:3 with water to an osmolality of 600 mosmol/l: give2-5mEq/kg

Indication:

Severe Metabolic acidosis Dextrose 1O%; give 0.5-1g/kg iv as 10-15% solution. (Severe asphyxia) Epinephrine.1:10,000 give 0.1 ml/kg iv or intracardiac during cardiac? Massage (severebradycardia). Calcium gluconate 10% solution 1-2 ml/kg/dose (bradycardia, poor cardiac out).

- Equipment needed for resuscitation -D / -Radiant warmer bed, blankets, -
- Endotracheal tubes with stylette: 2.5,3.0,3.5. –Nasogastric tube No 3.5 French and No 5F – Suction catheter, bulb syringe, -
- Flow-through anesthetic bag capable of delivering 100% oxygen –Infant masks of various sizes. –
- Umbilical catheters 3.5 and 5F –
- Scalpel, silk suture with cutting needle (No 000), umbilical tape, Penlight batteries, stethoscope, scalp vein needles No 23 and 25, ampule file, needles, and tourniquet. –
- Suction catheter A heated, warmed incubator with a portable oxygen supply. –
- A laryngoscope with size 00, 1 blade, extra laryngoscope bulb, tincture of benzoin,adhesivetape, Magill forceps, sutures, and various sized stilettos. -
- Emergency drugs and medications- Sodium bicarbonate 44 mEq/50 ml ampule.Calcium gluconate 10%, 1 ampule.
- Adrenalin 1;10,00C 0 ampule. Lasix 20mg;1 ampule

Bacteriostatic H2O - 1 bottle, 30m1NaCl 10%;2

ampnles,30m1

- Dextrose 10%;2 ampules, 50 ml
- Neonatal Naloxone:0.02 mg/ml ampules Potassium

  chloride, 2 mEq /kg- 1 bottle,10 mlHeparin 1000 u/mi 1

  bottle.

The subsequent carp of babies torn with perinatal asphyxia should include screening. For hypoglycemia during the first 24 hours (by dextrostix screening or laboratory determination) and hypocalcemia during the first 24 hours (by the laboratory and confirmed by ECE). Renal function should be monitored via urine output, or nu uber of voids, analysis and microscopic examinationof urine, and serial blood urea nitrogen determination.

COMPLICATIONS OF MECHANICAL VENTILATION

- *Infection,
- *Pneumothorax, pneumomediastinum, and subcutaneous emphysema.
- *Overcorrection of hypercapnia, with sudden changes in ph., cardiac arrhythmias, tetany, and soon.
- *Interference with venous return and a drop in cardiac output and blood pressure (sometimes because of a previously borderline hypervolemia condition) is especially worrisome in patients on CDAP.
- *Positive fluid balance.
- *Inappropriate ADH secretion.
- *Stiff lung

- *Accidental kinking or accidental displacement of the endotracheal tube into the right mainbronchus.
- *Tracheal inflammation, erosion, granuloma, formation, and later stenosis.
- *Oxygen toxicity; impairment of the defense mechanisms of the lung.
- *retention of the secretions above the cuff-or tracheal suction before deflating the cuff isessential to prevent aspiration.
- *Gastrointestinal; dilatation or bleeding, or both.
- *Psychological; dependence on mechanical respiratory, for example.
- *Exhaustion; lack of sleep due to constant intensive care.

Long-term complications of respiratory therapy:

Bronchopulmonary dysplasia chronic lung disease occurs in 5-30% of survivors of respiratory therapy for RDS, who often require prolonged treatment with oxygen and respirator• therapy because of the severe disease. Most recover some die of infection or corPulmonarynale slowly duringthe first year of life. Retrolental fibroplasia occurs in premature infants receiving oxygen. All premature infants treated with oxygen should have an eye examination prior to discharge. In verysmall premature (weighing under 1000g), RLF may occur, even if P02 did not exceed 100. To avoid vital impairment, close attention must be paid to oxygen concentration, and blood gases must be frequently assessed. Neurologic impairment occurs in 10-15% of survivors of respiratory therapy for RDS. Infants with less severe diseases are less affected.

UMBILICAL VEIN CATHETERIZATION

Umbilical vein catheterization (UVC)is used for emergency access to circulation and for exchange transfusion. It is not used for chronic care because of the risk of thrombosis and infection. Small premature (750g or less) may have to be managed only with UVC when X-ray confirmation must be made that the catheter is in the vena cava or right atrium before giving hypertonic infusions. After preparing, the vein is identified, the visible clots removed,and the vein dilated with iris forceps. Insert a saline-filled 5F (less than 1250g or 8F (more than1250g) catheter. A multi-hued catheter is used for exchange transfusion, and a single-holed catheter is for a long-term replacement. Never insert a catheter unless the free end is attached to a closed syringe since a low CVP combined with -ve intrathoracic pressure may drain air from the catheter into the vena cava (during shock), resulting in air embolism. When free blood flow isachieved (usually at 5-Ycm), the catheter is adequately placed for exchange transfusion (Catheter is positioned in the SVC at a level 04 above the diaphragm. Keep the catheter and the surrounding area sterile during exchange transfusion and maintain conditions. assterile as possible in the long-term placement. Following the exchange, place a purse-string silk suture around the vein before removing the catheter. For subsequent exchange, the cord must be soaked with warm saline until it is soft. The suture will assist in the identification of the vein and reinsertion of the catheter.

Umbilical artery catheterization (UAC) aids greatly in parenteraltherapy, monitoring blood gases and in, withdrawing blood samples, and arterial BP measurements via a pressure transducer. Indwelling artery catheters carry a great potential danger, including life-threatening infections and thromboembolism. UAC shouldn ‘t be used unless the infants under care are considered to have a 30-5 percent risk of mortality from their primary disease (gross prematurity BW 1000g RDS, severe aspiration pneumonia, and severe shock.

Complete sterility is required, including gloves, gowns,

and masks. Cut the cord 1-1.5 cm from the skin and tie the base with tape. Identify the arteries (gently insert the tip of the iris forceps into the lumen of one artery. Allow the forceps to expand and dilate the artery while holding the cordstump between the thumb and forefinger. Insert a saline-filled catheter (5F for infants more than 1250 g and 3.5F for those less than 1250g) into the artery for the appropriate distance. X-ray films should be taken after the placement of all umbilical catheters. This should be either at or below the level of 10-14 or just above the diaphragm (T6 -T10). The catheter is passed via the umbilical artery into the thoracic aorta proximal to the diaphragm. When adequate placement is assured, the catheter should be secured by a suture, as well as by adhesive tape. The umbilical stump should be covered with an antimicrobial agent (Betacaine sentiment) and left open to the air. The infusion solutions should contain a unit of heparin/M1 of infuscate arterial catheters. It should be removed as soon as possible. Use of the transcutaneous NO2 m monitors and heel stick blood gas determinations will include permutations.

HYPOVOLEMIC SHOCK IN THE NEONATE

Circulatory insufficiency may present at birth from prepartum, intrapartum, or postnatal causes.

PREPARTUM CAUSES OF SHOCK:

Fetuses-to-another transfusion detected by a Kleihauer Bekte smear of the mother's blood forfetal Hemoglobin); interdental transfusion in homozygous twins; and traumatic amniocentesis.

INTRAPARTUM CAUSES

Placenta previa or abruption, rupture of or avulsion of the umbilical cord, rupture of placental vessels (vasa previa), hematoma of the cord, or placenta; orincision of the placenta during the cesarean section.

POSTNATAL CAUSES OF HEMORRHAGE

Breech delivery leading to internal hemorrhage (retroperitoneal, adrenal, kidney, spleen, and liver) or fromcephalhematoma, intracranial hemorrhage, coagulopathy, and severe hemolytic anemia from very erythroblastosis fetal is.

Clinical features of shock:

Pallor, cyanosis signs of respiratory distress , shallow rapid or irregular respiratory, flaccidity, cold mottled skin tachypnea or bradycardia hepatosplenomegaly, and rarely convulsions. Edemaand hepatosplenomegaly may be due to erythroblasts.

The presumptive diagnosis of the shock should be considered in any infant in distress who is: pale with no hepatosplenomegaly. A hematocrit or Hemoglobin determination should be immediately taken and repeated in 6-12 hours to monitor the expected f fall after the hemodilution that followsthe acute loss of blood. Vital signs such as pulse, blood pressure, and respiratory, should be followed frequently during the first hours after birth.

Treatment: Treatment should be urgent to prevent irreversible damage or death. It includes blood volume expansion, correction of acidosis, and assisted ventilation. If the infant is pale andlimp, the airway should be cleared, oxygen administered or intubated if necessary, and an umbilicalcatheter or an Iv line inserted. Blood specimens from the mother and baby for type and crossmatch of blood should be obtained. Supportive treatment may be given with type 0-ve blood or electrolyte solutions until the results of cross-matching are known. In order of preference,10- 20ml/kg of Group 0-ve blood, plasma, 5% albumin, or isotonic saline. Repeat the infusion if further volume expansion is necessary. Oxygen should be administered, and correction of metabolic acidosis with NaHCO3 may also be indicated. Seizures secondary to dilutional hypernatremia may require prompt administration.3% NaCl solution by vein, followed by temporary restriction of water. Treatment of shock should improve the peripheral perfusion, which may result in increasing acidosis from the mobilization of accumulated metabolic acides4e. This should be corrected by sodium bicarbonate. Babies with severe acidosis. Who are hypovolemic and may have normal Bp because of peripheral vasoconstriction? Correction of acidosis, in some cases, may result in vasodilation and shock, which should becorrected immediately by volume expansion.

EDEMA IN THE NEONATE -

Generalized edema occurs in association with the most severe forms of Rhisominization, with homologous thalassemia, and in the infants of diabetic mothers. Some are premature and may have considerable edema. An apparent reason: those with RDS may become edematous even without. CCF. Edema of the face and neck may result from the pressure of the umbilical cord of the neck; transient localized swellings of the hands or feet may similarly be due to intrauterinepressures. Edema may be due to heart failure from CHD (even in the absence of a murmur. AA lag of renal excretion of electrolytes and water may result in edema when there has been a sudden large increase in intake of electrolytes with the feeding of concentrated mixtures of cow's milk. Edema may probably be related to low serum albumin or low Hemoglobin in older premature since plasma or blood relieves these. Edema is seen with anemia and vitamin E deficiency in premature infants. Idiopathic hypoproteinemia with edema lasting weeks or months may be observed rarely in term infants; the course is benign persistent edema of one or more extremities may represent congenital lymphedema

(Milroy 's disease) or, in females, Turner's syndrome. Generalized hypoproteinemia with edema may be seen in neonates with congenital nephrosisand rarely with Hurlers syndrome or after feeding hypoallergenic formulas to infants with cysticfibrosis of the pancreas. Another cause is scleroderma.

RENAL FAILURE IN THE NEONATE

The normal urine output of a neonate is 1-2ml/kg/h. After a severe intrapartum or neonatal asphyxia insult, there may be 2-3 days of anuria or oliguria, followed by polyuria and then gradualrecovery. If glomerular damage has occurred, urine will contain protein and RBC. If the damage isprimarily tubular, there will be abnormal urine flow rates and electrolyte imbalance. If the insult is due to hypotension or prerenal failure, treatment should be early to colloid administration followed by restriction of fluids to insensible water loss +urine output. The infant should be weighed every 8-12 hours. Excessive fluid administration will result in pulmonary edema, accumulation of extravascular water, and CCF. Hyperkalemia may lead to cardiac arrhythmias and death and must be treated with intravenous calcium bicarbonate, continuous insulin, glucose infusion, or cation exchange resin. Serial measurements of urine and serum electrolytes and osmolality will be extremely useful in determining fluid and electrolyte management. A problem of /LBW is glycosuria with obligate water and sodium losses and rapid dehydration. Therefore, infants weighing less than 1200g should be the star.

Ecchymotic discoloration or petechial may be present at birth. The edema disappears within the first days of life. Analogous swelling, discoloration and distortion, and distortion of the face are seen in face presentation. No specific therapy is needed, but if there is extensive ecchymosis, early phototherapy for hyperbilirubinemia may be indicated. Molding of the head and overriding of the parietal bones are frequently associated with caput succedaneum and become more evidentafter the caput has receded but disappears during the first weeks of life.

EPHALHEMATOMA

Ephalhematoma is a sub-periosteal hemorrhage, therefore limited to the surface of one cranial bone. There is no discoloration of the overlying scalp due to subcutaneous hemorrhage, and swelling is usually not visible until several daps' hours after birth since subperiosteal bleeding is a slow process. In 25% of the cephalhematomas, there is an underlying fracture of theskull, which is usually linear and not depressed. A sensation of central depression suggesting an underlying fracture or bony defect is usually encountered on palpation of the organized rim of a cephalhematoma. Cranial meningeal may be differentiated from cephalhematoma by pulsation, increased pressure on crying, and the X-ray evidence of the bony defect. Most cephalhematomas are absorbed within two weeks to 3 months, depending upon their size. They may begin to calcify by the end of the week. A few remain as bony protuberances for years and are detectable radio logically as widening of the diploid space; cystlike defects may persist for months or years. Despeciallyitee these residuals, cephalhematomas require no treatment. Since the introduction ofinfection is the only serious complication, incision, or aspiration of cephalhematoma is contraindicated.

SKULL FRACTURES

Skull Fractures may occur because of pressure from the forceps or against the maternalsymphysis pubis during oral promontory or ischia spines during birth. Linear fractures are the commonest; they cause no symptoms and need no treatment. Depressed fractures are usually indentations of the calvarium like a dent in a Ping-Pong ball; usually, they are a complication of forceps delivery. Such fractures should be elevated surgically to prevent corticalinjury. Fracture of the occipital bone with separation of the basal and squamous portions almost invariably causes fatal hemorrhage, owing to the disruption of the underlying sinuses; it may result from the traction of the hyperextended spine of the infant with the head fixed in the maternal pelvis during breech deliveries.

SPINAL CORD INJURY

Strong traction on the hyperextended spine, or when the spin directionof the pull is lateral or forceful longitudinal traction on the trunk while the head is firmly engaged in the pelvis when combined with flexion and torsion of the vertical axis may produce fracture and separation of the vertebrae. The injury is commonest at the level of the 7th cervical and the first thoracic vertebrae. Transection of the cord may occur, and out hemorrhage and edema may produce neurologic signs indistinguishable from those of transaction except that theyare not prominent. There is complete paralysis of voluntary motion below the level of injury, though the persistence of a withdrawal reflex mediated throughout spinal centers distal to the area of the injury is frequently misinterpreted as voluntary motion. The differential diagnosis includes amyotonia congenital and myelodysplasia associated with spinal Bifida occulta, severe spinal cord injuries usually cause death soon after birth, but if it survives, treatment is supportive. There is often permanent injury. In compression from a fracture or dislocation, theprogress is related to the time of elapsing before the compression is removed.

BRACHIAL PALSY:

Injury to the brachial plexus may cause paralysis of the upper arm with orwithout paralysis of the forearm or hand; such injury occurs when lateral traction is exerted on the head and neck during delivery of the shoulder in the vertex delivery or in the breech when the arms are extended over the head, or there is excessive traction on the shoulders. In Erb*Duchene palsy, the injury is limited to C5 and 6. The infant loses the power to abduct the arm from the shoulders to rotate the arm externally and to supinate the forearm. The characteristic position consists of adduction and internal rotation of the arm with pronation of the forearm. The power of extension of the forearm is retained, but the biceps reflex is absent the Moro reflex is absent on the affected side. There may be some sensory impairment on the outer aspect of the arm. The power in the forearm and the hand grasp is preserved unless it is fine.

The mild cases may not be detected immediately after birth. The paralysis from an injury to the brachial plexus may involve the entire arm; differentiation must be made from the cerebral injury, fracture-dislocation, or epiphyseal separation of the humerus, and fracture of the clavicle. The prognosis depends on whether the nerve was merely injured or lacerated. If the paralysis was due to edema and hemorrhage about the fibers, there should be a return of the function withina few months; if due to laceration, permanent damage may result. The involvement of the deltoidis usually the most serious; dropping of the shoulder may result from muscular atrophy. In general, paralysis of the upper arm has a better prognosis than paralysis of the lower arm.

Treatment of brachial palsy consists of partial immobilization and appropriate positioning to prevent the antagonistic pull of the non-paralyzed muscles. In the upper arm paralysis, the arm should be abducted 90. degrees, with external rotation at the shoulder and with full supination of the forearm and slight extension at the wrist with the palm turned toward the face.This may be done by pinning the sleeve of the infant's garments at the wrist to the undersheet. The restraint should be maintained for 2-3 hours at a time, alternating with short-term periods when the arm is free. In the lower arm or hand paralysis, the wrist should be splinted in a neutral position and padding placed in the fist. Physical therapy is a necessary adjunctto the treatment. If the paralysis persists, because of laceration of the nerve fibers, for 3-6 months, neuroplasty may offer partial recovery.

PHRENIC NERVE PALSY

Pherenic Nerve Palsy is suggested when cyanosis and irregular or labored respiratorys develop; breathing in thoracic in type so that there is no bulging of the abdomen with inspiration.The injury is usually unilateral and associated with homolateral upper brachial palsy. Breath sounds are diminished on the affected side. The thrust of the diaphragm, which often may be felt just under the costal margin on the normal side, is absent on the affected side. The diagnosis is established by screening examination, which reveals the elevation of the diaphragm on the paralyzed side and see-saw movements on the two sides of the diaphragm during respiratory.
There is no specific treatment; the infant should be placed on the involved side; oxygen may be needed; initially, IV feedings may be needed, but later, progressive gavage or oral feedings maybe started, depending on the infant's condition. Pulmonary infections are a serious complication. Recovery usually occurs spontaneously, but rarely surgical plication of the diaphragm may be done.

FACIAL NERVE PALSY

Facial Nerve Palsy is usually a peripheral paralysis that results from pressure over the facial nerve in utero, during labor, or from forceps during delivery. Rarely is it nonobstetric resulting from the nuclear agenesis of the facial nerve. When the infant cries, thereis movement of the normal side only, while on the affected side, the eye cannot be closed, the nasolabial fold is absent, and the corner of the mouth droops. The mouth drawn towards the normal side of the forehead will wrinkle on the affected side with central paralysis since only the lower 2/3 of the face is involved/Prognosis depends upon whether the nerve was injured by pressure or whether the nerve fibers were torn. Improvement will occur within a fewweeks if there is pressure injury, but if the paralysis is persistent, neuroplasty is done. Care of theexposed eye is essential.

LIVER RUPTURE

Liver is the only internal organ, other than the brain, which is frequently injured during birth; the damage usually occurs from pressure on the liver during delivery of the headingbreech presentation. Large infant size, IU asphyxia coagulation disorders, and hepatomegaly are the contributing factors. Overzealous artificial respiratory or extrathoracic cardiac massage is less frequent causes of liver rupture. Rupture of the liver occurs, leading to a subcapsular hematoma, which may be large enough to cause anemia. Shock and death may occur if the hematoma breaks through the capsule, reducing pressure and thus allowing fresh hemorrhage. Surgical repair of the laceration may be needed; otherwise, supportive therapy may suffice. Rupture of the spleen may occur with that of s liver.

FRACTURE CLAVICLE

Fracture Clabicale occurs more frequently during labor and delivery than any other boneand is especially vulnerable when there is difficulty in delivery of the shoulder in vertex presentation and of the extended arias in the breech presentation. The infant fails to move the arm on the affected side, and there is a spasm in it.

RESPIRATORY DISTRESS IN NEONATE

A variety of diseases can lead to respiratory distress in the neonate; the majority of neonates haveRDS with signs: and symptoms of respiratory distress , including retractions (subcostals, intercostal, and substernal) flaring of the alae nasi, tachypnea, expiratory grunting, cyanosis, pallor, and diminished breath sounds. Blood analysis should include blood gases, glucose, bilirubin electrolytes, hematocrit, and osmolality, X-ray of the chest and abdomen is the single most important lab test in evaluating respiratory distress . A radiopaque nasogastric tube should be placed just prior to the X-ray examination to confirm patency to the stomach, thus excluding canal atresia, esophageal atresia, and most instances of TE fistula. The radiograph should be read for the presence of the thymus, the size and configuration of the heart and pulmonary findings, and any bony abnormalities that may be the cause of respiratory distress . Repeat x-rays are indicated if the baby 's status changes or if the diagnosis is uncertain. The width of the intercostal spaces, the angle of the ribs with the vertebral columns, the position of the diaphragm, and the degree of aeration on the chest X-ray assist in differentiating diseases characterizing increased lung volume and functional residual capacity (aspiration syndromes, persistent fetal circulation) from those of decreased lung volume and functional residual capacity (RDS and atelectasis).

Patchy infiltrates are characteristic of aspiration syndromes, while diseases such as RDS and persistent fetal circulation are characterized by diffuse findings. Fluid in the interlobular tissue and peripheral streaking are characteristic of transient tachypnea of -a, newborn (wet lung syndrome). The presence of vascular markings (seen in congenital heart disease with L-R shunt and total anomalous pulmonary venous return) or their absence (persistent fetal circulation, meconium aspiration) may help in establishing the cause of rasp distress. The presence of air in the thorax with the collapse of the lung is evidence of pneumothorax. Mediastina shift usually indicates a tension pneumothorax, which requires immediate evacuation of the extrapleural air. Air shadows around the heart and thymus, which can be seen in the AP view, and substernal air in the lateral view are diagnostic of pneumomediastinum.

With a diaphragmatic hernia, the bowel will be seen on the left side of the chest with a shift of the heart to the right side (if no air is present in the bowel, the left side of the chest may be opaque). Measurement of the blood gases is important because pH, P02, and pCO2 cannot guarantee tod be assessed by physical examination. Normal pH at birth is 7.2 or more. In the normal fall-term infant, the pH approximates. 7.4 at 2-4h after birth (4-oh for the premature infant). The normal arterial p02 is 50-8O mm Hg and the normal pCO2 is approximately 40 mm. With normal peripheral circulation and no edema, a capillary heel stick sample is adequate for pH and pCO2. In-room air, a capillary p02 of more than 50mm is normal. But if supplementary oxygen is being administered, p02 should bemeasured only in arterial blood. Capillary heel stick serapes are not adequate because they tend to provide a minimal value for p02, which is potential damage that rotates because of the development of retrolental fibroplasia with hypoxemia. Monitoring the change in paCO2 in Response to breathing room air versus.100% O2 is helpful in differentiating heart from lung disease in a baby who is hypoxic (Pa02 less than 50mm) in room air. Often the PaCO2 is elevatedin lung disease and normal or decreased in heart disease. In heart disease (R-L shunts-decreased pulmonary perfusion), the Pa02 will remain less than 100 MM in 100% oxygen and be less than 50 mm in the room with lung disease (alveolar hypoventilation or abnormal ventilation/perfusion where perfusion of the alveoli is normal, but ventilation of the alveoli is. diminished), Pa02 will rise to more than 250mm in 100% 02 and be less than 50 mm in room air. Exceptions to this will occur in cases of an R-L shunt through the ductus arteriosus with the site of sampling distal to the

Ductus (as within umbilical artery catheter), the left innominate arteries arising distal to the ductuswith the arterial sample taken from the left upper limb, and intrapulmonary R-L shunting as RDSwith diffuse atelectasis. An ECG is indicated as an aid in the diagnosis of cardiac and electrolyte abnormalities. Treatment is directed towards the specific disease, providing supportively measured, such as temperature maintenance, fluid and nutrition, drugs, and oxygen. Establishing the diagnosis is of primary importance since. The mechanical causes, choanal atresia, pneumothorax, TE fistula, and diaphragmatic hernia, are usually amenable to surgery. Themetabolic causes such as hypoglycemia, hypocalcemia, drugs, hypovolemia, anemia, and polycythemia can usually be rapidly corrected.

A list of common causes of distress is found in Appendix 4.

HEART FAILURE IN THE NEWBORN

,

Heart failure in the neonate is difficult to recognize because the signs and symptoms are differentfrom those seen in older infants. The infant with earl; failure will show only an increased heart rate, excessive weight gain, and irritability. As the heart failure worsens, sweating, anxiety, and poor feeding occurs. Auscultation of the lungs rarely shows evidence of pulmonary edema. Abnormal heart sounds and murmurs are often not diagnostic. Ray will show cardio mega Increasing liver size is important to sign, and an enlarging or enlarged size in the absence of other dosage is good evidence of heart failure. Liver size should also be followed as a means: of evaluating the effectiveness. The treatment. Peripheral edema is frequent in preterm infants but is rarely a sign of heart failure. When it occurs in heart failure, it isa late and ominous sign. In general, peripheral edema reflects excessive sodium and water intake rather than heart failure. ECG is important for showing axis and atrial or ventricular dilatation or hypertrophy. Echocardiography enables one to perform the serial examination of critically ill infants without any gross manipulation of the infant. (It is useful for assessing the strength of myocardial contractions, facilitating the early diagnosis of various congenital anomalies of the heart, and providing an estimate of left atrial size through measurement of left atrial-aortic route diameters).

If structural anomalies are suspected, cardiac catheterization may be indicated (Treatment is the same, whatever the cause of the CCF: restricting water intake (to the number of evaporative basses and eliminating sodium intake. If water restriction is coupled with complete sodium restrictions, hypernatremia will not resume even if potent diuretics such as furosemide and ethacrynic acid are used. His regime can be instituted along with a single dose of frustrated and digitalization of the Infant after 12-24 hours; water and sodium intake can be increased, with the degree of sodium and water administered as per the course of the infant. The specific lesion should be sought and treated; for cyanotic CHD or persistent CCF, a palliative procedure or major CVS surgery may be needed. The mortality rate (of infants with cyanotic CHD undergoing surgery approaches 65%, with deaths being due (mainly to cardiac arrhythmias and reek failure diteintensive care support. The long-term effects on the survivors are delayed growth and development. The most serious squeal is severe neurologic dysfunction due to hypoxia, ischemia, or emboli due to primary cardiac disease or major invasive procedures.

CONGENITAL ATELECTASIS

Atelectasis (the incomplete expansion of the lung or a portion of the lung) at birth is always present in infants who dye shirt/y after birth. Congenital atelectasis is the failure of the lung to expand at birth, while acquired atelectasis sis is the collapse of the previously expanded lung parenchyma due to many caws. The first few breaths were taken by the vigorous neonate at birthproduce complete expansion of all parts of the lung with air Etiology of the primary atelectasis (failure of the initial alveolar expansion) Failure of the lung to expand at birth may be due to –depression of the respiratory center due to damage by intracranial hemorrhage or maternalanesthesia, or over-sedation prior to delivery –

due to the relative inability of the thin-walled bronchioles, alveolar ducts lined with columnarepithelium, and thick-walled alveoli, which are characteristic of the immature fetus

due to obstruction of the air passages by aspirated amniotic fluid containing blood, mucus, andvernix caseosa. –

Commonly it is premature due to the immaturity of the diaphragm and other respiratory muscles, with hypermobility of the thoracic cage, other defects of the peripheral respiratory mechanism, or severe illness.

Secondary atelectasis (alveolar collapse after initial expansion by air) may occur as a gross ormicroscopic lesion in all types of pulmonary disease in the neonate. Thus, it may occur with mechanical pressure of pleural effusion, chest deformity, enlarged heart or diaphragmatic herniation, etc.

Pathology: In stillborn infants, lungs are uniformly beefy red; histological of the interstitialtissues are congested, and the alveoli present the appearance of a crumpled sack. The degree of crumpling varies inversely with the expansion of the alveoli by fluid formed in the lung and bythe aspirated amniotic fluid. With sudden anoxia in utero, there may be more vigorous therapy inspiratory movements.

There are varying degrees of alveolar distension. If there has been vigorous inspiration natural orartificial), irregular areas of alveolar overdistension may be found. Rupture of the distended alveoli may result in interstitial emphysema and sometimes pneumomediastinum and pneumothorax.

CLINICAL FEATURES:

Cardinal signs of primary atelectasis are persistent cyanosis, rapid shallow respiratorys (poor reapeffort), grunting and apnea, and poor air exchange. Respiratory may be irregular, with periods of apnea and intermittent cyanosis, especially where there is an injury to or depression of the CNS. Small (800-1200g) premature infants with extensive atelectasis may have chronic pulmonary insufficiency; these infants are often well, with minimal signs of respiratory distress until the 2nd-3rd day when they develop frequent epistles of prolonged apnea and cyanosis that may become progressively severe and terminate in death or may gradually resolve over the next 2-3 weeks.

The signs include impaired percussion note over the lung portion involved, and decreased breath sounds with fine crepitation eventually heard; if the atelectasis is unilateral, the mediastinum is shifted to the affected side, in which case blockage of the main bronchus should be suspected, and bronchoscopy is done. The signs of secondary atelectasis usually merge with those of the underlying pulmonary problem. The infant with obstructive atelectasis may make vigorous efforts to breathe; there may be Respiratory distress, cyanosis when out of oxygen, rapid breathing with retractions, and grunting. X-RAY the chest will show the shift of the trachea and mediastinum to the affected side with raised diaphragm on the same side. Thus, cardinal signs in primary atelectasis are persistent cyanosis with poor Respiratory effort and air exchange, and in secondary atelectasis, Respiratory distress, cyanosis, rapid shallow breathing, with retractions and grunting. Treatment is mainly symptomatic and supportive; the air passage should be clear d by means of a tracheal catheter; the infant is put in a highly humidified 02 tent with an oxygen concentration not exceeding 40%, and the position of the baby is changed frequently; antibiotics as penicillin 100,000 units bhourly + kanamycin 15mg/kg in 2 doses; underlying conditions should be dealt with. Prevention ofpremature labor, fetal and neonatal anoxia, intracranial hemorrhage Respiratory distress syndrome, and pneumonia will eliminate most of the causes of atelectasis.

MECONIUM ASPIRATION (Fetal asphyxia of post-maturity)

Meconium may be passed in utero, and the infant may aspirate amniotic fluid containing meconium before or during birth. Bronchioles may be plugged, gas exchange interfered with, pulmonary resistance raised, and signs of severe reap distress may occur. Due to the irritating property of meconium, chemical pneumonitis or secondary bacterial infection of the lung mayfollow. There is a 10-20% incidence of pneumothorax or pneumomediastinum associated with meconium aspiration. X-ray shows localized areas of atelectasis associated with consolidationand emphysema.

Evaluation and diagnosis: The amount of and the thickness of the meconium is directly proportional to the severity of the disease. If tachypnea or respiratory distress increases, evaluation should include a chest x-ray, arterial or heel stick blood gas determination, andmeasurement of blood sugar, Mg, and Ca levels. If infiltration is seen on an x-ray, chest culture ofblood urine, skin nasopharynx, and trachea are indicated (as meconium enhances the growth of bacteria), and differentiation of infective pneumonia from meconium aspiration is difficult. Arterial desaturation due to R-L shunts is likely to be more of a problem than CO2 retention.

Prevention of Meconium aspiration -

Prevention of meconium passage in utero; can be done by STRESS-testing (oxytocin challenge test), non-stress testing with fetal monitoring, or scalp pH sampling must be done in all pregnancies with evidence of uteroplacental insufficiency. High-risk pregnancies include those with toxemia or hypertension, heavy smoking, chronic maternal disease, poor fetal growth, and post maturity.1/2 of the infants with meconium-stained amniotic fluid have meconium in the trachea on suction; such infants frequently post mature or have suffered intrapartum asphyxia. When thick particulate or pea-soup meconium is present, the obstetrician should finish.

The tube must be introduced into the trachea under direct laryngoscopy and sucked by mouth as it is being withdrawn. Usually, 2-4 intubations are sufficient, -Oxygen by mask should be administered after the trachea has been cleared. -To the extent possible, the airway must be cleared, and ventilation initiated before significant bradycardia occurs. Once the child has had a few breaths, meconium in the airway has moved from the trachea to the smaller bronchi, andextensive attempt to remove it at that point are unwise. similarly, no positive pressure should be used until after the trachea is sucked. The trachea should also be suctioned in infants with thin meconium and Apgar score of b or less.

Treatment -Infants with significant aspiration often have severe difficulty. Respiratory physiotherapy and or pharyngeal suction every 30 minutes for the first 2 hours at 1 hour for the next 8 hours. The trachea must be suctioned if a tube is in place. The infants may be acutely asphyxiated within an associated metabolic acidosis, which may tie corrected with its carbonates if FIO2 requirements are more than 40%. A trial of positive pressure end-expiratory pressure (PEEP) in the range of 4-7cm of water might be instituted use of antibiotics is indicated on an individual basis if an X-ray chest shows an infiltrate; antibiotics are used empirically after cultures have been obtained

TRANSIENT TACHYPNEA OF THE NEWBORN

TTNB or wet-lung syndrome is characterized by transient tachypnea lasting 24-36 hours cyanosis less often), good air exchanges, no acidosis or hypercarbiaonlycm signally requires supplementary oxygen, in concentration rarely exceeding 4010. It follows. in deliveries where there is no labor, elective cesarean section due to slow reabsorption of fluid by the lungmay follow normal delivery. X-ray of the chest may show central perihelia streaking and fluid inthe interlock bar fissures, suggesting that the syndrome is secondary to slow resorption of lung fluid; the increased respiratory rate may require discontinuance of oral feeding to avoid the risk of aspiration.

RESPIRATORY DISTRESS IN THE NEONATE

Respiratory Distress in the Neonate can be broadly divided into 3 categories; - Those with increased or normal pulmonary expansion, hilar infiltrates, rales, or rhonchi; wheezingmay be present; chest X-ray shows a slightly enlarged heart and streaky infiltrates radiating from the hilum of the lung following the general pattern of the lymphatic and venous drainage of the lung the peripheral lung fields are clear. Areas of infiltration or atelectasis may be present. These include congenital bacterial pneumonia, wet lung syndrome, transient tachypnea of the neonate, and amniotic fluid or meconium aspiration. –

Disorders with normal lung expiration, relatively clear lung fields, and marked hypoxemia arecommonly associated with persistent fetal circulation. Any congenital heart lesion with inadequate pulmonary blood flow also has these findings. Though shock-lung has a clinical spectrum comparable to that of a wet lung, occasionally, it may follow a severe hypoxic and hypotensive episode and have the features of persistent fetal circulation. -

Hyaline membrane disease is characterized by marked hypo expansion of and reduced lung volume and involves all lung fields so that an inspiratory chest X-ray has the appearance of an inspiratory film. Physically the findings consisted of decreased lung volume and included tachypnea, marked intercostal retraction, suprasternal retraction, and grunting.

Air entry is poorthroughout all lung fields.

PERSISTENT FETAL CIRCULATION

Babies with persistent fetal circulation (PFC)are characteristically full-term and present with marked cyanosis and signs of Respiratory distress within the first 12-14 hours after birth. Systemic bloodpressure is usually normal, but a systolic murmur is heard' frequently. Severe hypoxemia resultsfrom pulmonary hypertension and R-L shunt at the foramen ovale and ductus arterioles. The shutcan be documented by a greater rise in Pa02 in the temporal artery than in the umbilical artery in 100% oxygen compared to room air. Associated morbidity includes hypoplasia.

When the transient persistence of the fetal circulation is very severe, ventilation or support, muscle relaxation, and pulmonary vascular dilatation with tolazoline (1-2mg/kg iv) may be needed. Tolazoline is a general alpha-adrenergic blocking agent and has histaminic activity and reduces pulmonary arterial pressure and vascular resistance to some extent (potential side effects of tolazoline are hypertension, hypotension, renal insufficiency, intestinal hemorrhage, and abdominal distension). Assisted ventilation is used to drive arterial PCO2 to low levels in severely affected patients. Since topazine will cause vasodilation in other vascular beds also, and severe and irreversible shock may occur if colloid in the form of plasma or blood is not given at the same time as thiazine. Mean arterial blood pressure should be carefully monitored during andfollowing tolazoline therapy.

BRONCHOPULMONARY DYSPLASIA

An iatrogenic disease caused by the exposure of the surface of the reap tract to high concentrations of inspired oxygen(rather than by a high Pa02),it may be unavoidable in those infants with severeRDS who require high oxygen tenses-concentrations to ensure acceptable arterial oxygen tensions bronchopulmonary dysplasia is the end result of many factors as positive pressure assisted ventilation, endotracheal or nasotracheal intubation, and prolonged exposure to high concentrations of oxygen. The disease is characterized by a specific serial X-ray appearance of the lungs (opaque to cystic to fibrotic) accompanied by clinical signs (tachypnea, retractions, rales, and cyanosis) and by the prolonged need for supplemental oxygen. Thesebabies demonstrate an exquisite sensitivity to the small decrement of oxygen (as little as 2%) during the long process of weaning from supplemental oxygen-Some babies may have persistent abnormal pulmonary function for years. This condition is only rarely reported following assisted ventilation using a -ve pressure respirator and no tracheal intubation.

PNEUMONIA (PNEUMONIA IN THE NEONATE)

The respiratory system of the infant may get infected in utero, during passage through the birth canal, or at any time during the neonatal period. Pneumonia is found histologically at autopsy of infants dying of respiratory distress of any cause.

About 10% of neonatal deaths are attributed to pneumonia.

ETIOLOGY

Congenital pneumonia occurs during the first few days of life; it is especially common when there is premature rupture of membranes, prolonged labor, premature labor, maternal fever, or fetal distress. The presence of chorioamnionitis in most cases suggests aspiration of infected vaginal amniotic fluid as its cause. Aspiration of infected— vaginal secretions during delivery may also be a cause. The 2nd type of pneumonia, beginning after the first few days of life, is usually acquired through contact with adults or children with reap infections or through bacteremia. Coliform organisms, nonhemolytic streptococci, and staph avenues aurous are the mostfrequent causes for both types of pneumonia.

Enterococci klebsiella, pseudomonas proteus, and salmonella also tend to be more frequent pathogens than in the older child. Group B beta-hemolytic streptococci and strep galactic may alsobe associated with early septicemia and pneumonia. Pneumonia in early infancy is usually bronchopneumonia; only occasionally, it is interstitial or lobar.

CLINICAL FEATURES:

The first signs of pneumonia in the newborn are usually nonspecific; they include loss of appetite listlessness, poor color, which may or may not be definable as cyanosis, a rise or sudden fall in body temperature, abdomina distension, sudden loss or gain in weight, tachycardia, and a general impression In the part of the mother that the batty is not doing well Cough is inconstant,but almost always means pneumonia when present. A significant increase in respiratory rate, usually to about 80, is a constant and early finding alarming of the alae nasi accentuation of the normal irregularity of breathing and reap distress may be present. Pneumonia must be suspectedin infants with tachypnea, cyanosis, and retractions. Often no physical signs are elicited; though careful auscultation may reveal fin crackling rales most commonly in the peripheral areas posteriorly; they may be localized in any part of the lungs. The baby should be auscultated crying as well as quiet, since frequently crepitation is heard only at the end of the deep inspirations which come only with crying in the newborn. Areas of the hyper resonance may indicate compensatory emphysema. Blood gas determinations will show hypoxia, and in severe cases; progressive evidence is available.

Treatment includes ventilatory support of respiratory failure occurs, appropriate antibiotics, and percussion, drainage, and suction therapy to keep the airways clear. Prognosis in group B streptococcal and listeria pneumonia ranges from a fulminating course leading to death within hours in 50% cases to slow but complete recovery. In survivors, recovery of normal pulmonary function is anticipated since the infant can entirely regenerate normal lung tissue. In general, infants with conditions with infiltrates (pneumonias, wet lung, translucent tachypnea, and aspiration pneumonia) will not require to reap support, but for infants with reap failure, CPAP and ventilator support may be necessary to improve oxygenation while avoiding the risk of excessive high concentrations of aspiratory oxygen.6ince diseases in this group, in their earliercourse can't be distinguished from congenital bacterial pneumonia especially group B streptococcal, all of them should Be given antibiotics.

ASPIRATION OF FOREIGN MAPERIALS (ASPIRATION SYNDROMES)

Aspiration syndromes are seen generally in the term infants, and frequently follow perinatal asphyxia. During prolonged' labors and difficult deliveries, infants often attempt to breathe in utero, owing to interference with the supply of oxygen via the placenta. Under such circumstances, the infant aspirates amniotic fluid containing such debris as vernix caseosa, epitnelial celle, meconinm, or materials from the birth canal. His debris blocks the smallest airways and interferes with the alveolar exchange of oxygen and carbon dioxide. Pathologic Bacteria frequently accompany the aspirated material, and when pneumonia also ensues, Respiratory distress is usual. Aspiration of meconium Is brie most dangerous. Meconium staining of the amniotic fluid occurs in 5-10% of pregnancies, and incident of clinical illness from aspiration is about 1% of all births. In the presence of thick meconium, nasopharyngeal suctioning after the birth of the head and direct tracheal suctioning after birth decreases morbidity. The disease is characterized by increased lung volume and an increased AP diameter of the chest. Characteristic Xray findings are a depressed diaphragm, hyperaeration land large coarse patchy densities. The obstructive character of the disease leads to a high incidence of pneumothorax (10%) accompanied by a sudden and dramatic deterioration in the baby 's condition. A pneumothorax kit (a large 50-50 ml syringe. A 22-gauge needle.5-way stop-cock, antiseptic pledgets, and petrolatum gauze should be at the bedside of all infants born with meconium-stained amniotic fluid. Immediate treatment consists of the evacuation of the air and the insertion of a chest tube on the affected side. Other situations in which pulmonary aspiration of foreign material may contribute to serious consequences in the newborn infant include TE fistula esophageal and duodenal obstructions, improper feeding practices, the administration of medicines, and improper handling and placement of infants in their cribs. The contents of the stomach should be aspirated through asoft rubber catheter just before operation or other procedures requiring anesthesia. Procedures that may disturb the infant and especially those which involve changing the infant to the head down position, such as jugular and femoral punctures, LP, and SD taps, should be performed at least 2 hours after feeding.

STAPHYLOCOCCAL PNEUMONIA

Staph pneumonia: should be suspected in any infant who shows even slight and untoward nonspecific signs and who has been exposed to staph skin infections. Staph pneumonia in infantsis becoming common now. Empyema and pneumothorax are frequent complications-The latter constitutes such an immediate threat to the infant's life that infants with staph pneumonia should be etched closely for acute onset of Respiratory distress, so that treatment by closed thoracotomy drainage can be carried out without delay. Transmission is airborne or by personnel contact.

CLASSIFICATION OF PNEUMONIA IN THE NEONATE

Congenital pneumonia

1. Transplacental agents include Torch infections, enteroviruses treponema palladium, listeria modbcytogenes, mycobacterium TB genital mycoplasma, and pneumococci.

2. Maternal vaginal causes include Group B streptococci E. cloil and other Gm. venteric bacteria, staphylococca, pneumococcal anaerobic organisms, zhlamydia, mycoplasma, and herpesvirus.

i. Pneumonia acquired during birth, especially in immature, weak, or anoxic infants, due to the maternalvaginal flora, but may not be present until a few days after birth.

ii. Pneumonia is acquired after birth (by postnatal airborne infections), got from it.

3. Intrauterine infection particularly occurs in cases of premature rupture of the membranes, wheninfected amniotic fluid is aspirated. General debility with the refusal of feeds is often seen at the outset. There is an increase in respiratory rate associated with cyanosis and dyspnea. Fever and cough may or may not be present.

4. The physical examination will show fevers, lethargy, tachypneas grunting, flaring of nasal alae, retractions, irregular breathing, rales, and cyanosis may be present. Diagnosis is made by the presence of physical signs; a chest X-ray is often decisive and shows pulmonary infiltrates. Chest percussion is of little help. Diagnosis is difficult and careful auscultation of the entire chest always necessary in order not to miss the area of pulmonary consolidation, which may be very small. The presence of fine crepitation in conjunction with cyanosis and dyspnea is suggestive. CBC chest X-ray for the evidence of palm infiltrates or pleural effusions and gastric aspirate for gram staining and culture (the presence of neutrophils is correlated with pneumonia more than is the finding of bacteria), cultures and Gil stains of blood urines CSF, and tracheal aspirate are the investigations needed. If pleural fluid is present tap must be done, and if necessary direct lung aspiration (lung tap) is indicated. Treatment includes general supportive measures (fluids electrolyte and acid-base balance; maintenance of hematocrit, blood volume, and blood pressure; nutrition,

temperature control, feeding by nasal tube may be needed); respiratory support (respiratory physical therapy-02 may be needed; intermittent pressure ventilation; drainage of pleural fluid if the fluid is compromising the respiratory; changing the position of the regularly to improve pulmonary circulation, or in case of aspiration pneumonia, to facilitate drainage) antibiotics depending on the C'S Prognosis is generally grave, but the earlier theonset of therapy, the better. Many cases: of bronchopneumonia in the neonate are part of generalized septicemia.

AIR LEAK IN NEONATES (Pulmonary interstitial emphysema, pneumomediastina sternums, and pneumothorax)

Asymptomatic pneumothorax (unilateral or bilateral) is estimated to be occurring in 1-2% of all newborn infants, but symptomatic ones are less common. It is more common in males than females and more common in term and post-term infants than in premature infants. But the incidence is increased in the neonates with RDS and –aloe receiving artificial ventilation especially if a continuous elevation of end-expiratory pressure is contained. The commonest case is over-inflation of the alveoli, leading to alveolar rupture or dissection of the air into the pulmonary parenchyma outside the branching tree. Rupture of the alveoli may be spontaneous or idiopathic or be due to resuscitations, mechanically assisted ventilation, underlying pulmonary disease such as lobar emphysema, rupture of a congenital or a pneumonic cysts trauma to a bivalve type of bronchial or bronchiolar obstruction resulting from aspiration. If the ruptured alveoli are on the pleural surfaces, pneumothorax without pneumonic mediastinum occurs; if not, pulmonary interstitial emphysema occurs. Air in the interstitial spaces of the lungs dissects along the per bronchial andperivascular connective tissue sheaths to the root of the lung. The pulmonary veins may be compressed at the hilum, and cardiac output is severely reduced with belated compression. If the volume of the escaped air is great enough, it may follow the vascular sheaths to cause mediastinal emphysema or a rupture of- with subsequent pneumomediastinum pneumothorax and subcutaneous emphysema (air in the SC tissue of the neck and chest). Rarely there may be increased mediastina pressure and interference with the venous return to the heart. Tension pneumothorax occurs if an accumulation of air within the pleural space is sufficient to elevate intrapleural pressure above the atmospheric pressure. Not only is ventilation impaired in the collapsed lung by a unilateral tension pneumothorax but in the normal lung may be compromised by mediastina shift to the other side. Compression of the vena cave and torsion of the great vessels may interfere with venous return. Those who are at a special risk of developing air leaks are infants who have RAS or pneumonia, who have required resuscitation at birth, and those who have sustained meconium aspiration.

CLINICAL FEATURES

The physical signs in asymptomatic pneumothorax are hypersensitive-resonance and diminished breath sound over the involved side of tit (chest. When symptomatic, clinical signs of pneumothorax develop rapidly with moderate to severe respiratory distress (respiratory distress varies from only.

There is a shift of the heartbeat since the organ is displaced towards the opposite side, and thediaphragm is displaced towards, as is the liver with right-sided pneumothorax. Both sides are affected in 10% of cases. Therefore, the symmetry of the findings does not rules out pneumothorax.

Pneumomediastinum occurs in 25% pts, and the degree of Respiratory distress is age-independent ofthe amount of trapped air. If it is great, there is bulging of the midthoracic area, the neck veins are distended, and blood pressure falls. Distension of the neck veins and low BP is due toblockage of circulation by compression of the systemic and pulmonary veins. A dramatic changein BP or percussion indicates a shift of the mediastinum or dissection of the alt along the peraorta. Pneumomediastinum may manifest as SC emphysema, and subcutaneous emphysema in the neonate is pathognomonic of pneumomediastinum Pneumopericardium will cause immediatedeterioration of BP, heart rate, and arterial oxygen; and will lead to death, if not diagnosed quickly. Pneumothorax and pneumomediastinum should be diagnosed in any infant with respiratory distress, other Respiratory signs or restlessness, or irritability. Ray establishes Use the diagnosis, and cross-table lateral X-ray films to help in the differentiation of air/leak from other causes: of respiratory distress. Or acute evaluation of an infant who deteriorates dramatically, a fiberoptic transilluminator may be used to diagnose pneumothorax. Tilts dyspnea, cyanosis, brown chest, and circulatory collapse will suggest the dial miss, and an X-ray chest (lateral or apt) will establish the diagnosis.

TREATMENT

Patients with uncomplicated pneumothorax-Infants who have no underlying pulmonary disease or complicating therapy like PEEP and who are not in respiratory distress (asymptomatic cases of pneumothorax or mildly symptomatic), in which there is no continuing air leak, will require only conservative therapy, i.e., observation in an incubator -frequent small feedings which prevent gastric dilatation and minimize crying, which could further compromise ventilation and worsen the pneumothorax. -a follow-up X-ray -The air will usually resolve within 24-46 hours. The use of 100% oxygen accelerates the resorption of the free air in the pleura by reducing the nitrogen tension in blood with a resultant nitrogen pressure. There is a shift of the heartbeat since the organ is displaced towards the opposite side, and thediaphragm is displaced downwards, as is the liver with right-sided pneumothorax. Both sides are affected in 10% of cases. Therefore, the symmetry of the findings does not rule out pneumothorax.

Pneumomediastinum occurs in 25% pts, and the degree of Respiratory distress is an independent on the amount of trapped air. If it is great, there is bulging of the midthoracic area and the neck veins are distended, and blood pressure falls. Distension of the neck veins and low BP is due to blockage of circulation by compression of the systemic and pulmonary veins. A dramatic changein BP or percussion indicates a shift of the mediastinum or dissection of the alt along the Pneumomediastinum, may manifest as 6C emphysema, and subcutaneous emphysema in the neonate is pathognomonic of pneumomediastinum Pneumopericardium will cause immediate deterioration of BP, heart rate, and arterial oxygen; and will lead to death, if not diagnosed quickly. Pneumothorax and pneumomediastinum should be diagnosed in any infant with respiratory distress, other Respiratory signs of restlessness, or irritability. Ray established the use of the diagnosis ap, and cross-table lateral X-ray films to help in the differentiation of air/leak from other causes: of respiratory distress. Or acute evaluation of di infant who deteriorates dramatically, a fiberoptic transilluminator may be used to diagnose pneumothorax. Tilts dyspnea, cyanosis, brown chest, and circulatory collapse will suggest the dial miss, and an X-ray chest (lateral or apt) will establish the diagnosis. Treatment Pat with uncomplicated

pneumothorax-infants who have no underlying pulmonary decrease or complicating therapy as PEEP and who are not in respiratory distress (asymptomatic cases of pneumothorax) mildly symptomatic), in which there is no continuing air leak, will require only conservative therapy, i.e., observation in an incubator -frequent small feedings which preventgastric dilatation and minimize crying, which could further compromise ventilation and worsen the pneumothorax. -a

follow-up x-ray. The air will usually resolve within 24-46 hours. The use of 100% oxygen accelerates the resorption of the free air in pleura by reducing the nitrogen tensionin blood with a resultant nitrogen pressure grabbing from the trapped airline blood, but for the danger of retrolental fib neoplasia, it is not recommended generally). With severe respiratory distress or circulatory embarrassment, emergency need: aspiration may require he needed. This may occasionally occur in the infant who has n (underlying pulmonary problem or continuing air leak (P/ace the infant in a sitting position, if possible-Attach, a 25-gauge needle to a 50m1 syringe via a 5-way. Place a hemostat about 1cm from the needle tip to prevent deep penetration. The needle should enter the pleura through the interspace in the anter1(r axillary line lateral to the pectorals major muscle. Hit the rim with the needle and slide it over thetop to minimize the chance of bleeding from the lute coastal artery. If the infant is breathing or crying after the visceral. Pleura opposes the parietal pleura; the needle tip may cause a bronchopleural fi6tala. Ibis is not common, but it is prudent to remove the needle as soon as possible.: Chest tube placement: If needle aspiration is unsuccessful in maintaining relief: of distress, or if there is adequate time, closed thoracotomy is done. Infants who have a continuing air/weak underlying pulmonary disease causing continued distr sour are in respiratory therapy or PEEP, they need chest tube placement and suet: on; the tube is connected to a water trap so that air may escape but not end (the chest. In asymptomatic pneumomedastinum is present and there is no continuing leakier only mediastinum is present, neonly conservative treatment is employed.
Pneumopericardiumrwhen symptomatic may be drained using a 20-gauge,13 inches nee (le attached via a 3-way stopcock to a 10-20m1 syringe (Following surgical preparation, insert a needle at the sub-xiphoid region, aiming for the posterior left shoulder, andwith suction on the syringe, advance the needle until air appears. When the air stops flowing, withdraw the needle. Often a single aspiration result

is in clinical improvement. About 25-40% patients will have a recurrent symptomatic pneumopericardium, treated as above. Infrequently, the pneumopericardium will act as if constant air drainage into pericardial space has occurred. Placement of a 16-gauge intricate into the pericardial space is appropriate in this situation

It occurs in 10-20/1000. live births (hut the incidence is highest in LBW infants; especially those weighing less than 1000-1600g, where the incidence is as high as 550: 1000 LBW babies and themortality is as high. as 60-70% in them. The special risk groups for RDS are premature infants, infants of diabetic mothers, infants born of cesarean section, infants subjected to IU distress, andantepartum vaginal bleeding. The disease is rare in full-term infants.10-35%) of all premature have RDS.

Etiology: The exact cause of the RDS is still unknown. There are many mechanisms that are ard to the development of PDS—

Deficiency or absence of surfactin; this surfactant is a surface-tension lowering lipid formedin the walls of the alveoli and present in term infants but deficient in premature infants. The lungs deficient in surfactant tend to collapse since the surface tension is high. Surfactant is most. Probably lecithin (a phospholipid, dipalmitoyl phosphatide choline. There is no surfactant prior to 20 weeks; by 24 weeks, synthesis occurs by methylation of phosphatide ethanolamine, and by 34-55 weeks, functional surfactant is synthesized by an active phosphatidylcholine pathway combining cyst dine phosphocholine with diglycerides (Choline phosphoglyceride=lecithin). Thus, RDS is strongly associated with prematurity as well as other factors which affect lung maturity. Pulmonary maturity is achieved at 35 weeks of gestation.

The absence of these pathways or the degradation or alteration of lecithin, can be the cause of the deficiency of surfactant could result in atelectasis, decreased lung compliance, increased work of breathing, and eventually insufficient ventilation with asphyxia, hypoxia, and acidosis. These latter events can produce pulmonary arterial vasoconstriction with increased vascular resistance and shunting through the foramen oval and ductus arteriosus. Pulmonary blood flow would thusbe reduced, with ischemic injury to cells producing lecithin and injury to the vascular bed resulting ìnan effusion of proteinaceous material into the alveolar spaces.

Hypo perfusion therapy hypothesis is that intrauterine or neonatal asphyxia with hypoxia and mixed respiratory(placental)and metabolic acidosis leads to increased pulmonary vascular resistance and systemic hypotension. As a result, venous blood bypasses the lungs through the foramen oval and ductus arteriosus., which leads to ischemia of the alveolar lining cells that produce surfactant or lecithin further compromising surfactant productions with resultant atelectasis and hypercarbia from a deficiency of surface tension-lowering lipids and with. Effusion of plasma and red cells from injured capillaries, leading to the formation of fibrin in the airspaces (thus left heart failure with subsequent conversion of fibrin from the effusion from pulmonary capillaries is thought to be responsible for the formation of hyaline membrane). –

Certain diseases such as maternal diabetes (class A, B, C) and severe Rherythroblastosis are 'associated with a delay in pulmonary maturity. Other maternal diseases may accelerate lung maturity as chronic hypertension, chronic placental insufficiency, and possible PROM. 8-10% ofall cases of RDS result from elective surgery or elective intervention with normal pregnancy (Cesar or induction); therefore, assessment of fetal pulmonary maturity should be done prior to such intervention.

Pathology: The lungs appcar dccp purplish rcd and are liver-like in consistency) Histologicallythere is extensive atelectasis, with engorgement of the interalveolar capillaries and lymphatics. Several alveolar ducts, alveoli, and respiratory bronchioles are lined with acidophilic homogeneous or granular membranes. The presence of osmophilic inclusion bodies characteristic of phospholipid storage in type II alveolar lining cells correlates with the time of the appearance of surfactin. Amniotic debris, intraalveolar hemorrhage, pneumonia, and interstitialemphysema are additional but inconstant findings; interstitial emphysema may be marked whenan infant has been ventilated with a method employing an increased end-expiratory pressure (PEEP). This characteristic membrane is rarely seen in infant dying earlier than 6-6 hours. after birth. Intracranial hemorrhages are common in infants of VISW (less than 1250g) but is probably associated with anoxia or prematurity rather than RDS.

Postnatal evaluation of RDS

The disease is characterized by decreased alveolar surfactant resulting in diffuse pulmonary atelectasis, leading to diminished functional residual capacity and compliance, hypoventilation, even ventilation/perfusion ratio, occasional hypercarbia, and acidosis. These cause pulmonary vasoconstriction and decrease pulmonary blood flow, resulting in capillary endothelial damageand leakage of blood intercostal, snbcostal or sternal retractions, expiratory grunt or Whining, nasal flaring, and cyanosis. The course is characterized by increasing evidence of air hunger and fatigue from the excessive respiratoryeffort. There is a tendency for hypothermia and hypotonia as the condition worsens, dyspnea, pallor, and cyanosis increase. On auscultation, air exchange may seem to be normal or diminished; on deep inspiration, fine rales are often heard, especially over the lung bases posteriorly. There may be hypotension. edematileus and oliguria. In addition to signs of respiratory distress , there are signs of fatigue the frog leg posture, flaccidity, and a declining respiratoryrate.

LAB FINDINGS

Lab findings include progressive hypoxemia and acidosis; there is a fall in pH, a rise in CO2, byperkalemia, hyponatremia other lab data should include hematocrit Ca, total proteins, biliruhin; ECG and several blood pressure measurements; culture of the skin, nose, throat, ear canal, umbilicus spectrum, gastric aspirates urine, blood, CSP, if the conditionallows dastric aspirate should de be obtained during the first hours of life and processed for gram stain for neutrophil and bacceria neutrophils per HPF or the presence of bacteria in the first hr of life are associated with infection.

–

A gastric aspirate snake test is done to assess the amount of pulmonary surfactant in the newborn infants' lungs if the L/S ratio is not known. (0.5ml of absolute alcohol is added to 0.5ml of gastric aspirate in a small glass tube and the test tube capped by the thumb is vigorously shaken for 15 sec, and allowed to stand for 15 min. Readings

-ve no bubble

1+ very small bubbles in meniscus extending 1/3 or less of distance around the test tube (amagnifying glass is required to differentiate small bubbles from particles)

2+ A single rim of bubbles extending 1/3 to all around the test tube (a magnifying glass is notneeded)

3+ a rim of bubbles all the way around the test tube.

The negative test shows a high risk of RDS,5+ shows little chance of the disease, and 1-2+ shows intermediate risk. The test has. 10% false -ves and only 1% false +ves rate. A premature infantwith grunting respiratorys, rapid Respiratory rate, and hypoxia starting within 2 hours of birth usually has RDSbut otter causes of Respiratory distress should also be considered. Tachypnea beginning later suggests conditions other than the RDS.

Prognosis: Mortality is 20-30%; the death rate is lower among the more mature and heavier infants. Most deaths occur within 72 hours of birth, with the smallest infants dying within 24 Jarsunless artificial respiratory and intensive care are given. The condition may progress to death within a few hours, but in milder cases, the symptoms reach a deal within 3 days after which. Gradual improvement sets ii Signs of asphyxia wH711 secondary to periods of apnea or partial respiratoryto: dupe occur when there is a rapid progression of the disease. When recovery occurs, the prognosis is generally good though permanent, persistent pulmonary disease with fibrosis and recurrent pulmonary infections do occur in a small percentage of infants. The chronic pulmonary changes maybe oxygen related. Neurologic residuals are probably related more to intracranial haemorrhage, anoxia, hypoglycemia hyperbilirubinemia and other complications of immaturity than to RDS. Death is rare after 3 days, except in infants whose natural course of the disease has been altered using a respirator when death can occur later also. Long-term follow-up suggests that they don 't have an increased incidence of mental disabilities when compared to the general population with the same weight and gestational age but no disease.

Prevention of RDS (and prenatal evaluation)

The prevention of prematurity avoidance of unnecessary cesarean section, and careful management of the diabetic mother and the erythroblastosis are the most important factors• in the prevention of Respiratory distress syndrome. - In timing cesarean section, assessment of the degree of lung maturity is done by the L/S ratio, and estimation of fetal head: circumference,and the creatine concentration of amniotic fluid, decreases the chances of delivering a prematurebaby. -.

Measurement of the L/S ratio in the amniotic fluid is a reliable index of fetal lung maturity in pregnancies that are not complicated by maternal diabetes or Rh sensitization. The incidenceof RDS is under 2% if the L:S ratio is more than or equivalent to 2:1(a high LS ratio). Ratios of 1.5 or less is indicative enough.

Prompt treatment of or prevention of severe acidemia by iv $NaHCO_3$ may be helpful in reducingthe severity of respiratory distress though the course and prognosis of the disease are not altered. –

The use of maternal corticosteroids in preventing RDS by affecting the surfactant metabolism and thus accelerating the maturation of lungs has been recommended. Thus if an infant of fewer than 33 weeks gestation with evidence of pulmonary immaturity (1:S less than 2:1) must be delivered, alleviation of pulmonary immaturity may be accomplished by administration of glucocorticosteroids to the mother. In a study when an infection of 6mg betamethasone phosphate and 6 mg of betamethasone acetate was. Given, and repeated once 24 hours later; in gestations under 32 weeks and in the absence of maternal oedema, hypertension, or proteinuria, theirappeared to be a decrease in the incidence of RDS and in the mortality from the RDS and intraventricular haemorrhage among infants delivered between 24hours to 7days after the first dose. A full course of dexamethasone (4mgim 8hourly for 48 hours or betamethasone 12mgim 24 hr for 48 hours) must be given to ensure a beneficial effect. If the infant remains undelivered formore than 7 days after the course of steroids, And gestation is still less than 55 weeks; a repeat course must be given).

X-RAY PICTURE: The classical picture is a reticulogranular appearance or ground-glass appearance (black dots on a white background) and the presence of air bronchograms in the peripheral parts of the lungs.(The air containing bronchi is visible by virtue of surrounding nonaerated). There is an apparent cardiac enlargement (In contrast, fetal distress syndrome shows a coarsely granular pattern with irregular aeration typical of aspiration of materials such as Vx caseosa, epithelial cells, and meconium. Contained in the amniotic fluid). The findings of RDS arealso found with early onset of bacterial sepsis, especially with group B beta-hemolytic streptococci (GBBS). Therefore all babies with prolonged respiratory distress should have systemic cultures drawn (blood, urine, CSF) and be given antibiotics.

Treatment: Treatment of RDS is supportive. The prevention of immediate treatment of asphyxia at birth and maintenance of the baby 's normal body temperature from the time of birth can diminish the severity of RDS.Regardless of the etiology of respiratory distress , the basic defect in the pulmonary exchange of oxygen and carbon dioxide, metabolic acidosis is a secondary manifestation. The infant tries to overcome his ventilatory problem by increasing Expiratory grunting, usually an early feature of the diseases may serve the physiological function of increasing alveolar ventilation by decreasing the tendency of the alveoli to collapse from the highintrathoracic pressure transmitted to compliant airways at the beginning of the expiration.
Grunting decreases or disappears as the disease progresses. –

The mechanical use of +ve end – ve expiratory pressure does the same as grunting does physiologically. Continuous positive airway pressure (CPAP) normally begins at 4-6 cm of

water. CNP (continuous -ve pressure) reduces the air pressure surrounding the lungs. And thorax.Both these use spontaneous respiratory.CNP and oxygen are more effective than oxygen singly in improving oxygenation and in reducing the duration of exposure to high oxygen concentrations and the need. For respiratory therapy in infants with severe RDS. An increase in the end –ve expiratory transpulmonary pressure may also be achieved during artificial ventilation by providing positive end-expiratory pressure (PEEP) or continuous +ve pressure ventilation (CPPV). If positive pressure ventilation is required, lower pressures can be used to achieve adequate oxygenation if inspiratory-expiratory ratios of 1 or more are used. Peak inspiratory pressures greater than 24-25 cm water and rates greater than 20-30/min are rarely required. –

Sufficient oxygen should be given to maintain Pa02 greater than 50mmHg (generally about 60- 70mm). The lowest concentration required to maintain adequate arterial saturation should be used whenever arterial oxygen tension is less than 50mm. Oxygen should be full but not excessively warmed and humidified, and the humidity the chamber should be changed daily to avoid bacterial growth. Oxygen should be administered via oxygen-air blenders that allow precise control over the concentration of oxygen. The oxygen concentration being administered should be checked at least every hrly. If an infant requires oxygen and it is given, Pa02 should be checkedno less than 6 hrly4A Pa02 over 100 tore' are unnecessary and hazardous to the retina and pulmonary parenchyma). If hypoxemia persists with the fraction of inspired air (Fi02) exceeding o.5(i.e., 50%), then continuous positive airway pressure should be used(by mark nasal prongs or endotracheal tube).

-Chilling causes pulmonary vasoconstriction and an increase in the metabolic need for oxygen and the production of CO2. Both hypoxemia and acidemia both result from and cause pulmonary vasoconstriction, oxygen, and a better form of the best treatment. Chilling should be avoided. When the skin temperature of the premature is kept between 36-37C/Chilling is avoided, and oxygen consumption is minimal. Temperature control is best accomplished by special. Thermo regulatingequipment controlled by a thermistor taped to the skin of the abdomen. if such equipment is not available, an incubator temperature between) d and40 at a relative humidity of 80-90% is usually necessary to maintain the thermal stability of the infant. Relative humidity of .70-60, i(is adequate when special Thermo regulating equipment is used, out in its absence, heat loss is less ata relative humidity of 00-90%. Nebulized water mist offers an advantage in cases where the nose is bypassed (in tracheal intubation or tracheostomy if an ultrasonic nebulizer is used, care must be taken lest too much water be inhaled. The lungs. The temperature of the nebulized water should be near that of the ambient air in the incubator. –

Frequent gastric suction during the acute phase of the disease to prevent aspiration of gastric contents. Acommon complication of RDS is paralytic ileus. Oral readings during tachypnea may lead to aspiration and lead to fatigue. Intravenous feeding is continued, as 5-10% dextrose in half-strength saline if the course of the disease prolongs. IV feeding is also required for the buffer, and the sodium required may be given via the vein as NaHCO3.Fluid balance and status. of hydration require frequent evaluation. Hematocrit must be maintained above 40% while respiratory support is provided. Infant needs a minimum of 100-120cal/kg/d for adequate growth.Gavage feeding can be attempted if the infant is stable, even if on the respirator. They may require the circulatory support with Iv infusion with colloid or crystalloid solutions. –

Periodic monitoring of oxygen and carbon dioxide tension and of the pH of arterial or arterialized (by wrapping in a warm wet compress for 5 minutes) capillary; blood is important (essential with assisted ventilation). Pa02 is conveniently measured in blood drawn from the temporal artery or from an indwelling plastic catheter threaded through one of the umbilical arteries so that its tip lies just above the bifurcation of the aorta or above the; the position should be confirmed radiologically. PaCO2 and pH may also be measured from the arterial blood obtained from the above methods; the umbilical artery catheter may be used forte administration of fluids and drugs. –

Hypothermia increases the demand for oxygen by increasing oxygen consumption. In order to attain high oxygen and constant supply, • plastic hood may be used that is just large enough to accommodate the infant's head, and through which oxygen flow can be maintained and adjustedon the basis of the periodic measurement of the oxygen content. Of the atmosphere within the box. The airflow in the incubators can 't be maintained at a high and constant atmosphere of oxygen. –

When assisted ventilation is to be used, it can be done by the intermittent use of a mask and bag respirator for 5 minutes out of every 20 minutes or another regime individualized for the infant. A patient-cycled positive pressure or con. Oiled volume respirator with a nasotracheal tube in place is used but it leads to serious upper respiratory complications. Fitted plastic nasal prongs areused to administer oxygen under pressure; in some, avoiding the use of more traumatic end tracheal intubation. A well-fitting gas mask can be used. Negative pressure respirators heed neither masknor an endotracheal tube but are not usually effective. For infants weighing less than 1500g –

Monitoring of the aortic BP through an umbilical artery catheterer and central venous pressure bya catheter passed through the umbilical vein may provide guides for shock like state, which may occur during the first hour or so after premature birth of an infant who has developed respiratory distress . -Owing to the frequency of pneumonia accompanying the RDS and of infection complicating assisted ventilation and indwelling vascular catheters, routine administration of antibiotics to the neonate is recommended by some, others believe that cultures should be taken antibiotics started, and if after 48 hours the cultures are -ve, the antibiotics can be stopped. Pencillinor ampicillin with kanamycin or gentamicin suggested (25000 units. OOf penicillin or 50mg ampicillin, 7.5mg kanamycin, or 2.5mg gentamicin/kg every 12 hourly until recovery is assured - Acidosis is the real hazard in RDS; serial monitoring of pH pCO2, bicarbonate, base deficit, and electrolytes land for correction of abnormalities is needed, The heart rate and ECG should be continuously recorded to identify arrhythmias if they occur. Mortality is not affected by the correction of acidosis with buffers; the severity of the disease appears to be lessened, and the risks ofvicious.

The pH should be maintained above 7.25 to ensure pulmonary perfusion and adequate Hemoglobin saturation. This may require the use of IV $NaHCO_3$.With respiratoryacidosis or a substantial respiratoryacidosis, combined acidosis), bicarbonate is usually infused at a rate of 65ml/kg/d (ofa 5-10% solution): as follows. If the pH of the arterial blood or arterialized capillary blood is 7.10-7.20, the concentration of $NaHCO_3$ should be 1 OmEq/100ml. If less than 7.1,150 Eg/100ml of glucose other formula is Wt in Kgx0.4 (bicarbonate space of the body) base excess (nomograms are used):1/2 of a such calculated dose is given slowly. It may be needed to infuse bicarbonate more rapidly when distress is severe, especially when there is an impending shock also insuch cases 3-40 g/kg of a solution containing 0.5mEq/ml may be infused over a 20-30 min period. A PĂ, bicarbonate concentrations, and estimation of the base deficit should be obtained immediately after such infusions and subsequently at intervals. More than 12mEq/kg/d of sodium bicarbonate should rarely be given unless the serum sodium is normal and the output of urine adequate. In the presence of hypernatremia with edema, oliguria CCT, an infusion of 0.3 molar THAM (tris-hydroxymethyl amino methane) infused at a rate of 1ml/min to provide 1.0ml/kg for each pH unit below 7.40 is preferred to bicarbonate. Rapid infusion of both these through an umbilical catheter into Ć portal vein leads to liver necrosis; this risk is increased by the circulatory stage at the time of rapid fusion; therefore, caution should be taken to maintain adequate BP bycareful external cardiac massage if needed, while they are being given.

-Occasionally, it may be needed to increase the rate of water and glucose in fusion substantially above 65ml/kg/d to avoid dehydration due to water loss from tachypnea and diuresis; Parenteral fluids should be given through a superficial vein in an extremity. Umbilical catheters used shouldbe radiopaque, and their position should be checked radio logically after insertion. Placement and supervision should be ensured, and catheters removed as soon as the indication for their use has gone. Improved therapy and better survival have resulted in an increased rate of comp] actions such of RDS, such as PDA, bronchopulmonary dysplasia, and pneumothorax (incidence is 3.5% with no associated ventilation, 11% with CPAP, 35% with artificial respiratory and CPAP).

COMPLICATIONS OF INTENSIVE CARE

*The most serious complication of nasotracheal intubation is cardiac arrest during intubation orsuctioning; other complications include bleeding from trauma, difficult extubation requiring tracheostomy), ulceration of the nares from the pressure of the tube, tube, permanent narrowing of the nostril due to tissue damage and scarring from the irritation of infection around the tube, evulsion of a vocal cord, laryngeal ulcer, papilloma of a vocal cord, subglottic stenosis, and pe resistant hoarseness, stridor or oedema of the larynx. Measures to reduce the incidence of the complications are the use of pol vinyl endotracheal tubes (which don't contain tin that is toxic to thecells), the use of a tube of the smallest practicable size in order to reduce the local ischemia and necrosis, avoidance of a motion of a tube in situ, avoidance of the too frequent or vigorous suctioning,8 avoidance of infection through cleanliness and sterilization of all apparatus that is attached to or passes through the tube Use of the anaesthetic gas mask in selected patients avoids all these complications. The use of a -ve pressure respirator eliminates the need for either tube or mask but is less desirable than a patient-cycled positive pressure machine, eap for infants who require assisted ventilation only; Negative pressure respirators are ineffective for infants less than 15008. + Risks of umbilical catheterization include Vascular embolization, thrombosis, spasm and perforation, ischemic and chemical necrosis of abdominal viscera, infection, accidental hemorrhage, impaired circulation to the leg with subsequent gangrene, rate of complication with umbilical vessel catheterization is on an average 3-5%. Aortography shows that clots form in or about the tips of 95% of catheters placed in an umbilical artery; the risk of complications is greater with venous than with arterial placement. Transient blanching of the leg may occur during umbilical artery catheterization due to reflex arterial spasm; the incidence is lessened using the smallest available catheter especially in a very small infant. The catheter should be removed immediately, and the catheterization of the other artery may be attempted.

Persistent spasms after removal of the catheter may be relieved by warming the opposite leg. Intermittent severe spasm may, or unrelieved spasms may respond to the cautious iv infusion of tolazoline (10-25mg injected). Serious hemorrhage on the removal of the catheter may rarely occur; the catheter should not be removed for bars after any heparin is infused through c, to avoid bleeding Thrombus may form in the artery or in the catheter use of an STHLO tipped catheter reduces the Incidence of itīromosis(the catheter should have only one hole at the end of the tube, and rinsing of the tube with a wild saline solution containing 10 units of heparin/ml or by continuously infusing a solution containing 1 unit/ml of heparin. The risks of thrombus formation with potential Vascularocclusion can also be reduced by removing the catheter when there are early signs of thrombosis, such as narrowing of pulse pressure and disappearance of the diuretic notch. Some use umbilical chatter for blood sampling only, leaving the catheter filled with heparinized saline between the samplings.

USE OF OXYGEN IN THE NEONATE AND ITS TOXICITY

is needed for infants whose arterial oxygen tensions fall below 50-60mmHg(=hypoxemia). Cyanosis is not a reliable indication for arterial oxygen levels and cannot be used as a guide forcontinued oxygen therapy. Blood gases must be monitored. Hypoxemia results in metabolic acidosis from anaerobic metabolism, with its accumulation of lactic acid and pyruvic acid.

Acidosis reduces the production of surfactant, leading to respiratory distress syndrome, and potentiates the development of kernicterus by dissociating the albumin-bilirubin bond. Hypoxia also causes pulmonary vasoconstriction, which diminishes pulmonary blood flow, further impairing alveolar-capillary gas exchange. The final effect of hypoxemia is tissue death and permanent brain damage. Oxygen should be warmed, humidified, and given through an air blender, so that the desired concentration may be carefully delivered. The concentration being delivered into the incubator or hood should be monitored by an oxygen analyzer located near theinfant's nose. This level of inspired oxygen should be measured and recorded each time a blood gas sample is drawn. Arterial oxygen tension should be maintained at 60-Coming. If blood gas measurements are not available, oxygen supplementation may be administered in concentrationsjust high enough to relieve cyanosis PaO2 up to 80mm is not harmful Retrolental fibroplasia (RIF)is secondary to partial pressures of oxygen above the normal range in the blood and the riskvaries inversely with the maturity and weight of the infant. The blood of a healthy fetus or newborn infant can be 80-90% saturated at PO2 of about 35mm and a pH of 7.4. The oxygen tension of the blood under normal circumstances while breathing air progressively increases in thenewborn period from fetal levels to 80-100mmHg; while breathing 40% oxygen, it is usually 140- 150mm. Therefore, the partial pressures of oxygen in the arterial blood should be monitored in thepink infant receiving oxygen and kept below 80 mm and above 50 mm. The oxygen tensions in the cyanotic infant are well below. If blood gas measurements are not available, oxygen supplementation may be administered in concentrations just high enough to relieve cyanosis.

Infants with gestational ages of less than 36weeks who have received oxygen therapy should have an eye examination at a time before discharge for evidence of RI Hy peroxemia (levels exceeding 80mm) leads to RLF in the premature infant by a series of events involving retinal vessel dilatation, retinal arteriolar vasoconstriction, neovascularization, proliferation into the vitreous, hemorrhage, scarring, and at worst retinal detachment. The duration of hypoxemia sufficient to initiate RLF is unknown, but the process may continue and progress ditethe discontinuance of supplementary oxygen. The process may spontaneously regress or may continue to complete retinal detachment. RLF is a disease of prematurity, with its preppertie- incidence proportional to gestational age; it may occasionally be seen in full-term infants (though rare) and has been reported in neonates who never received any supplementary oxygen. Oxygen excess is injurious to the lung also. Unlike RLF, where hypoxemia leads t changes, lung changes are the direct result of hyperopia, especially if administered by a positive pressure respirator. Factors associated with the development of bronchopulmonary dysplasia (BPD)include an increased F102, endotracheal intubation, artificial, ventilation positive pressure ventilation, and duration of the oxygen therapy. Prolonged exposure to high ambient Oxygen will cause this disease. Instead of showing improvement on the 3rd or 4th day, consistent with the natural course of the disease in survivors, some infants who have been on prolonged intermittent positive pressure breathing using high concentrations of oxygen have X-ray evidence of worsening and continue tobe cyanotic without oxygen in high concentrations. The chest X-ray changes from a picture of total opacification with air bronchogram to one of small, round, lucent areas alternating with areasof irregular density resembling a sponge (this picture is similar to bubbly lung syndrome of some per mucosa fibrosis and Widespread metaplasia of the bronchiolar mucosa, thickening of basement membranes and separation of the capillaries from the alveolar epithelial cells These hazards necessitate frequent monitoring of both the concentration of oxygen delivered(maybe about 40%), and the arterial oxygen tension(which should be kept between 50- 80mm). Oxygen analyzers can monitor Fir2 by continuous (or intermittent) readout. Arterial PO2can be determined by blood sampling from a u umbilical or peripheral catheter, percutaneous arterial puncture, or intra-arterial oxygen electrodes. The transcutaneous oxygen electrodes are less invasive but do not always accurately reflect the true arterial PO2. All infants receiving supplementary Oxygen should have a fundoscopic examination following completion of oxygen therapy and at 3, 6, and 12 months. Recently possibility of oxygen toxicity for cerebral blood vessels has been suggested. Therefore, as little oxygen as possible for the shortest possible time be adhered to in the therapy of infants.

WILSON MIKITY SYNDROME (INTERSTITIAL PULMONARY FIBROSIS OFPREMATURE.

A pulmonary syndrome of premature infants (usually less than 52 wk gestation) and LBW infants (birth weight of less than 1500g) characterized by the insidious onset of dyspnea, tachypnea, retractions, and cyanosis during the first month of life (rare cases have been seen in full-term infants, usually with b/o meconium aspiration C oxygen administration). Some infants have respiratory distress at birth, occasionally very severe, resembling RDS, and requiring oxygen, others have no early symptoms, and the onset of symptoms is at several weeks of life. Coughing, wheezing, and rales may develop, but fever occurs only with concomitant infection. There may be the collapse of a lobe or lung; other complications are right-sided heart failure, osteoporosis, and rib fractures. The symptoms usually increase over 2-6 weeks, with increasing oxygen dependencypersisting for several months, followed by a gradual resolution of the progression of respiratory or cardiac failure. The most characteristic features of this syndrome are X-ray features. Early, there are bilateral petieuteerakuter reticular streaky infiltrates and often overexpansion of the lungs with small areas of emphysema which develop into multisystem lesions. Subsequently, the cysts enlarge and coalesce to give a hyper lucent bubble appearance (Bubbly lung). The X-ray tends to clear over months to several years. In fatal cases, the lung has a hobnail appearance, with cystic and emphysematous areas in the parenchyma and thickened fibrosis septa. Microscopically the alveolar walls are thickened, with the proliferation of capillaries, and infiltrate nuclear cells. Differentiation must be made from pneumonia due to Pneumocystis carinii and cyst fibrosis. Treatment consists of supportive measures of oxygen for cyanosis, digitalization diuretic forcardiac failure, acid-base correction, and assisted ventilation when indicated. The mortality is 25%

LUNG CYSTS

Most lung cysts in the neonatal period are acquired because of rupture of alveoli by overinflation or infection, often staphylococcal; congenital cysts are rare. They may be solitary or multiple, air-containing, or filled with fluid. And are believed to be the result of a developmental anomaly of the bronchial buds. In: ants with congenital or acquired cysts. May be asymptomaticor present with tachypnea and dyspnea at birth or any time thereafter, or with recurrent or persistent pneumonia, Air-filled cysts on the surface of the lung, whatever their origin, sometimes rupture and cause pneumothorax. This is especially true of multicystic disease. Since most cystic areas discovered by X-ray will disappear spontaneously, surgical removal is reserved for those which cause severe respiratory distress .

PULMONARY HEMORRHAGE

Pulmonary hemorrhage can have many causes and may occur in association with acute pulmonary infection, severe anoxia, RDS, hemorrhagic disease of the newborn icterus Gravis or kernicterus, cold injury, prematurity, and intracranial hemorrhage may be found in both premature as well as in full-term infants. The reporter incidence is 1-4/1000 live births. About 4 of hthe patients are welding less than 2500g avvirun massive pulmonary hemorrhage 18 presents in about 1 5o of premature infants, and 454 of mature inrantewao come to autopsy in Cue first 2 weeks of life.in the majority of PTO, bleeding into the other organs is seen at autopsy, but bleedingother than in rough the nose and mouth is relatively rare during the start at the time of birth or be delayed for several days. There is the subnormal temperature of the body, edema of the extremities, and detectable hypoglycemia. 1/2 of the patients cough up or regurgitate material containing old or fresh blood from the nose and mouth, and this is the most important diagnostic finding. X-ray findings are varied, ranging from minor streaking or patchy infiltrates to massive consolidation. Treatment is by repeated small blood transfusions, simultaneous warming of the body, glucose to combat hypoglycemia, antibiotics to prevent secondary infection, and vitamin K in the case of hypothrombinemia. The prognosis is grave, and death occurs within the first 48 hours of life in 3 of the infants who come to autopsy.

CONGENITAL PULMONARY LYMPHANGIECTASIA

Rarely occurs among full-term infants with respiratory distress at birth. Cyanosis is marked and [illegible] rapidly progressive Death is usual during the first month of life, often within hours of birth. Rarely symptoms abate, and patient may survive for some time. The day shows a general haziness or diffuse reticulogranul pattern with hyper aeration, prominent fissures, and occasionally pleural effusion.

CHOLTHORAX

Rarely occurs within the first days of life with cyanosis and signs of unrelated al or bilateral pl effusion. The fluid is clear, initially becoming opalescent due to fat globules after milk feeding isestablished with chylous ascites and lymphedema elsewhere, presumably due to congenital formations of the lymphatic system Treatment is by thoracentesis repeated as necessary or by continuous drainage of the affected pleural spaces. About 1/2 of the patients recover within 30 days; protein depletion may be a problem if large amounts of the fluid (protein content=2-4g/dl) must be removed.

APNEA

Apnea is defined as cessation of respiratory for 20 seconds or longer and is usually seen duringREM sleep. It is accompanied by cyanosis and bradycardia. Apnea can be a sign of very serious significance in the neonate. Apnea can occur at any time during the neonatal period, particularly in very immature infants. About 25% of babies less than 1800g at birth will have apneic episodes during the first days (10 days), and the episodes may continue until the equivalent of 34-36 weeks gestation. Therefore, all babies weighing 1800g or less should have apnea monitoring for the first 10 days. In contrast, in the full-term infant, 25% of sleep time in REM sleep, the premature baby spends 60% in REM sleep. Obstructive apnea, when the tongue blocks the airway and, diteapparent movements of respiratory, the lungs arenot aerated, also occurs in premature sleep. Obstructive apnea, when the tongue blocks the airwayand, diteapp: rent movements of respiratory, the lungs are not aerated, also occurs in prematureinfants. Virtually any illness can lead to apnea episodes. When episodes occur, associate diseases should be considered as metabolic deficiencies such as hypoglycemia or hype calcemia, sepsis, respiratory conditions such as RDS, pneumonia, aspirations, hypotension

PDA, anemia, changing temperature especially, rapid rewarming and overheating, intracranial hemorrhage, CNS disease, must be excluded. Though in some cases, apnea apparently unassociated with any metabolic or physical illness may occur, usually serious associated diseases are to be sought. Therefore, panic attacks in any infant need careful evaluation with special attention to any infection or CNS disorder. Severe apneic attacks in a previously well infant may be an indication for an EEG because seizures in the newborn infant may present as apnea only. Apneic episodes in infants with neonatal seizures will often stop when seizures are successfully controlled by anticonvulsants. If idiopathic apneic episodes are frequent, an oral loading dose of theophylline, 5mg/kg, can be given; a blood level reading should be obtained 2 hours. after administration of the loading dose, at which time the drug level is likely to be at its peak. A maintenance dose is adjusted based on blood level readings but is generally in the range of 1- mg/kg every 12 hours, given orally. Lower the ambient temperature provide intermittent stimulation by gentle ribbing of the skin, use a rocker bed or an oscillating waterbed, or music.If apnea continues, employ intermittent bagging with) 2. Low levels (3-4 cm of water) pressure) nasal continuous positive airway pressure (CPAP) may be used. Xanthines Tanffnina and honnhy174nalohanla ho cart alone with monitoring of serum conc. Apnea must be differentiated from periodic breathing, in which apnea is brief (usually less than 10 seconds and is not accompanied by cyanosis or bradycardia Respiratory rates, normally 40-60/min in the full-term infant, are progressively and lower with decreasing birth weight. The respiratory pattern in 1/2 of premature infants is periodic breathing.

PERIODIC BREATHING

Periodic breathing is common in newborns and young infants. It is usually not clinically significant, but in some cases (especially premature), prolonged respiratory pauses may be associated with cyanosis and bradycardia. Periodic breathing is rarely seen during the first 24 hours after birthad occurs during a wakeful state. It usually continues for several days and may persistently intermittently until the equivalent of 36 weeks gestation. It is more common at higher altitudes. Irregular respiratory patterns may be due to changes in respiratory drive or effective respiratory timing. Stimulation of laryngeal chemoreceptors may result in slowing or cessation of respiratory. Careful monitoring has shown that active and quiet sleep states may not develop normal cycling and regulation in some premature and term infants...

NECROTISING ENTEROCOLITIS

Necrotizing enterocolitis (NEC) has been reported in 1–10% of premature infants, often occurringin clusters in nurseries.

AETIOLOGY

Aetiology is unknown, but associated factors are the presence of an umbilical catheter, hypoxemia especiallyfrom RDS, perinatal asphyxia, sepsis, polycythemia, PDA, hyperosmolar formulas feeding, ischemia, bacterial invasion, absence of normal colostrum, and some medications as neomycin leading to mucosal damage. There I suggestive evidence to support the inference that breastfeeding may protect against the development of NEC.

Evaluation and diagnosis

Signs and symptoms include those of infection (temperature instability, jaundice, lethargy, apnea) and gastrointestinal abnormalities (abdominal distension, gastric residue, and vomiting with bile), progressing to shock, and disseminated intravascular coagulation. Bloody diarrhea in asmall premature, with abdominal distension and bloody or bile-stained gastric aspirate, suggests NEC. Mucosal slough may be passed per rectum. Lab studies include a flat X-ray of the abdomen (may show pneumatics cystoids intestinal, free peritoneal gas or gas in the portal venous systemoften seen with the presence of an umbilical catheter and a persistent and unchanging dilated loop of the small intestine), the culture of blood and stool should be obtained; Impaired carbohydrate absorption may be an early sign of the disease and monitoring fecal reducing substance and decreasing feeding may prevent severe disease and perforation. The presence of reducing substances and occult blood in the Stoll often precede the clinical signs of NEC and should be utilized as screening procedures in infants at risk for NEC.

Treatment

NPC and nasogastric tube drainage of the stomach and parenteral fluids are instituted. Parenteral alimentation may be needed. Serial X-rays are obtained at 6 hourly intervals if the infant is ill.All umbilical lines should be discontinued. Systemic and oral antibiotics are used. The patient is treated as having a case of sepsis. If symptoms improve, treatment should be continued for 7-10 days. If the baby worsens, surgical removal of any necrotic bowel may be necessary; if early feeding is needed; breast milk is preferable. Progressive deterioration with bowel perforation is an indication of surgery. More than 70% of babies survive, although they are at risk for the development of stricture formation and obstruction during subsequent months.

CYANOSIS IN THE NEONATE

Cyanosis usually indicates respiratory insufficiency, which may be due to pulmonary conditions (when breaths tend to be rapid and may be accompanied by retraction of the thoracic cage) or may be due to intracranial hemorrhage or anoxic injury to the brain (breath tend to be irregular and weak and often slow). Cyanosis persisting for several days when unaccompanied by obvious signs of respiratory distress is suggestive of cyanotic CHD or methemoglobinemia. Central cyanosis is often transitory within the first 20 min after birth because of the incomplete circulatory and respiratory adjustments to the extrauterine life. Occasionally acrocyanosis may occur at the inception of a disease that is ultimately characterized by central cyanos18. Causes of cyanos18: Diffusional impairment diseases associated with a barrier to absorption of oxy and en from inhaled air (meconium aspiration, pneumonitis, pulmonary edema) - Congenital heart disease with an R-L shunt - Hypoventilation as CNS depression from hypoxia, trauma, or maternal sedation, -Ventilation-perfusion imbalance. This occurs in connection with diffusion impairment and refers to an imbalance between the capacity of the alveoli to permit the caliber of proximate blood vessels to perfuse these alveoli and acquire oxygen from them. Thus, in RDS, there is an impairment of the hyaline-lined alveol1 and alveolar ducts to diffuse oxygen and a lack of blood flow due to pulmonary arteriolar constriction, which limits the pickup of oxygen by the RBC. At times, partially functional alveoli, capable of delivering oxygen,are effectively passed by constricted arterioles, while in atelectasis, unaerated alveoli are adequately perfused by the blood that has no access to oxygen. In effect, there is intrapulmonary shunting of blood. This imbalance results in worsening PaO2 and decreasing på.

Some disorders that are especially problem for premature Those affecting the respiratory system: Appeand, RDS, and Wilson-Mikity syndrome. PDA has an increasing incidence with increasing prematurity (77% of babies at 28-30 weeks gestation compared to 21% at 34-36 weeks gestation and less than 0.07% at full term). The ductus arteriosus, in Response to the normal increase in arterial oxygen tension in the transition from intrauterine to extrauterine life,functionally closes within hours to days. This Response to oxygen is related to gestational age. Hypoxemia, especially in preterm infants with RDS, delays or prevents closure of the ductus. Signs andsymptoms of PDA occur earlier in the premature infant because of pulmonary Vascular resistance and the earlier appearance of the L-R shunt through the ducts. Over hydration may be an additional factor causing PDA in this group. A systolic murmur, hyperactive precordium, and bounding pulses, especially in an infant recovering from RDS, begin to deteriorate, and are suggestive of PDA. Signs of COF appear with tachypnea, tachycardia, and increased pulmonary vascularity. Echocardiography demonstrates an increased left atrial to aortic root ratio greater than1.3 while normal is less than 0.27 is diagnostic; If COF is present, fluid restriction, diuretics, and digoxin with monitoring of se Treatment.

Indonethacin, a prostaglandin inhibitor, is effective in the closure of PDA (50-85% effective). If the PDA persists, surgical Liga ture may be considered, especially in a baby who is notimproving. Necrotizing enterocolitis is common in them. A VLBW baby is at high risk for bilirubin encephalopathy. These babies have developed kernicterus at peak bilirubin levels of Img/dl, especially due to diminished albumin binding capacity from lower serum albumin levels), and increased incidence of potentiating factors. Bilirubin production in these tiny babies is greater, compared to that of the full-term infant, because of the proportionately larger blood volume, shorter span of RBC, and greater immaturity of the liver. Gastric mobility is diminished, and thedelays in the initiation of oral feeding and in the development of intestinal flora increase the enter hepatic circulation of bilirubin and contribute to the higher concentrations of bilirubin. The frequent complications of prematurity (perinatal asphyxia, hypoxemia, acidosis, cold stress, infection, and hypoglycemia) potentiate the development of the kernicterus at lower levels of bilirubin in this group of infants. Prophylactic phototherapy has been recommended beginning after birth and continuing for 2-4 days or longer if necessary. Exchange transfusion is recommended at a serum bilirubin concentration of 10g/dl in a sick 1000g baby.

Many of the metabolic problems that complicate the course of a premature baby can be explained by functional immaturity or by the lack of stores that are normally laid down during the last trimester of pregnancy. (as subcutaneous fat, hepatic glycogen, and minerals such as calcium, iron, and magnesium). The overall rate of transient neonatal hypoglycemia in the premature baby, which is appropriate for gestational age, is 15%. The more immature the infant, thehigher the risk. The risk for babies of less than 30 weeks. Gestation is 75%. Hypoglycemia while receiving parenteral glucose is reported in IVLBW babies. The incidence of hyperglycemia (blood glucose exceeding 125mg/dl) in infants of BW less than 1100g receiving IV.

Each rise of 10mg/dl in glucose concentration raises the serum osmolality by
1 mosm/l; the resultant hyperosmolarity leads to osmotic diuresis, which in turn results in greaterwater loss but may cause osmolality increases more than 25-40 mosmol/1 (=glucose concentration exceeding 500-800mg/dl). A higher incidence of hyperglycemia in tiny babies necessitates frequent monitoring of blood glucose and of urine for the presence of glucose, Hypocalcaemia is common in premature, and up to 50% of IVLBW infants develop hypo calcemia early (less than 72 hours) although fewer are symptomatic. Potentiating factors (asphyxia,obstetric trauma, or buffer therapy) are frequently present in these babies who are already sick and at risk. The high incidence of hypocalcemia in them demands serial screening of serum calcium and ECG measuring of the Q-TC a and Q-oT'c intervals.

ANEMIA IN THE NEWBORN INFANT (Full-term and Premature)

Anemia at birth is manifest by pallor or shock. -Anemia is usually caused by hemolytic disease of the newborn but may be due to the tearing of or cutting of the umbilical blood cord during delivery or of hemorrhage from the fetal side of the placenta, which may be due to accidental incision of the placenta in the course of Cesarean section or by transplacental hemorrhage, where bleeding from the fetal into the maternal circulation is probably more common than is generally recognized, but is not usually sufficient to cause clinically apparent anemia at birth. Anemia at birth may also be seen in one of the twins with conjoined placental circulation, in which case, the anemic twin bleeds into the other twin.
Acute blood loss before or during delivery can occur in the maternal circulation, the amniotic sac into a twin fetus in the twin, or into the vagina. Acute blood loss after the delivery may be external (as gastrointestinal, circumcision, site, or umbilical stump or internal (fracture site, cephalhematoma, CNS or pulmonary hemorrhage, soft tissue hematoma, injured internal organs).Scalp blood sampling for fetal distress may result in anemia.

Anemia appearing in the first few days after birth is most frequently due to hemolytic disease of the newborn; other causes are a hemorrhagic disease of the newborn, bleeding from an improperly tied or clamped umbilical cordlar hematomas, intracranial hemorrhage or subcapsular bleeding from the rupture of the liver Rapid decreases in kb Hemoglobin or hematocrit values during the first few days of life may be the initial clue to intracranial hemorrhage or rupture of the liver.[1] Frequent blood sampling in patients

[1] Due to advancement the original notes did not distinguish between Rh Hemolytic Disease and General Hemolytic disease.

with RDS can lead to anemia.

Later in the neonatal period, delayed anemia from the hemolytic disease of newborn (with or without exchange transfusion) may be seen. Vitamin K in large doses may cause anemia in premature, characterized by inclusion bodies (Heinz bodies) in the erythrocytes. Congenital hemolytic anemia (spherocytosis)occasionally makes its appearance during the first month of life; hereditary nonspherocytic hemolytic anemia during the neonatal period can occur secondary to deficiency of G6PD its appearance during the first month of life; hereditary nonspherocytic hemolytic anemia during the neonatal period can occur secondary to deficiency of G6PD and pyruvate kinase. Bleeding from hemangiomas of the upper GIT or from ulcers caused by aberrant gastric mucosa in a Meckel's diverticulum or duplication is a rare sourceof anemia in the newborn. Repeated blood sampling of infants needing frequent monitoring of blood gases and chemistries may produce anemia.

The degree of bleeding which occurs in the process of delivery at different sites, including muscle and skin, is frequently underestimated, and whenever there is doubt about the extent of bleeding, patients blood volume should be expanded with plasma expanders or whole blood since a further physiologic decrease in RE and Hemoglobin content is to be expected in all neonates, treatment of any significant anemia (less than Og of Hemoglobin Kal)present at birth or shortly after birth consists of elimination of cause and small infusions of packed red cells(10-15 ml/kg; 2ml/kg raises Ha aboutby 18/01). Early feeding of red meats or IM iron is effective in enabling anemia infants to increase rather than decrease their RBC and Hemoglobin concentrations before the 2nd-grd month of life for chronic severe anemia or acute hemolysis, exchange transfusions with small volumes of sedimented RBC is given (small volume LT to avoid overloading Vascular space). -ANEMIA INTHE PREMATÜRE: #" common causes of anemia in the premature alle vitamin E deficiency, anemia of prematurity or iatrogenic. Iatrogenic anemia 18 due to frequent blood sampling; common in sick in are receiving respiratorysupport. The use of transcutaneous oxygen monitoring helps to decrease this cause. Serial hematocrits or Hemoglobin should be done to help determine the time when the transfusion should be given in babies receiving ventilator support, and the hematocrit should be maintained at over 40-50%. After birth at the earliest to avoidhemolysis. Since Hemoglobin begins to fall after the first 24 hours and continues to do so during of fall and the lowest concentration of Hemoglobin CO relates with gestational age (Infants of birth weight of 1200g or less may normally have a Hemoglobin concentration of as low as 6.0g/dl within 406 weeks after a birth coma to more than 10g in the healthy full-term neonate).

The anemia of prematurity is due to diminished total body iron content of the preterm infant, rapid somatic growth a 10008 baby of 28 weeks gestation more than doubles the birth weeks within the first 8-12weeks) with the expansion of blood volume, and proportionately 1 less hematopoiesis Reticulocytosis often appears when the Hemoglobin falls below 10g.in some IV Low, a haemoglobin concentration May 1 dl below 75 ceiore leukocytosis appears. Transfusion for anemia of prematurity may be indicatedif the Hemoglobin falls below 7-8g and the baby becomes symptomatic (lethargy, apneic, spells, or signs of CCF). Calculation of the volume of the transfusion can be made as follows; 1ml of packed red blood cells/kg BW will raise the hematocrit by 1 volume%. 2-3ml packed RBCR$ will raise the Ab level by 18% Volume of packed RBC = (desired Hemoglobin-actual Hemoglobin) x Wt in kg x blood volume 75-85 -'m1/kg 22g / 100ml In babies who are sick especially, those with respiratory distress , maintenance of a sufficient HD concentration is important. The oxygen Hemoglobin dissociation curve is shifted to the left with fetal Hemoglobin. The functional significance of this is decreased provision of oxy gets to the tissues. Transfusion with adult red cells causes a rightward shift of the curve. Increased incidence of RLF has been reported in IVLBW who have received transfusion or exchange transfusion using adult blood. Iron supplementation is essential after 1 month in the preterm infant. Babies of BW greater than 1500g should be given 2-4mg/kg/d of ferrous iron and those less than 1500g 4-6mg/kg/d.

BLOOD IN THE VOMITUS OR STOOL

Swallowing maternal blood during delivery is not uncommon if enough must be ingested, the infant may vomit bright red or dark blood or may pass stool containing dark or bright red fresh-appearing blood. Clinical evidence of acute blood 1088 is lacking, but a transient rise in blood urea may occur. Blood of maternal origin can be differentiated from infant blood by testingfor fetal Hemoglobin, which is resistant to alkali denaturation 's mall amount of red blood stool, or vomitus is mixed with 5-10 ml of water and centrifuged To 5 parts of pink supernatant, add 1 part 0.25N sodium hydroxide if fetal Hemoglobin is present the solution remain and pink if adult Hemoglobin is present, it becomes brown. GIT bleeding in the newborn may be due to trauma, peptic ulcer, duplication of Wilson Meckel's diverticulum, intussusception, volvulus, hemangioma or telangiectasia of the bowel, poly rectal prolapse, anal fissure (a common cause of blood in small amounts), infection especially salmonella and shigella), systemic bleeding disorders (especially hemorrhagic disease of the newborn) and tumors. For maternal blood, no treatment is needed if fetal, it is treated as acute blood 1066 with blood transfusion and supportive care, till the cause is found and treated. The most commoncause of intrinsic bloody vomitus is a gastric ulcer (which seldom causes massive bleeding and perforation), and bleeding can be managed with frequent oral milk feedings alone. If blood loss has been significant, but transfusion is not necessary, iron supplementation may be required during first few months.

VOMITING during the first few days of life suggests obstruction in the upper digestive tract orincreased intracranial pressure. Ap and lateral upright firm of the abdomen should be taken, followed by barium studies if the diagnosis remains in doubt. Vomiting also may be nonspecific,as in septicemia. It is a common manifestation of overfeeding, pyloric stenosis, milk allergy, duodenal ulcer, stress ulcer, adrenal insufficiency and a reflection of a nervous mother, or emotional upset in the parents. infants placed in body casts for orthopedic treatment often vomit transiently, as a manifestation of frustration of physical movement, Vomitus containing dark blood is usually a sign of life-threatening illness, whatever the cause bile-stained vomitus suggests obstruction below the ampulla of Vater.

SOME OTHER SYMPTOMS IN THE NEONATES

Pallor may be due to anemia, hemorrhage, hypoxia,

hypoglycemia, sepsis, or shock.

EVALUATION OF INFANT WITH RESPIRATORY DISTRESS

BILATERAL CHOANAL ATRESIA

If only one side is affected there is no severe difficulty , but if both nares are blocked by a membranous, cartilaginous or bony Beptum, obvious symptoms occur in most but not all babies,some infants are unable to breathe through their mouth e begele- when both pares are blocked, while others can Those who are unable to breathe through their mouths make increasingly vigorous efforts at inspiration, with a suckling in of their lips, become cyanotic quickly and may soon die. Infants able to breathe through their mouths have trouble only 10 sucking and swallowing and become cyanotic as they attempt to nurse. Bilateral occlusion should be suspected in a newborn infant who persistently breathes through his mouth. Or is cyanotic when at rest with his mouth closed but returns to normal when he cries, Unilateral obstruction is usually asymptomatic until the first respiratory infection, at which time the diagnosis may be suggested by unilateral nasal discharge of disproportionately severe nasal obstruction. The obstruction is demonstrated by the falling of the first catheter or probe to pass into the nasopharynx.01 her diagnostic method is installation of a radiopaque substance through a cat) enter into each nostril while the infant is lying on the back. The anterior nasal cavity will be outlined, and the block readily seen on ray with bilateral choanal atresia, prompt establishment of an 18 urgent. In an emergency this is done most readily by propping the jaws open with any suita bile device or by 1DBerting an airway from the lips into the nasopharynx. The infant can then be fed by gavage until such time (2-3 weeks) as he learns to eat and breathe without the airway. Surgery may be done immediately or postponed even to years in patients who adapatient well to the obstruction.

CONGENITAL ABNORMALITIES OF THE LARYNX

Except for atresia, laryngeal malformations are characterized by the development of aweak, sometimes hoarse cry and varying degrees 66 of stridor. Congenital obstructive laryngeal lesions Ray cause symptoms of primarily inspiratory obstruction from the time of birth, or the infant may be relatively free of symptoms until the first upper Respiratory infection. The additional airway darrowing due to the infectious inflammation of the Respiratory epithelium bay precipitates significant respiratory difficulty. The clinical findings in patients with congenital laryngeal ma 1 formations are likely to include inspiratory Stridor, intercostal and supraclavicular retractions that are worse with crying, and hoarse cry. The diagnostic evaluation should include a careful history and physical examination, AP, and lateral chest X-rays, lateral soft tissue rays of the neck and fluoroscopic examination of the neck, and fluoroscopic examination of the upper airway and of the contrast fi 11 ed esophagus to rule out an anomalous V688el that might be compressing the upper tracheae. Pulmonary function tests performed on patients with Nixed upper airway Dar rowing who are old enough to cooperate more than 6 years- demonstrating decreased peak flow rates, moremarked on inspiration than of respiratory. The definitive diagnoses are made by direct laryngoscopy or bronchoscopy. Inspiratory obstruction due to a wide variety of cameos is likelyto be ameliorated by placing the infant. Other congenital cause of inspiratory stridor is macroglossia, micrognathia, upper airway cysts, nasal obstruction, and congenital subglottic stenosis or subglottic hemangioma.

CONGENITAL LARYNGEAL STRIDOR

Congenital laryngeal stridor is a usually benign entity due to minor developmental variations of the larynx. It is usually due to relaxed vocal cords or a flabby epiglottis that causes more than theusual amount of collapse on inspiration.

Noisy crowing respiratory sounds (Usually associated with inspiration) are relatively common in the neonatal period and r during the first year of life. Some infants have merely noisy breathing others have a laryngeal crowing, hoarseness, or aphonic, dyspnea, and inspiratory retractions in the supraclavicular, intercostal, and subcostal spaces. If inspiratory retractions are severe, deformity of the thorax may result. Infants with severe dyspnea frequently have difficulty in nursing so that undernutrition is common. Cyanosis is rarely observed. Respiratory infections tend to exaggerate all the symptoms. In the first few days of life, it may be difficult to distinguishbetween the congenital disturbances of the larynx and transient disturbances, such as laryngospasm of tetany of the newborn or laryngeal edema secondary to trauma or aspiration of irritant substances at birth The h/o aspiration at birth, hoarseness or aphonia, and laryngoscope examination establish the presence of postnatal laryngeal edema.

Stridor persisting or appearing after the first few days of life results from disturbances in or adjacent to the larynx. The most common of these is congenital deformity or flabbiness of epiglottis and subglottic aperture (laryngomalacia). Developmental malformations may be present or there may be merely an exaggeration of the normal omega-shape of the infantile epiglottis. Unusually shaped and long epiglottis, which falls posteriorly during inspiration. Causingpartial obstruction. Anomalies of the larynx may include malformed laryngeal cartilages (as unusually mobile arytenoid cartilages that move forwards during inspiration and cause an obstruction), intraluminal webs, and malformations or duplication of the vocal cords. A particularly' short aryepiglottic fold may lead to obstruction. Sometimes generalized chondromalacia of the larynx and trachea may be observed. In such instances the lamb and the trachea tend to collapse with inspiration and to expand with expiration. Congenital tumors as fibromas of the larynx are rare. Mucous retention cysts, branchial cleft cysts, and thyroglossal dust remains are other infrequent causes of stridor.

Strider may also be produced by extra laryngeal causes. Hypoplasia of the mandikyle permits thebase of the tongue to displace the epiglottis posteriorly and cause laryngeal obstruction. Macroglossia from hypertrophy of the muscles, hemangiomas, lymphangiomas or cysts may have the same effect. ln Pierre-Robin syndrome, a combination of the hypoplasia of themandible, pseudomagroglossial and glossopteris is; responsible for laryngeal stridor. And dyspnea. Compression of larynx by congenital goiters has been, reported. Congenital vascular anomalies may also cause stride or. Direct laryngoscopy is diagnostic in congenital laryngeal stridor. Abnormalities of the epiglottis, the vocal cords and other parts of the larynx can be seen. Congenital laryngeal stridor accounts for more than 75% of all laryngeal problems of infants. The onset of the laryngeal stridor is usually within the first week of life but may be delayed for months. It is a beginning and self-limited disorder, and the stridor disappears by 12-18 months. But may persist for years. Such infants have stridor crowing inspirations, sometimes with marked dyspneabut there is no hoarseness and only rarely become cyanotic. There are feeding problems as vomitingafter feeding, and an increased incidence of early speech problems. Extra laryngeal causes of stridor are established often without laryngoscopy; vascular anomalies: that partially occlude the trachea or esophagus can-often be-detected by fluoroscopic observation during a barium swallow. The most common cause, of laryngeal stridor (laryngomalacia) rarely requires treatment, and symptoms progressively become less severe, generally disappearing by 1 yr of age. Some infants may require hospitalization at the time of an URI due to increased severity of the rasp: obstruction in the very unusual case, tracheostomy may be needed because of the chronic upper airway obstruction usually during the2nd year of life. Cysts, webs tumors and malformations of the larynx need various specialized procedures as excision, devastation, laryngoplasty or tracheostomy. Particula attention must. Be given to the feeding of these infant's aspiration is a real danger, also the respiratory efforts preclude normal. Sucking, and swallowing in some infants. Slow, careful feeding from a small nipple or by a dropper or glass are usually adequate feeding by gavage or even. Gastrostomy maybe needed. Infants with strider must be protected from the reap infections.

LARYNGEAL WEB

Laryngeal web is a triangular membrane often. Concave posteriorly, in the anterior portion of thelarynx, and the membrane is usually attached to the superior surface of the true vocal cords. In others apparent fusion of anterior part of the true or false cords produces a web like structural theweb is large, the onset of stridor is usually, at birth. Affected infants have weak hoarse cries inspiratory stridor, and mild dyspnea (with incomplete web), with complete weir there is quick asphyxiation unless immediately perforated. Larngeal atresia is associated with exophthalmia sometimes. Direct laryngoscopy is diagnostic, as well as affords treatment. A series of dilations is done, but dilatation may precipitate increased laryngeal edema and further obstruction and may necessitate tracheotomy after dilatation. Thus, it may be necessary to insert atracheostomy tube while a series of dilatations is carried out. Direct laryngoscopy incision excision or removal of a web is always followed by prompt. Reformation and thus rarely, successful. Anterior division of web. Is followed by introduction of a a thin sheet of Teflon silicone or some other nonirritating metal within the larynx between the leaves of the divided web is attached to thyroid cartilage and allowed to remain in -place until complete epithelization has occurred is helpful when the patient has reached the age of 8-10 years.

LARYNGEAL CYSTS

A laryngeal cyst may present as a localized swelling in the neck that increases with crying or may impinge on the airway from the laryngeal ventricle leading to inspiratory obstruction anddysphagia. These are removed surgically.

LARYNGOTRACHEOESOPHAGEAL CLEFT

An unusual congenital anomaly that results from the failure of posterior cricoid fusion during the embryologic formation of the tracheoesophageal septum, leaving the larynx and part of the trachea open posteriorly. There is inspiratory stridor due to poor laryngeal support and frequentaspiration of secretions and food; the cry is weak. There are frequent cyanotic episodes due to aspiration -and recurrent or persistent pneumonitis, poor weight gains due to severe feeding problems, and chronic lung disease. The diagnostic studies include a barium swallow and fluoroscopy -direct laryngoscopy esophagoscopy, and bronchoscopy. These pts. are fed by a gastric tube, their nutritional status is improved, and intensive pulmonary therapy is instituted pt. may he needing gastrostomy or tracheostomy, and corrective surgery may be done

Vocal Cord Paralysis

VC paralysis may be unilateral or bilateral and. congenital or acquired.VCP at birth is usually a.laryngeal manifestation. of a significant anomaly of another organ system; bilateral VCP may rarely be an isolated finding, but generally, it is associated with birth trauma, ceretral agenesis, severe retardation, or myelo-menin gocele. Unilateral VCP of any origin is more common on the left than on the right side (because of the long course of the left recurrent laryngeal nerve in the thorax and its anatomical proximity to major thoracic structures. Clinically it is just like any other congenital obstructive lesion of the upper airway; the amount of the obstruction depends onthe, the severity of the paresis or paralysis. With bilateral and sometimes unilateral palaces artificialairway is needed. Direct laryngoscopy is Bilateral diagnostic paralysis that leads to dyspnea, also

BIRTH THRUM TO THE LARYNX:

Larynx during birth may result in dislocation of the cricothyroid or cricoarytenoid articulation leading to hoarseness, wheezing, and fluttering. Laryngoscopy is diagnostic as well as. Palliativebut tracheostomy may be needed. During instrumental delivery unilateral or bilateral recurrent laryngeal nerve paralysis may be caused; when only one cord is paralysed, there is hoarseness with stridor, and usually no dyspnea, but with bilateral paralysis, there is dyspnea with stridor.

Direct laryngoscopy is diagnostic; tracheostomy is necessary for bilateral. paralysis. The older child may wear a valvular cannula a laryngoplasty with lateral fixation of one VC may be doneto improve the airway and permit decannulation unless. Breathing through the larynx has improved spontaneously.

POSTNATALLARYNGEAL TRAUMA

Laryngeal fractures and soft tissue injuries in children are usually the result of the child being hurled against the dashemoglobinard of a car, during sudden deceleration. If the larynx is crushed, the airway may be completely obstructed so that only immediate tracheostomy' can prevent death. Once the child survives the immediate post-injury period careful observation is necessary during the ensuing 48 hours. since edema and expansion of hematoma may-compromise the airway. Afterthe airway is established, debridement is done and lacerations. Closed For the normal function to be restored. Reduction of laryngeal fractures should be done and treatment. she should not be conservative. Any trauma such as a fall over a hard object may produce acute or chronic stenosisof the larynx as may high tracheotomy and prolonged intubation. With any signs of obstruction immediate tracheostomy should be done.

LARYNGEAL STENOSIS

1. Acute laryngeal stenosis may be due to any infection that is acute or diphtheria or no diphtheritic, which leads to oedema of the andabsinthe region or epiglottis is and arytenoids, or maybe due to inflammation following the inspiration of a vegetal FB such as a peanut and especially. After instrumentation in the removal of such an object from edema resulting from allergic factors or cardio-renal disease; or from a FB lodged in the larynx. Airway should be promptly provided byintubation or tracheotomy and appropriate

treatment. of the underlying condition.

2. Subglottic stenosis: Narrowing of the subglottic airway (from the level of cricoid cartilage up tojust below the VC) can be congenital or acquired. Infants with congenital subglottic stenosis usually have inspiratory stridor since birth (though mild cases may have only recurrent attacks of croup), voice and cry are normal Acquired subglottic stenosis is secondary to trauma associated with insertion or presence of an endotracheal tube. There is an increased risk of developing stenosis when the traumatized subglottic area is infected also. The risk can be minimized also by using a small endotracheal tube gentle intubation using an endotracheal tube made of polyvinyl chloride and providing optimal tube stabilized and mouth care.

3. Chronic laryngeal stenosis frequently follows a high tracheostomy in which the first trachealring or cricoid cartilage has been damaged.

4. Resulting in perichondritis and subsequent overgrowth of cartilage or fibrous tissue. This complication can be avoided if damage to these 2 structures is avoided; laryngeal disease may beresponsible for chronic stenosis as diphtheria, syphilis, TB, burns_X-ray or radium), and external trauma. Scarring and stenosis most often develop in the subglottic area, and at times there is necrosis of cartilage. Ciinically, there is the inability to decannulate the tracheotomized patient. Or to extubate the intubated pt; but neither intubation nor tracheotomy had been done, there will be dyspnea with audible. Stridor, indrawings at the suprasternal notch and at the supraclavicular and intercostal spaces. Palpation of the larynx, direct laryngoscopy, and X-ray establish the diagnosis.In the milder casea, the tracheostomy cannula is replaced by a smaller one, and occlusion (first partial and then complete) by a cork of this tube will reeducate the paticnt to brcathc through the mouth and permit removal of the cannula. If this is not successful, dilation through a direct laryngoscopy may be done, repeating ii as desired,

cauterization of the narrowed airway, and if these fail, resection of the area with or without the use of at indwelling mold. The prognosis for eventualcure is good but it may take even years.

GLOTTIC and SUBGIOTTIC TUMORS

Papilloma and subglottic hemangiomas are the commonest tumors of the larynx in children. Bothmay present at birth and present with inspiratory stridor. Subglottic lymphangioma can also occur but is very rare. Papilloma is the commonest tumor in childhood larynx, most often presents between ages 2-4 years, may grow profusely from any part of the larynx (but usually arise from VC), is histologically benign, consisting of proliferation. Of stratified epithelium with a. central core of connective tissue and very little vascular supply. There are usually multiple papillomata, and they typically disappear after puberty, and if these remain into adulthood, spontaneous remission_ is unlikely and malignant degeneration may ensue -Most commonly, VC and the anterior commissure may- is involved but may extend to other glottis and subglottic structures; occasionally may go farther down the airway. Initially, there is. Only hoarseness and croupy cough, but there is progressive evidence of upper airway obstruction, and when papilloma persists an extensive, and finally, dyspnea in unrecognized cases, asphyxia has occurred. The condition can be diagnosed even during the hoarseness: stage in infants as pinkish warty tumors which scalp off easily when grasped off with forceps) and confirmed by histology. Treatment is by repeated superficial excision. Until the problem spontaneously subsides. There is a rapid recurrence but ultimately cure is: achieved. If recurrence is too rapid to be controlled. By excisions, tracheostomy may be needed if asphyxia threatens, and a cannula should be left in place while the tendency to recurrence occurs. Radical excision or intensive irradiation is contraindicated ultrasound treatment, cryosurgery, and laser surgery are used often, there has been a fear that ultrasonic therapy may inhibit the normal growth of the larynx.

Subglottic hemangiomas are usually subglottic in infants and tend to present early in life with signs of airway obstruction usually without hoarseness. It is sessile:180ft and compressible, andmore than 90% present within first 6 months. In 1/2 cases, of subglottic hemangiomas there are associated skin hemangiomas. Most subs/attic hemangiomas tend to regress during first. Few years but tracheostomy may be required while waiting for the hemangiomas to regress spontaneous. These have been successfully treated with CO2 laser.

FOREIGN BODIES IN THE LARYNX, TRACHEA, AND BRONCHI

Children between: 6 mon-4years are at particular risk for aspiration of any small object to which they have access such, as seeds, grasses, nuts, heads, pins or pebble There is usually a sudden onsetof coughing and wheezing, followed by chronic cough. The changes produced by FB depend upon their nature and upon the degree of the obstruction of the air passages. A sharp or irritating object lodged in the larynx will produce severe edema and later. Supportive perichondritis. In the broach us a non-obstructive FB may produce little pathologic changes, whereas an obstructive FR will cause atelectasis and later bronchiectasis, pulmonary abscess, or empyema. A vegetal object as a peanut may immediately produce a. generalized inflammatory condition involving not only the portion of tracheobronchial tree but also the entire respiratory tract.

Clinically there is a sudden onset of choking, gagging, coughing, and wheezing, which in some casesis associated with severe Respiratory distress, depending on the location of the FB in the airway. If the FB is not removed or coughed out, a symptomless period or an interval with minimal symptoms follows, lasting for days.

Lasting hours, days to weeks, followed by recurrences of wheezing and persistent cough. The secondary symptoms may give clue to the site of the lodgment of the FB, can also point whether it is lodged in the food passage or in the air passage. But occasionally dysphasia may occur from the FB swelling that resulted from the lodgment of the FB in the region of larynx, and a FB in the upper esophagus may cause symptoms referable to the air passages by compression or by the overflow of food or secretions from the esophagus into the larynx. Trapping of secretions behind.The FE may occur, and they may become infected. Recurrent or persistent. Pneumonia always recurring in the same area of the lung may be due to a retained FB. If the FB remains in the airway for a long time with persistent pneumonia, bronchiectasis or lung abscess may develop in the distal airways. Physical examination of the chest will usually reveal asymmetric auscultatory findings as decreased breath sounds. Over the affected lung, often associated with inspiratory rhonchi and expiratory wheezing, particularly during first few hours after aspiration. There may be increased or decreased resonance to percussion] over the affected area, due to over-inflation or decreased air entry lodging, in the larynx or trachea will cause severe respiratory distress , and when the FB comes to rest in the lower Respiratory tract, there may be tracheal shift and asymmetric cheat movement and aeration.

LARYNGEAL FB

A FB in the larynx causes hoarseness, a cough which is soon changing (into a croupy cough, and aphonia; hemoptysis, dyspnea with wheezing, and cyanosis may occur. Obstruction resulting from the FB or the combination of it and the inflammatory reaction may prove fatal if treatment is. Delayed. Direct laryngoscopy, as well as X-RAY, show the FB, if it is. Lodged anteriorly, it is obviously in the larynx, and when it is behind the soft tissue's shadows of the larynx, it is in the hypopharynx or the cervical esophagus (on lateral X-ray). The plane in which the FB lies is another differential point; if it lies in the sagittal plane, it is in the larynx. If it is in the coronal planes, it is in the food passage. Even if the FB is not opaque, ray will provide indirect evidence of its presence. Films should be taken in both AP and lateral projection. In some cases. Insertion of a little opaque material can be helpful. Direct laryngoscopy is both diagnostic and curative,affording access for instrumental removal of the FB. When there is severe dyspnea, tracheostomyshould precede the direct laryngoscopy.

- TRACHEAL FB The characteristic findings are the audible slap and palpable thud due to momentary expiratory impaction at the subglottic level, and asthmatic wheeze, but it may causecough, hoarseness, dyspnea and cyanosis. X-ray chest may help but, in most cases, definitive diagnosis is made on bronchoscopy.

- BRONCHIAL FB: The initial symptoms are like the FB in larynx or trachea in addition to cough, blood steaksand sputum and metallic taste in the case of a. metallic FB. The degree of theobstruction produced determines the symptoms and pathological changes no obstructive nonirritating FB may cause few symptoms even after prolonged stay, but an obstructive FB quietly leads to signs and symptoms. When there is a slight obstruction only, wheeze is heard. Obstruction of a greater degree leads to obstructive emphysema or obstructive atelectasis; if sit her is allowed to persist, chronic bronchopulmonary disease may be caused. When both main bronchi are obstructed, others may be severe dyspnea and even asphyxia. If the FB is vegetal (peanut), vegetal or archaic bronchitis will result, which is a severe condition characterized by cough septic type of fever and dyspnea. When a' bronchial FB has been presentfor a long time, chronic pulmonary suppuration may be expected.

The symptoms of the bronchia/ FB depend upon the stage in. which the patient it is seen. A FB should be considered in all acute and chronic pulmonary lesions whether there is h/o a FB accident. Or not-The physical signs include limited expansion, decreased vocal fremitus, impaired (atelectasis), or hype resonant (emphysema). Percussion notes, and diminished breath sounds distal to the FB. When there is complete obstruction, with atelectasis or atelectasis, there is absence of the vocal resonance and vocal fremitus (leading to an erroneous diagnosis of emphysema). Varying degrees of tympani are noted over the areas of obstructive emphysema which may persist for some time. Rales are more likely on the healthy side than the involved side. In a first-degree obstruction there is a bypass valve type obstruction, allowing the passage of air in both directions with-slight interference only; it leads to wheeze. In the 2nd type is sufficient interference to the passage of air so that only one direction is available; a check-valve action depends primarily on the physiologic expansion of the bronchus on inspiration and its contraction on expiration. If the obstruction is to expiratory phase but air passes freely during theinspiratory phase, air will accumulate with obstructive emphysema if the blockage of the bronchus is complete by corking of the bronchus by the object or the FB+inflammatory reaction of the bronchial wall, a stop-valve obstruction results so that the air in the distal lung gets absorbed, leaving an area of obstructive atelectasis.

FB is usually radiolucent. And can ‘t be seen on chest x-ray. If such an obstruction causes bypassobstruction, it can ‘t even be detected on screening. Fluoroscopy is a very useful method to detect and localize the FB in the bronchial trees. With a check-valve obstruction, there is obstructive emphysema which allows to localization of the obstruction (whether radiolucent or radiopaque). The obstructed lung will remain expanded during expiration, while the heart and the mediastinum will shift to the opposite side as the unobstructed lung empties. The diaphragm is low, flattened, and fixed to-then the obstructed side while its excursion is will free and exaggerated on the normal side. The differences between the lungs are much more evident in the expirations than ininspiration.

For a permanent record, two films are taken, one during full inspiration and another at the end of a full expiration, a ball-valve obstruction, a chest X-ray is almost normal if taken. After full inspiration, but a film during forced. expiration will show localized hyperinflation with greater latency) with mediastina away from the affected side. A forced expiratory film can be obtained In patient of any age by, manual pressure on the abdomen during a spontaneous expiration.

With complete obstruction, obstructive bronchitis results (after the FB remains for several weeks), the heart and mediastinum are drawn towards the obstructed side and remain there during both phases of respiratory. The diaphragm on the obstructed side remains high, while thatof the normal side moves normally. Film taken at the end of the inspiration and expiration show only the slight difference restating from the filling and emptying of the normal lung. Opaque FB are clearly revealed on the x-ray, and both AP and lateral fins should be taken. Sufficient exposurein the AP view is needed to show a FB behind the heart.

PROGNOSIS: 2-4% of FB are coughed up spontaneously -about 99% can. Be removed safely by the bronchoscopy.1f the patients survive the initial episode and the FB is. Removed promptly chances of complete recovery are excellent. FB that remains in place for many weeks leads to distal bronchiectasis, or lung: abscess FB that are not removed prove fatal sooner or later.

TREATMENT:

All patients with suspected acute FB aspiration. Should be hospitalized. Bronchoscopy is safely employed for the. Majority of casea, but bronchoscopy for. FB in cases of children a difficult - procedure and. should be performed by a FB experienced bronchoscopist.A. FB impacted near the carina steed's immediate removal by bronchoscopy. When the FB is impacted in. a main stembronchus, bronchoscopy should be done within hours. Attempted. to dislodge the FB by cheat. Physiotherapy may to complete obstruction by the FB at the level of main. Stem bronchus and lead to extreme respiratory. Insufficiency or it may get impacted at the level of trachea et subglottic area leading to asphyxia. But once the FB has been removed. Pulmonary physiotherapy Should be continued: until the physical examination and chestx-ray- Show that thelungs have returned to full physiological and anatomical Status.

ANATOMIC NARROWING OF INTRATHORACIC. TRACHEA and BRONCHI

The intrathoracic airway can be narrowed by intrinsic tumors, granulation tissue, inflammatory tissue, acquired or fixed congenital stenosis, extrinsic compression by aberrant vessels, or dynamic. Compression from transdermal pressure gradients across the airway wall due to primaryobstruction of the more peripheral airways. Mediastinal masses also cause extrinsic airway obstruction. Superior mediastinum-cystic hygroma, vascular tumors, neurogenic tumours, thymic tumor, teratoma, meningioma, mediastinal abscessoortic aneurysm, intrathoracic thyroid, oesophagal lesions. Middle mediastinum-lymphoma, granuloma, hypertrophic lymph nodes, bronchogenic cyst, gastrointestinal tract duplication, metastases, pericardial cyst, aortic aneurysm, anomalies of great vessels, Anterior mediastinum-thymoma, thYmic hyperplasia,thymic cyst, teratoma, vascular tumors, lymphoma, intrathoracic thyroid, pleuropericardial cyst, lymphadenopathy. Posterior mediastinum-Neurogenic tumors, gastrointestinaltract duplications, thoracic meningocele, and aortic aneurysm.

Clinical features. Patients with fixed narrowing of the larger intrathoracic airway: may present with acroupy cough, which is generally associated with more expire tory than inspiratory difficulty there is an expiratory wheeze. There is often a hike recurrent pneumonia, often localized to the area distal to the obstruction and increased respiratory distress with apparently mild infections. Cheat X-ray may show localized or diffuse parenchymal infiltrates and a mediastinal mass. All mediastina masses: don 't cause airway narrowing. Airway tomography, CT scan, and high kilo voltage X-ray better delineate the tracheobronchial tree and thus may demonstrate a localized airway narrowing. Pulmonary function test show decreased maximal inspiratory and expiratory flow rates. With fixed narrowing, but with narrowing due to dynamic compression, the peak expiratory flow will be decreased much more than the inspiratory flow. Bronchoscopy, bronchography, esophagography or angiography may also be helpful.

MALFORMATIONS OF THE TRACHEA, BRONCHI, and LUNGS

Tracheo-esophageal fistula is the most important anomaly of the trachea; Rarely, there may be tracheal stenosis. Tracheal compression. May he be produced by an anomalous aortic arch or another large vessel? The trachea of the young infant is significantly more complaint because of the incomplete development of the airway cartilage and other supportive tissue. Tracheal collapse may occur in any patient with obstruction in smaller airways that necessitates forced expiration to empty the lungs. The positive pressure developed causes dynamic compression of the larger intrathoracic airways. Other causes of tracheal compression are vascular compressing ring. Theremay be rare defects. Of one or more tracheal rings that can cause a truly isolated tracheomalacia

Cysts. of the lungs are occasionally present in infants early in the neonatal period and. may be localized or distributed in. 2 or more lobes. It is presumed that those with an epithelial lining arecongenital and these without such a lining are the

result of the postnatal destruction...Cysts of congenital origin have been seen in association with adenomatous malformations of the lungs.
The lesion, which is usually limited to one label may initially appear on the X-ray as a sold structure. The bronchi are malformed. As the lote is irregularly' aerated during the first few days of life, air accumulates in the potential structures. These enlarged progressively and may cause severe respiratory distress . In the left lower lobe, the condition can be confused with diaphragmatic hernia. Most cystic structures during the neonatal period or later are acquired and result from. Destruction of the pulmonary architecture; this may occur during artificial respiratoryand occasionally may be responsible for an accumulation. Of air within one or more lots. Partial blockage of air a bronchus with creation. Of a ball-valve type of mechanism will permit the retention of an increasing amount of air. Undersuch circumstances. Whether the condition is inflammatory or purely mechanical and whether it is in or extra-bronchial, a retention cyst is caused in other circumstances connection with the tracheobronchial tree is broken, alveolar sacs are ruptured, and the accumulation of air remains for a long time before it is finally absorbed, and the architecture of the: lung is realigned. Many factors can. Be responsible for such obstructions of the bronchi (some are congenital), but the majority are probably the result of postnatal disturbances, usually inflammatory. An unusual association with cytomegalic inclusion disease has been recorded. The cysts may be filled entirely with air or fluid or with a combination of them.Host cysts disappear eventually without interference, but when a tension cyst continues to expand and compress other lobes, it is usually necessary to remove the lobe containing it. Even such cysts may establish an equilibrium with the normal portions of the lung, become closed andeventually disappear. The degree of respiratory embarrassment and its progression determine the need for surgical removal.

VASCULAR RINGS

Congenital abnormalities of the aortic arch and its major branches result in the formation of vascular rings around the trachea and esophagus with varying degree of compression. The most common type is due to persistence of both right and left 4th aortic arches they arise from the- a branching of the ascending aorta, encircle the esophagus and trachea, and join posteriorly to formthe descending thoraaorta. The commonest anomalies are -double aortic arch, right aortic arch with ligamentous arteriosum, anomalous subclavian(right)artery arising as the last major thoracic branch of a normally placed aorta, anomalous innominate artery arising to further to the left on the arch than usual, anomalous carotid artery arias further to the right than usual, and passing anterior to the Archaea, and anomalous left pulmonary artery(vascular sling)-this abnormal vesselarises from the an elongated main pulmonary artery or from the right pulmonary artery; it course between and compresses the trachea and esophagus. Tracheobronchial compression will by anomalous or enlarged blood vessels will usually cause symptoms during the first year of life if at all. There may be associated congenital cardiac disease. Clinical patterns are variable, and there may be no symptoms at all (as for instance with an anomalous right subclavian artery) But if vascular ring compresses trachea and esophagus, symptoms occur during infancy. The symptomsof obstruction are a persistent expiratory wheeze and noisy breathing; the wheezy respiratorys are aggravated by crying, feeding, and flexion of the neck. Extension of the neck tends to relive the noisy respiratorys; therefore, the child prefers to keep the head hyperextended which reduces the tracheal compression. There is coarse stridor (predominantly expiratory), and there may be brassy cough; vomiting is common and feeding difficult. There may also be recurrent pneumonias and persistent brassy cough. Patients may assume an opisthotonos position to facilitate the airway.

Rarely there may be apneic episodes. ECG is normal, X-ray of cheat may show persistent or recurrent increased Broncho vascular markings, and occasionally there may be evidence of airway indentation. Barium swallow reveals typical esophageal indentations. Air- or Lipoid filledtrachea also discloses the anomaly.

Bronchoscopy and angiography with injection into the ascending aorta establish the diagnosis inmost cases. With minor symptoms there is no danger to life, but with severe symptoms they may be endangered; the infant may be in severe respiratory distress . Severe respiratory difficulty may lead to death from aspiration and pneumonia. All the symptomatic infants with radiological evidence of compression of trachea or esophagi should undergo surgery and cases of double aortic. Arch one of these is divided. In those with. Right aortic arch accompanied by left ligamentous arterlosum or PI An anomalous right subclavian artery is divided at its on from the aorta. Anomalous innominate or carotid arteries can be divided and the compression is relieved by attaching the adventitia. Of these vessels to the sternum. Anomalous left pulmonary artery it divided. At its. Origin and. anastomosis to the main pulmonary artery after the anomalous vessel has been brought lint front. Of the trachea Many infants have: prolonged persistence of symptoms. Of expiratory obstruction even: after surgical correction, it suggests a permanent abnormality, Of airway development, possibly secondary to the initial presence of the vascular anomaly.

BRONCHOPULMONARY DYSPLASIA

This consists of the chronic requirement of increased inspired oxygen in infants, usually following severe acute RDS. Bronchopulmonary dysplasia occurs in 20-30% of babies with clinical RDS who require mechanical ventilation. There is 4 stat -Stage 1 lasts. For 1-3 days;4s a period of acute hyaline membrane disease with a characteristic chest X-ray revealing air-Broncho gram andreticular granularity of the Lunt: fields; during this period, there is tachypnea, hypoxemia due to shunting through the areas. Of wide specially read. Alveolar atelectasis, and often hypercapnia. As a result of the deficiency of the surfactant that causes diffuse micro-atelectasis, the lungs are stiff, and functional residual capacity is low. Histologic fly there is the diffuse collapse of the terminal air spaces, but the larger airway: are normal. Most patients with. RDS begin to improve within 3 days and are normal by 5-10 days. But those who are going to develop Broncho pulmonary dysplasia are likely to continue to worsen over the first several days of life, requiring mechanical ventilation. –

Stage 2 lasts for 4-10 days and is the period of initial regeneration; there it is marked. There is a marked increase in oxygen requirement and failure to improve clinically. X-ray shows nearly complete bilateral opacification (this picture is characteristic but may be eliminated by therapy using +ve pressure ventilation). Histologically there is early regeneration and metaplasia of thealveolar epithelized and some necrosis of the bronchiolar epithelium. –

During stage 3, which lasts 10-20 days, the period of transition to chronic disease is reached; oxygen dependence persists though the patient no longer needs mechanical ventilation. Chest X-ray demonstrates a Honey-comb lung with multiple small, round radiolucent areas. Histologically, their id, regeneration of and metaplasia of the bronchiolar epithelium, with increased airway mucus secretion and inflammatory cell Response . There are alternating areas of emphysema and atelectasis. –

Stage 4 starts after 4th week and is the period of true lung disease. There is a requirement for increased oxygen for several months although there is usuall2 a progressive slow decrease of thisrequirement. Clinically there are diffuse rales and wheezing, chest wall retractions, increased chest circumference due to expiratory obstruction. The chest X-ray typically shows enlargement of the previously small radiolucent areas, beginning in the lung bases, with. progression to the generally radiolucent hyperinflated lung fields with fibrous and atelectasis streaks. The histology during this phase shows alternating areas of atelectasis and emphysema, metaplasia of the bronchiolar epithelium, hypertrophy of the medic smooth muscle in the pulmonary arterioles,and dilatation of pulmonary lymphatic' There may be interstitial edema and eventually fibrosis. The stages are not distinct, and the lung shows different stages in different areas at the same timein many pts, stages 2,3,4 appear only as nonspecific streaky markings on x-ray,with areas of atelectasis alternating with area, of emphysema-bronchopulmonary dysphasia should be distinguished from chronic lung disease that may follow some viral infections, especially adenovirus infections, and occasionally may follow chronic CCE due to a PDA,both are clinically and pathologically similar to Bronchopulmonary dysplasia.

PREVENTION OF BRONCHOPULMONARY DYSPLASIA

High positive airway pressure(barotrauma), high inspired oxygen concentrations (oxygen toxicity), and pulmonary immaturity contribute to the development of the iatrogenic disease; therefore, great care should be taken during the treatment of acute clinical RDS to minimize the patients exposure to high airway pressure, i.e., more than 30 cm water and high oxygen concentrations i.e., more than 60% infants with bronchopulmonary dysplasia. Are likely to require several re-hospitalizations for increasing respiratory distress and increased. Oxygen requirements. Often precipitated by a mild viral infection.

Some such infants, even in absence of signs of heart failure may benefit from the diuretic therapy especially during acute exacerbations of the disease. This is because of an increased permeability of pulmonary capillaries that leads to pulmonary edema. Since excessive airway secretions and necrotic cellular debris. May contribute to airway obstruction and since normal lung clearance mechanisms are not likely to be functioning properly, Chest percussion. And postural drainage may help them. It is important to maintain an adequate Hemoglobin concentration (morethan 14g) in. patients requiring chronic oxygen therapy to minimize the oxygen requirement by maximizing the oxygen-carrying, capacity.ECG should he followed for signs of increasing RVH, which may indicate increasing hypoxemia. Increased serum carbonate may indicate chronic hypercapnia. Adequate nutrition is also important. Chronic bronchodilator therapy may help some pts. Most patients shows slow but progressive improvement of lung function over the first few years of life.

BRONCHITIS OBLITERANS (Bronchiolitis Fibrosa Obliterans)

It is quite rare in children and is due to a major insult to the lower respiratory tract, and may follow inhalation of toxic gases, lower Respiratory tract infections, such as influenza pertussis adenovirus type 21, or inhalation of FB, and in some cases, the cause can be found. There occurs extensive damage to the bronchiolar wall with obstruction to the lumen by organized exudate and polyploidy masses of granulation tissue. Distal to the bronchiolar, there may be air-trapping or marked accumulation of the fat-filled phagocytes. Ultimately the installer and bronchioles may bereplaced by fibrous acara. There may be a dissipated, associated interstitial pneumonia. The commonest symptoms are interracial pneumonia

The commonest symptoms are cough, dyspnea chest pain malaise sputum production andsometimes hemoptysis. Rales are commonly heard on chest auscultation. Chest X-ray abnormalities are variable and may include modular densities, alveolar abnormalities or occasionally hyperinflation. Pulmonary function. Tests show restrictive or obstructive disease. Diagnosis is only by microscopy of the lung tissue. Some are benefitted with steroidtherapy sent in some cases antibiotics are indicated.

BRONCHIAL AND PULMONARY LESIONS SECONDARY TO ASPIRATION OF FOREIGN MATERIALS

Aspiration syndromes that occur during the childhood period are – aspiration of toxic fluids as gastric acids hydrocarbons meconium –aspiration of bacteria.
Aspiration of particulate. Material as food or meconium.

The most frequent aspirations are the aspiration of particulate matter and the aspiration of toxic fluids. Aspiration of gastric acid is most common. During periods. With impaired consciousness disorders of the esophagus or cardio oesophagal sphincter... Hydrocarbon aspiration.is common during childhood and should be suspected In a patient who has ingested hydrocarbons. Hydrocarbon.Aspiration typically produces. A generalized chemical pneumonitis, whereas other forms of aspiration generally involve. Primarily- the dependent portions of the lung. In the supine position, this would include the posterior segments of the upper lobes and superior segments; Lower lobes; in the upright position, the basements ape- of the lower lobes are dependent.

Debilitated, newborn, or premature infants. May aspirate baby powders, formula, or food or regurgitate and then aspirate the regurgitated contents. This is specifically easy to do during supine position pneumonitis may result, especially in the right upper lobe and may be a lipoidpneumonia if the aspirated contents contained milk or some other fat-containing substance.

Lipoid pneumonia may also result from aspiration of oily

nose drops. Or vitamin preparations. Signs and symptoms will vary with the type and amount of aspiration and X-ray is nonspecific. Often widening hilar densities are present- Secondary infection is. Common, and adrenal steroidsare beneficial if used. Early. Aspiration of zinc stearate Aspiration of zinc. Stearate powder usedfor infants leads to severe respiratory distress immediately following the inhalation. There is generalized obstructive emphysema with an expiratory dyspnea; respiratory embarrassment is due to an inflammatory reaction caused by the irritation of the zinc stearate. Due to the extreme lightness of the powder lit is immediately drawn into the finer bronchioles, therefore bronchoscopy aspiration is of no value except in removing the sections which subsequently accumulate. Immediate treatment is by oxygen in high timidity atmosphere; bronchoscopy aspiration may be done if there is large accumulation.

ASPIRATION OF GASTRIC ACID

The aspiration of gastric acid may be subclinical and recurrent, especially during sleep, producing a chronic obstructive bronchitis that may progress to pulmonary fibrosis this is associated with achalasia and gastroesophageal reflux or there may be a single large aspiration that produces the rapid onset of fever, tachypnea, diffuse rales, and severe hypoxemia, in which cases there will be cough cyanosis, wheezing, apnea and shock. The severity of this clinical syndrome is related to the acidity and volume of aspiration. And general condition of the patient and specific lung capabilities. Rapid onset of symptoms differentiates it from other types of pneumonia. X-ray abnormalities develop within the first 24-36- hr; and include diffuse or 'Localized mottled. Infiltrates with or without atelectasis A small percentage of affected patients die soon after the aspiration -but others sin rapid clinical and radiological improvement within 2-5 days of aspiration, while others develop secondary infection when there is clinical deterioration with increasing: lung infiltrates, reappearance of fevers leukocytosis, and recovery of pathogens from tracheal aspirates. Treatment includes humidified oxygen to maintain adequate oxygenation, immediate (tracheal intubation and suctioning if aspiration is significant, vigorous pulmonary physiotherapy, and mechanical ventilation in severely affected pts. Broncholi later therapy may be helpful; in some cases corticosteroids are helpful. Antibiotics are used for secondary infections. With no further aspiration prognosis excellent in the maturity provided theis no secondary infection, where it is worse. Since recurrent subclinical aspiration due to achalasia may cause chronic lung, disease may benefit from surgery of incompetent cardio esophageal sphincter. Finding of fat-filled macrophages in. tracheal aspirate material suggests chronic recurrent aspiration.

ASPIRATION OF FOOD

Infants. with obstructive lesions such as TEF and duodenal obstruction and weak debilitated infants who have no obstructive lesions aspirate or regurgitate and the' aspirate an amount of food sufficient to cause significant. Pulmonary damage. Aspiration may rarely be the immediate causeof death by asphyxiation, but more frequently, the irritated mucous membrane becomes a site for bacterial invasion. Prophylaxis is of paramount importance care should be taken to avoid amounts of feeding that over distend the stomach especially in the patients who are gavage fed.

After the infant is fed, he should be placed, on the abdomen or on his right side. If he is in the supine position his head should not be lower than the rest of his body but when the infant is lyingdown on his abdomen drainage from. The lux can he materially aided by lowering the head of thebed.

HYDROCARBON ASPIRATION(KEROSENE):

Hydrocarbon aspiration may cane immediate choking coughing dyspnea cyanosis intercostal retractions and fever developing, shortly thereafter. Coughing and vomiting follow the in gestational most immediately Temperature rises to

100-104F, and the child may be drowsy or comatose. Respiratory symptoms develop within the fix a few horal there may be symptoms at all. Chest findings may be diminished resonance on percussion, diminished. Lacrosse or tubular breathing sounds and rale Pneumonic involvement is disclosed more frequently by X-ray than clinical finding, and chest abnormalities on X-ray appear within first. 12 hours. Occasionally X-ray findings may' he minimal a few hours after ingestion only to progress rapidly thereafter initial X-ray may show mottled' peripheral densities with. Extension into the midlung fields, basal pneumonitis, or atelectasis. With passage of time, the mottle dirties may be coalesced into larger patchy infiltrates. There may be peripheral obstructive emphysema and. ultimately development of pneumatoceles and lungs cysts. The stormy clinical course lasts 2-5 days, but the majority recover as the clinical and X-ray abnormalities. Clear complication 's will include pneumothorax, SC emphysema of the chest wall and pleural effusion. Since the kerosene reaches the lungs during swallowing, vomiting, or gastric lavage, because of this gastric lavage and vomiting after the ingestion of kerosene should not be attempted When only small amounts of kerosene have been ingested, and several hours. Have elapsed, gastric lavage should not be done. But if large quantities of kerosene or other hydrocarbon have been ingested lavage should be done, with great care to avoid aspiration. The administration of an oil apparently decreases absorption from GIT but is not useful in practice. If there is dyspnea or cyanosis, the child shouldbe placed in an oxygen tent; Humidified oxygen, vigorous pulmonary physiotherapy and mechanical ventilation are appropriate. The occurrence of secondary infection of the affected lung can be readily detected by the reappearance. of the fever on. The 3rd day-5th day, and penicillin or another suitable antibiotic can be used. Steroids have no beneficial effect on the course illness. Some have benefited from bronchodilator treatment.

ASPIRATION OF LIPID MATERIAL

Lipoid pneumonia is a chronic interstitial proliferative inflammation resulting from aspiration. Of lipoid material and occurs principally in debilitated infant Aspiration of oil may follow intranasal instillation of medicated oils, any condition whichinterfere, with the swallowing act such. As: cleft palate, debilitating or a horizontal position during feeding, and forced feeding and the administration of cod-liver oil, castor oil or mineral oils to crying children. The severity of pulmonary reaction depends on the y type of the oil inhaled.

Vegetable oils are the least irritating (thus olive -cottonseed and sesame oil cause no inflammation but chaulmoogra oil produces extensive damage), animal oils on the other hand owing to their high fatty acid content, are the most damaging, as Cod-liver oil. Liquid petroleum.Is chemically inert and not so irritative as so some of the other oils but acts as a foreign body.
The reaction within the lung begins as an interstitial proliferative inflammation with which theremay be exudative pneumonia. In the 2nd stage, there is diffuse chronic proliferative fibrosis, and acute bronchopneumonia may be superimposed at this stage; in the 3rd stage, there are multiple localized nodules (tumor-like carcinomas). Microscopically there are numerous macrophages in the involved_ areas with giant cell formation of the: FB type; the lipid substance is both intra andextra-cellular. The oil-laden cells may be carried through lymphatic channels to the hilar lymph nodes. Clinically there is a cough, and. in severe cases, dyspnea unless there is a superimposed infection, there is no. fever Or any physical sign. With extensive involvement, there may be someimpairment to percussion, increased or decreased breath sound. Secondary bronchopneumonia infections are commons. The only characteristic finding is seen. On X-ray with mild involvement, there is Only an increase in the

density and the extent of the hilar shadows with increasing involvement there is. Greater density of the. Perihelia shadows with widening all directions, and few instances, the pulmonary changes have been limited to the right lung, ending in the recumbent infant, most changes are seen. In the right. Upper lote. There is no specific treatment, but the infants. the Position should tee changed frequently to lessen the chances of hypostatic pneumonia Prognosis is guarded and depends on the extent of the pulmonary damage and avoidance of intercurrent infections.

SILO FILLERS DISEASE

This is an acute interstitial pneumonia seen in some farm children. It is due to inhalation of nitrogen oxide(N02), a gas generally encountered only in freshly filled silos. Immediately afterexposure cough and dyspnea occurs, followed by a period of no symptoms, but then the patient experiences chills and fever associated with progressive cough, dyspnea, and cyanosis.

Auscultation of the chest reveals rales throughout both lungs; radiologic examination shows Widespread pulmonary infiltrations. There is no effective treatment, and the disease leads rapidlyto death.

HYPERSENSITIVITY TO INHALED GAS

Many pulmonary diseases are supposed to be due to hypersensitivity to various inhaled substances such as maple bark (maple bark strippers' disease), sugar cane bark (bagassosis)» redwood tree mark, pigeon dropping and feathers (pigeon breeders' disease) inhalation of moldy hay lung), and the dusty output from, the air conditioners. Clinical, features of all these are almost identical »several hours following the exposure there isacute onset of chest pain, fever, and dyspnea; occasionally there is wheeze and crepitations. X-ray is normal usually but may show minimal emphysema. If there is no further contact, symptoms abate over a period of several days, but if the exposure continues, symptoms progress to severe dyspnea and cyanosis, also dated with a diffuse, usually rather fine, infiltrate on chest x-ray.

Histologically this infiltrate consists of sub-acute granulomatous inflammation with the accumulation of plasma cells, lymphocytes epitheloid cells, and giant cells of the Langhans type. With continued exposure, inflammatory lesions are replaced by fibrosis. Hypergammaglobulinemia develops With the elevation of lgG. IgM and IgA fractions, which show the immunologic basis of the lesions, specific precipitins to the antigen occur in the serum of the affected pt. And the intradermal injection of this antigen causes a vigorous delayed hypersensitivity Response . Treatment consists of immediate removal of the pi from the offending environment in which the antigen occurs. Corticosteroids usually results in promptbreraission of symptoms, and the continued use of these drugs for 1-6 months may prevent sut sequent development of pulmonary fibrosis in the more chronic cases. Hypersensitivity pneumonitis is the result of a type immediate IgE mediated or type3 (Arthus allergic Response to an inhaled organic antigen. The acute form is characterized by the sudden onset of a nonproductive cough, chest tightness, fever, chills, malaise, and dyspnea beginning within 4-6 hours after the exposure. After recurrent exposures weight loss can also be there. Cyanosis, tachypnea, and basilar rales are found without wheezing usually. There is leukocytosis. Most of the X-ray findings (small diffuse nodules or patchy interstitial infiltrâtes) begin to resolve within 12-24 hours after the termination of antigen exposure.

Chronic hypersensitivity pneumonitis is characterized by progressive dyspnea with eventual cyanosis and digital clubbing, which will occur after prolonged and intense exposure. Chest X-ray shows a progressive increase in interstitial markings, and ultimately, theremay be a cystic appearance with decreased lung volume.

EOSINOPHILIC PNEUMONIA

A combination of pulmonary infiltrates (wide specially read, transitory pulmonary infiltrates which vary in size and may even resemble miliary TB) and eosinophilia
infiltrates in the lung on histology and which may be accompanied by blood eosinophilia (whichmay be as high as 70%). All 5 types represent some form of hypersensitivity reaction. The clinical course is not severe, may vary from a few days to several months, and consists ofparoxysmal attacks of coughing, dyspnea, pleurisy, and little fever. In many cases, in infants, there is. Associated hepatomegaly, while a biopsy of the liver shows multiple focal areas of necrosis, granuloma formation, and eosinophilia infiltration; they have hyperglobulinemia due to hepatic dysfunction and parasitic invasion of the tissue. Eosinophilic infiltrations are seen in the lungs and other organs. Localized pneumonic consolidations with associated eosinophilia may be seen.

Löfflers syndrome (simple pulmonary eosinophilia) consists of migratory pulmonary infiltratesassociated with minimal respiratory symptoms and mild fever. Duration of symptoms is less than 1 month:

- Prolonged pulmonary- eosinophilia lasts for over 1-2 months and is usually associated withhigh fever, malaise, productive cough, and chest pain

- -During chronic asthma, transient or prolonged eosinophilia infiltrations may occur
  which may last from. 3 months to years

- -Tropical eosinophilia. Consists of fever, expiratory obstruction, and weight loss with diffuse, finely nodular X-ray infiltrate. there is marked peripheral eosinophilia caused by severaldifferent helminths. Including filarial and paragonimiasis

- -Pulmonary eosinophil associated with polyarteritis nodosa and Wegener 's granulomatosis primarily pulmonary blood vessels are involved, but others may also be involved, and the symptomsare very severe and the outcome fatal.

Löfflers syndrome is not a clinical entity but an unusual allergic manifestation to a variety of antigens. In children, it would appear to be most often a manifestation of helminthic infections. Toxocara catis and cati Ascaris lurabricoides, strongyloides stercoralis, and hookworm can cause this syndrome.

Excepting in the case of tropical eosinophilia (best reacted with diethylcarbamazine), others can be controlled with corticosteroids which should be used if the symptoms are severe

PULMONARY ALVEOLAR PROTEINOSIS

A rare asedisease characterized by fever, dyspnea, productive cough, chest pain, and poor wt. Gain in an Infant below one year; there may be yellow sputum production, and cyanosis in the older child. Death occurs within a. few months of onset. Physical findings are sparse (but there may be scattered fine rales, clubbing, and eventual cyanosis). but chest X-ray shows bilateral, fine, diffuse,symmetricalinfiltrates radiating from the hilus to the peripheral in a typical butterfly fashion. Other pets may show bilateral lower lobe infiltrates; others show nodular densities That progress to complete lobar consolidation). Diagnosis is confirmed by lung biopsy, which shows alveoli and bronchioles distended by accumulation of a fine, granular eosinophile PAS-positive material. Silver staining is done to rule out P carinii infection,

This PAS-staining material and birefringent crystals may be present in sputum also. Patients show various sorts off immunologic deficiency states including thymicalymphoplasia, therefore variousfungal and bacterial superinfections. Treatment is unspecific neither corticosteroids nor lung lavage by heparinized saline alters the relentless progressive course; most children die of respiratory failure within 12 months of onset and the maximum. Period of survival till now has been only 2 years. The adult form though more common has a much favorable prognosis.

IDIOPATHIC PULMONARY FIBROSIS

Idiopathic pulmonary fibrosis of the lung consists of a continuum of the disease characterized by varying combinations of cuboidalization of alveolar lining, cells, and the presence of large mononuclear cells within the alveolar spaces and thickening of alveolar walls by fibrosis and inflammatory cells-Alveolar process represents the Initial stages but later the process, is primarily interstitial Different stages have previously been described under different headings asdesquamate interstitial pneumonitis —interstitial pneumonitis and Hamman Rich-syndrome (idiopathic diffuse interstitial fibrosis of. the lung) -In moat pediatric cases –the cause is unknown but previous infections may initiate this process in some parts; in adults drug exposureor connective tissue disorder may be the causative factors, IN fact, desquamative pneumonitis hassometimes been classified as one of the collagen diseases

In the desquamative stage, pathologic changes consist of massive proliferation of and desquamation of alveolar cells with thickening of the walls of the distal air spaces; Hamman-Rich syndrome isa chronic, more severe fatal disorder; pathologically, there is cellular infiltration of the walls of the alveoli, alveolar ducts, and per bronchial tissue by lymphocytes, plasma cells, and occasionally eosinophils which later progresses to the extensive and diffuse proliferation of fibroustissue throughout all the lobes of the lungs, association with the organization of intra-alveolar exudate

Clinical features; are progressive pulmonary insufficiency resulting from interstitial fibrosisand alveolar-capillary block. Onset is insidious;, and there is progressive dyspnea which first occurs with effort only but later occurs at rest also; tachypnea, nonproductive or bloody cough, weight loss, no fever, poor weight gain or weight loss, anorexic, fatiguability; finally there is cyanosis, clubbing, of fingers, and evidence of right-sided cardiac failure Pulmonary hypertension, respiratory failure - and cardiac failure occur- in more severely affected pts(generally Hamman Rich are the more severely affected pts). Pulmonary function tests show decreased vital capacity and total lung capacity, indicative- restrictive, lung disease. And diminished pulmonary diffusing capacity. The amount of hypoxemia indicates the extent of the pulmonary fibrosis. Lung compliance has decreased. Gallium scintigraphy and analysis of the cells obtained by Broncho alveolar- lavage may help in predicting the outcome and in selecting and assessing treatment. Chest x-rays shows diffuse ground glass, appearances of both lung bases, with poorly defined densities in the hilar regions and fine to coarse mottling; this progresses with appearance of peripheral linear markings; this progresses to the end stage picture. Progressive, increased linear markings associated with hyperlucent areas, particularly at the lung bases, widespread granular or reticular mottling or honeycomb appearance. The progression of this pattern generally extends over a period of 2-6 years. In severely affected patients cardiomegaly is evident on chest x-raying others ECG shows RVH.

Corticosteroids, prednisone 2mg/kg, given daily is given for 2 months; if there is improvement,prednisone is continued for at least l year and then withdrawn gradually. Corticosteroid therapy arrests the progress of the disease in early stages and may produce remission of symptoms. In later stages.it gives some symptomatic relief but does not alter the progression of the disease or improve the degree of pulmonary function.

Choloquine has been used in occasional cases- Cytotoxic drugs have been used.
The mean survival of reported cases Is 4-6 years.

PULMONARY ALVEOLAR MICROLITHIASIS

A familial disease of unknown cause characterized by extensive intra-alveolar deposits of calcium carbonate, seen on X-ray as fine, sand like mottling distribute uniformly throughout both lung fields. The X-ray appearance is likened to an overfilled normal bronchogram. The disease in childhood is usually asymptomatic, progresses slowly, and may lead to dyspnea, cough, cyanosis, clubbing, corPulmonarynale and cardiopulmonary failure during the middle adulthood. In rare cases, there has been h/o sand in the sputum which may point into the diagnosis.

WILSON - MIKITY SYNDROME

A clinical syndrome characterized by gradually progressive respiratory distress and Increased inspired oxygen, requirement in small premature infants, who have had no previous lung disease.Increasing, tachypnea, chest wall retractions, and cyanosis typically begins several weeks after birth.

Chest examination shows rales and wheezing; hut may be normal; chest X-ray shows a widespread reticular pattern resembling that of stage 5 of Broncho pulmonary dysplasia with small radiolucent areas or cysts scattered throughout the lung fields; these changes become moreprominent as the disease progresses further; lung biopsy shows thickened alveolar septa and mononuclear cell infiltration. Though thc course is prolonged, and there is extensive lung involvement, only 10-15% of the patients die of respiratory failure or right heart failure. The majority recover after a few months-The differential diagnoses includes, Bronchopulmonary dysplasia, viral pneumonia, PDA with pulmonary congestion due to increasing L-R shunts, and chronic pulmonary- insufficiency of prematurity which may be due to lung volume loss due toperiodic breathing of the prematurity.

PULMONARY EDEMA.

When the rate of accumulation of extravascular lung, water exceeds the capability of the pulmonary lymphatic system to remove this fluid-With the result the serous fluid, first accumulates in the interstitial space first in the area, surrounding. The vessels and. airways, laterit fills, the bronchioles and alveolar spaces. The development of pulmonary edema, from the escape of fluid from, the pulmonary capillaries is usually due to a change in the hydrostatic or oncotic pressure gradient across the pulmonary vessel wails or increased, permeability of the pulmonary capillary endothelium. It is usually associated with circulatory and neurocirculatory collapse. It can occur as a terminal event in many diseases, and is associated, with, heart disease,many infectious and toxic lung insults, including a. high level of inspired oxygen ,and hypoproteinemia is a common a manifestation of Myocardial failure in acute or chronic rheumatic carditis-,in congenital heart disease, or may be due to hypervolemia from, too rapid ortoo large an intravenous infusion ..It may be a manifestation of acute or chronic nephritis or rarely of pneumonia and other infections of substantial, degree of toxicity . Poisoning due to barbiturates, morphine.eoine0hrine.and alcohol. Inhalation of toxic gases as illuminating gas, ammonia and nitrogen dioxide, and ingestion of, with. Consequent aspiration, of highly volatile hydrocarbons, as lighter fluid can cause pulmonary edema. Neurogenic pulmonary edema follows severe CNS injury or insult.

CLINICAL FEATURES:

The onset is usually rapid in most cases. Mild pulmonary

edema may only cause tachypnea, mild rales., expiratory wheezes, and slight hypoxemia. Severe cases cause a sense of oppression or pain in. the chest, dyspnea, chest wall retractions, and cough with frothy, pink-tinged sputum; the pulse is rapid and feeble, and the child is very pale and may be cyanotic Chest examination reveals dullness to percussion, and: moist, bubbly rales are heard in the lower portions of the chest. Chest X-ray shows prominent pulmonary vascularity, often with diffuse haziness of the lung fields.
Pulmonary edema is ominous even in its mildest stage; the treatment depends on the stage of the pulmonary edema (the severity), the underlying disease, and age of the patient but will include oxygen, diuretics, restriction of the fluids, and salt intake, and in some cases morphine, phlebotomy rotating tourniquets on the extremities, placing the patient in a semisecret position, and. digitalis therapy for cardiogenic pulmonary edema. Management of myocardial failure, - nephritis,and various poisonings is done. Oxygen relieves chest pain; and. is best given by inter attentive pressure. Dyspnea can be relieved often with morphine sulfate»G-15rag/kg. If pulmonary edema is secondary to increased IV fluids or blood or due to cardiac failure, the application of tourniquets or inflated blood pressure cuffs to the extremities or the withdrawal of blood may be lifesaving.

PULMONARY EMBOLISM AND INFARCTION

Rare in children and usually due to venous stasis or trauma. Emboli most often arise from thrombi in the femoral and pelvic veins and are usually postoperative complications. Fat emboli are most likely derived from fractured bones, but occasionally may stem from necrotic tissue inthe bone marrow of patients inside cell d diseases. Multiple pulmonary infarcts resulting from smallemboli may be associated with severe dehydration in diarrheal disease, cyanotic heart disease, bacterial endocarditis, and long-standing nutritional deficiencies. lt may also complicate polycythemia, atrial fibrillation nephritic syndrome, or ventricular venous shunts for hydrocephalus Emboli-carrying bacteria may be responsible for multiple pulmonaryabscesses.

The clinical presentation depends on the extent of the pulmonary bed that is obstructed. Suddenobstruction of pulmonary artery or its larger branches will lead to sudden chest pain, usually substernal, but may be pleural and radiate to the shoulder, dyspnea, tachycardia, cyanosis chest splinting, large expectoration containing blood.

The chest findings are sparse often there are no findings, but if the infarct is sufficiently large (the base at the periphery, and the apex towards the midline at the point of infraction), there may be impaired resonance and a pleural friction rub. Breath sounds may be distant or absent, and there may be moist rales. The chest X-ray may be normal, or may show- a. peripheral infiltrate, small pleural effusion or elevated diaphragm ECG is usually normal but may demonstrate right. 1heart strain with large emboli. Lactic dehydrogenase is often elevated. A. lung perfusion scan will show a localized perfusion defect.

For prevention of pulmonary embolism- it is essential that venous stasis and- j prevented and good nutrition is maintained, especially in the bedridden children, Embolism of larger branches of the pulmonary artery Is a. medical emergency -The child is given morphine to induce quietness and allay fears. pt, should he keep in the oxygen tent for relief of dyspnea and cyanosis. Attempatients are made to prevent venous, stasis or any extension of the thrombosis by use of anticoagulant therapy (though it is of limited usefulness In children). Survival of the acrembolic period depends on the size of the embolus. Thrombolytic therapy may be considered in patients with, massive pulmonary embolism or unstable hemodynamics (systemic hypotension) due to pulmonary embolism. mortality is very high, but recovery may occur even in large infarctions Secondary infection may lead to abscess formation. The long, term prognosis is dependent on the underlying disease.

ADULT RESPIRATORY DISTRESS SYNDROME (SHOCK LUNG.)

It is a nonspecific reaction of the lung to a variety of severe insults. lt is characterized by severe progressive hypoxemia diteinhalation of oxygen in high concentrations as. a result of diffusely increased permeability of the pulmonary capillary endothelium causing pulmonary edema-The alveoli and small, airway is filled with oedema, fluid, tenacious, exudates, hyaline membranes, and blood, resulting in a marked right -to-left intrapulmonary shunting and very stiff lungs... Subsequently, there may be a proliferation of type II cells and eventually, thickening of the alveolar septa with inflammation and fibrosis-Some causes of ARDS are extensive viral pneumonia. Widespread fat emboli inhalation or aspiration corrosive chemical substances, near drowning severe shock, severe trauma, sepsis fluid overload, and oxygen toxicity ARDS develops in patients with no previous h/o pulmonary disease, and its onset is 24-48 hours after serious trauma or illness. The onset is marked by tachypnea, the retractions, and cyanosis. There is often relentless progression, despite therapeutic efforts, to acute respiratory failure –The essentials of diagnosis are acute Respiratory failure, severe progressive hypoxemia –and markedly decreased lung compliance (stiff lung). Blood gas determinations show hypoxemia and metabolic acidosis earlyin the course of the disease. As the process progresses, C02 detention develops. Calculated! Alveolar to arterial oxygen gradients will become progressively larger, reflecting an increasing, right-to-left shunt. Because of the marked pulmonary edema and surfactant deficiency, the lungs become very stiff and tidal volumes quite small-Initially the x-rays are normal, but with the onset of Respiratory failure bilateral patchy will appear and eventually coalesce as lung aeration deteriorates.

Optimal resuscitation and treatment of the underlying condition are imports in minimizing the risk of and severity of ARDS. General therapeutic measures should include careful monitoring of fluid intake and output to minimize the amount of extra. Vascular lung water (. minimizing intravascular volume when possible) careful monitoring of intravascular pressures, filtering of any blood administered through a filter (25-40 micro-m filter)to remove any macro aggregates, vigorous chest physiotherapy, and postural drainage, and maintaining caloric intake. Diuretics as furosemide may be useful. Aggressive ventilator support should be initiated when a patient requires oxygen in a concentration greater than 60% to maintain satisfactory p02. A volume ventilator is desirable since high pressures may be needed for adequate ventilation. Initially, continuous airway pressure may be sufficient to improve oxygenation. Short term corticosteroids may be used (use in high doses). Because of the severity of the pulmonary insufficiency and the often-severe associated precipitating insult, prognosis is generally poor, skillful use of ventilators, pulmonary physiotherapy, continuous positive airway pressure, and fluid management may improve the outlook. Patients recovering from the ARDS probably have persistence of some degree of interstitial lung disease although there is progressive normalization of lung volumes and compliance.

CONGENITAL PULMONARY LYMPHANGIECTASIS

Congenital dilatation of the pulmonary lymphatic causes respiratory failure and death within thefirst few days of life. Lymphatic dilatation of lungs is secondary to a primary developmental defect of the pulmonary lymphatic, pulmonary venous obstruction or occasionally as a part of a syndrome of generalized lymphangiectasia. Symptoms starts usually at birth, with cyanosis and respiratory distress , but may be delayed occasionally for a few days or weeks after birth.

The condition is twice more common in the males; and lung biopsy confirms the diagnosis by showing marked, irregular cystic dilatation of pulmonary lymphatic vessels and some interstitialfibrosis. Chest X-ray shows hyper aeration and diffuse nodular or reticular parenchymal lesions. If the patient survives for some time, X-ray lesions become bullous. The differential diagnosis includesRBS, aspiration pneumonitis, pulmonary hemorrhage, fulminant pneumonia, and in the patients who survive the newborn period, chronic lung disease, pulmonary edema, and cystic fibrosis. Oxygen, digitalis, diuretics may give some relief but there is no effective treatment.

NEUROMUSCULAR DISORDERS

Diseases that can cause weakness of the respiratory muscles can result in chronic hypoventilation and inability to effectively clear secretions and maintain n normal lung volumes and may ultimately progress to respiratory failure . These patients areespecially susceptible to get recurrent pneumonia -As the involvement becomes more severe, such patients have decreased breath sounds, rales, wheezes, and dullness to percussion at the lung bases. Chest X-ray shows elevated diaphragms and often increased Broncho vascular markings with infiltrates. Arterial blood gas will demonstrate hypoxemia and at a later stage, C02 retention with respiratory acidosis that may or may not is compensated. Pulmonary function, tests show decreased functional residual capacity, maximum expiratory flow rates, andlung compliance. It is important to measure the tidal volume or vital capacity of these points since a vital capacity less than twice the tidal, volume indicates that the patient will be unable to produce an effective cough and may require intubation for pulmonary toilet and prevention of respiratory failure . Patients benefit from vigorous chest physiotherapy at regular intervals with postural drainage and chest percussion. Various neuromuscular diseases that can cause respiratory failure include myasthenia gravis, Guillain Barre syndrome, muscular dystrophy cervical spinal cord injury, Werdnig-Hoffman disease. Poliomyelitis, and respiratory paralysis, associated with polymyxin therapy The prognosis depends on the underlying cause.

EMPHYSEMA

Emphysema is a distension or rupture of the alveoli. There is a loss of the elastic tissue- properties of the lung tissue, and thus distention of alveoli with or without destruction of alveolarwalls, resulting in air trapping. Emphysema may be generalized or localized, may involve part or all the lung, and maybeobstructive or compensatory. Compensatory emphysema occurs.

COMPENSATORY EMPHYSEMA

Compensatory emphysema occurs when the normally functioning lung tissue expands to fill thespace of the collapse or absent part of the lung. When for any reason, a sizable portion of the lungs is partially or completely airless (as in pneumonia, atelectasis, empyema, pneumothorax), the unaffected portion of the lung expands to compensate for the deficient tissue. Compensatoryemphysema may be acute or chronic.

OBSTRUCTIVE EMPHYSEMA

When there is a partial or complete obstruction to a bronchus or a bronchiole, there is a difficulty of getting the air out of the alveoli (but relatively lesser difficulty in getting the air in) there is gradually increasing accumulation of air distal to the obstruction. Therefore, there is a bypass orcheck-valve type of obstruction. Such obstruction can be bronchial or extra bronchial. Thus, anything that lets the air in but not out will cause obstructive emphysema.

1. Localized obstructive emphysema, in such a type, a whole lung, one lobe of the lung, or only one lobule may be involved. When thebypass obstruction partially occludes the main stem bronchus, the entire lobe is emphysematous if secondary bronchus is occluded, only individual lobules are affected. Localized obstruction that can cause localized emphysema are FB and inflammatory reaction to them, intrabronchial TB, TB or tracheobronchial lymph nodes, intrabronchial and mediastina tumors, vascular ring, local inflammation due to viral or bacterial infection. When most or all a lobe is involved, percussion note is hyper resonant over the area. And thebreath sounds decreased in intensity. The distended lung may extend across the mediastinum into the opposite hemi thorax Fluoroscopy, during expiration, shows that the emphysematous area does not decrease in size, andthe heart and the mediastinum shift to the opposite side (There is shift of heart and mediastinum towards the normal side during forced expiration.

2. Congenital or infantile obstructive lobar emphysema- It may lead to severe respiratory distress in the neonatal period, or

early infancy. Symptoms may appear in the neonatal period or be delayed up to 5-6 months. A part or usually all a lobe may be involved, the left upper lobe is most often involved. Check-valve obstruction is produced by defective cartilage In the bronchi, mucosal folds (which create a valve-like obstruction), bronchial stenosis, external compression by the aberrant vessel's tumors, and the like. With considerable distension, the emphysematous lung compresses the unaffected lung below or above it and the opposite lung by extending across the mediastinum, and the compression of the normal lung cause Respiratory distress. In most cases, lobectomy is indicated. Emphysema of the 3 lobes of the right lung, has been caused by anomalous location of the left pulmonary artery, which partially constricts the right main bronchus.

GENERALIZED OBSTRUCTIVE EMPHYSEMA

When there is widespread involvement of bronchioles. In a disease process, generalized emphysema occurs. This is more common in infants and occurs in respiratory infections: associatedwith cystic fibrosis acute bronchiolitis interstitial pneumonitis a typical form of acute laryngotracheobronchitis, aspiration of zinc stearate, chronic passive congestion secondary to a congenital cardiac lesion, and. miliary tuberculosis and in older child asthma is a frequent cause (while as in infants the aforesaid are common).

Emphysematous part of the lung is paler than usual light pink is distended and does not readily collapse. In chronic emphysema, there is a permanent loss of elasticity; many of the alveoli are ruptured, communicate with one another, producing distended saccules. As a result of the ruptureof the alveoli, air may enter the interstitial tissue (Interstitial emphysema) and result in pneumomediastinum and pneumothorax.

The cardinal feature of emphysema is dyspnea, usually an

expiratory type of dyspnea due to the greater difficulty in expiration inspiration, the air gets trapped in the alveoli, the lungs become increasingly over-distended, and the chest remains expanded during expiration. The reverse occurs in laryngeal obstruction, where there is interference with inspiration than expiration, and the lungs do not become fully inflated) Respiratory rate is increased, and there is rapid shallow breathing with decreased respiratory excursions because of the over-distension of the alveoli and their inability to be normally emptied through the narrowed bronchioles. Air hunger is responsible for forced expiratory movements. Overaction of the accessory muscles of the respiratory results in drawing; at the suprasternal notch, the supraclavicular space, the lower margin the thorax, andthe intercostal spaces. In drawings, comparatively are not so great as in the laryngeal and tracheal obstruction since the overinflated lung will not permit it.) There is scarcely any reduction in the size of the over-distended chest during expiration (there is a flattened chest during both inspiration and expiration in laryngeal obstruction). There is cough, tachypnea, cyanosis, and high-pitched wheeze; wheeze is especially present if there is associated emphysema. There are no hoarsenessand stridor as in laryngeal obstruction. Cyanosis is common in severe cases.

There is a hyper resonant percussion note, the breath sounds are decreased due to poor air entry,the inspiratory phase of the breathing.is less prominent than the expiratory phase, which is prolonged and roughened on auscultation, fine or medium, rales may be present. Increased resonance on percussion, shift of mediastinum, wheezing, or absence of breath sounds indicatesthat the airway involvement is sufficiently to cause air trapping.

X-RAY and fluoroscopy of the chest establish the diagnosis; the lung fields are less dense, the diaphragms are low and flattened, the ribs are farther apart than usual (widened intercostal spacesor horizontal ribs, decreased density and decreased lung markings, depressed' diaphragms

There is restriction in the movement of the diaphragm, on fluoroscopy-the normal deeming of the diaphragm during expiration is decreased, and the excursion of t the low, flattened diaphragmin the most severe cases is barely discernible. Another evidence of the retention of the air duringexpiration is a paradoxical increase in the horizontal diameters of the chest during this phase, suggesting that the lungs are merely being forced into different positions by the activity of the diaphragm (the abdominal Respiratory effort is stronger than the intercostal), and there is- no significant emptying of the trapped air.

While, aiming at the therapy, the cause should be eliminated if possible. Postural drainage and breathing; exercises should he instituted. Bronchoscopy is indicated if the condition does not clearin 8 weeks.

FAMILIAL EMPHYSEMA

Familial emphysema due to alpha-i-antitrypsin deficiency is characterized by an onset of emphysema „usually at early adulthood and progressive dyspnea in the absence of any clinical bronchitis. Probably absence of alpha-î-antitrypsin allows naturally occurring proteolysis enzymes, as well as proteolysis enzymes released from the leucocytes; destroyed during infection to slowly digest the structural protein of normal lung, leading to emphysema. Diffuse panacinar emphysema is seen on microscopy. Symptoms generally start at or after 3rd decade, but rarely adolescents or children may be involved. This is an autosomal recessive disease and heterozygotes may also have an increased risk of developing lung di diseased of the population carries the gene and 1:.2000 births are homozygous recessive, Associated juvenile hepatic cirrhosis may also be present. Diagnosis is by absence of the alpha-i-globulin peak in routine protein electrophoresis, and specific assay of antitrypsin activity and Pi (protease inhibitor) typingis most definitive. These patients should avoid pulmonary irritants such as smoking and environmental pollution.

BULLOUS EMPHYSEMA

Bullous emphysematous blebs or cyst and (pneumatoceles)result from the over distension of and rupture of alveoli during birth, or shortly thereafter, or they may be sequels of pneumonia and of other infections; they have been observed, in tuberculosis. Also, especially during treatment Rupture of distended alveoli form a sing or multiloculated cavities. At times, the cysts may assume large proportions and besides air –they may contain some fluid, and an air-fluid level may be seen on X-ray. The cysts, in most cases disappear spontaneously within a few months, but these may persist for a year or so. There is never any indication for inter fearing and unless there is severe respiratory distress or cardiac embarrassment no surgery or aspiration should be attempted.

SUBCUTANEOUS EMPHYSEMA.

Whenever free air finds its way into the SC tissue, it is SC emphysema and that may occur as a computation of a fracture of the orbit permitting air to escape from the nasal sinuses, in. the neck and over the thorax emphysema may follow tracheotomy ulcerations in the pharyngeal region- esophageal wounds or any perforating lesion of the larynx or trachea occasionally may complicate thoracic sis, asthma follow abdominal surgery and air may form in. in the SC.Tissue by gas-producing bacteria.

ATELECTASIS

Atelectasis in. the Imperfect expansion- or the collapse of air-bearing tissue of the lung, and thereby no aeration. of the part of a. lung. Atelectasis is common in pediatric practice. Collapse may be produced by any factor which completely obstructs the intake of air into the alveolarsacs and persists sufficiently longer to permit absorption of the alveolar trapped air into the bloodstream. In general, the causes can be divided into two groups-

1. External pressure, directly upon the pulmonary parenchyma or a bronchus or bronchiole.Atelectasis from external pressure can occur in the ways below.
2. Interference with the movements of the thoracic cage neuromuscular abnormalities as in the cerebral palsy, poliomyelitis, spinal muscular atrophy, myasthenia gravis osseous deformities asin. rickets., scoliosis., kyphosis; scleroderma. Splinting of the chest by casts, and surgical dressings.
3. Defective movement of the diaphragm, as in paralysis of the phrenic nerve, increasedabdominal pressure
4. Direct interference with expansion of the lungs, as in pleural effusion,pneumothorax, intrathoracic tumors, diaphragmatic hernia.
5. External compression of the bronchus completely obstructing the ingress of the air asenlarged lymph nodes, tumors, cardiac enlargement.
6. Airway obstruction due to extrinsic compression is usually due to an enlarged lymph node, usually associated with infection or cancer. Enlarged or aberrant vessels may occasionally cause marked extrinsic, compression of the airway sufficient to result in distal atelectasis. In addition, atelectasis can be due to direct local parenchymal compression, as secondary to lobar emphysema or pleural effusion chronic shallow respiratory due to diaphragmatic hernia or muscular from Intra bronchial or intrabronchial obstruction. Complete intrabronchial obstruction of a bronchus may be produced by a FB, neoplasm granulomatous tissue as in TB or by secretions as in cystic fibrosis, bronchiectasis, pulmonary abscess allergy chronic bronchitis, oracute laryngotracheal bronchitis. Thus, obstruction of a major airway may be caused by a mucousplug, tumor, inflammatory tissue, or aspirated food, foreign body or vomitus, and end bronchial TB. Atelectasis is a common

finding in cystic fibrosis and asthma. Allergic children have a tendency towards the right middle lobe atelectasis which may be chronic or recurrent. Atopy is the commonest cause of it. At right middle lobe, atelectasis. Postoperative atelectasis is also not especially when the anesthesia timeis prolonged or if the surgery involves a major abdominal operation. Obstruction of one more bronchiole in each area may be produced by many diseases, but the widespread bronchiolar obstruction is most often produced by bronchiolitis or interstitial pneumonitis and asthma. Generalized obstructive emphysema is the initial result; of such bronchiolar obstructions, but as the pathologic changes progress, some of the bronchioles my feet completely obstructed, and then is their interspersed areas of atelectasis and Patchy emphysema atelectasis is relatively common in acute bronchiolitis and asthma and is always present in advanced chronic diffuse infections such as the pulmonary infection associated with cystic fibrosis. Any factor is responsible for a continuously decreased amplitude of respiratory paralysis may be contributory. The flex stimuli may be the initiating factors. Pulmonary embolism, intraabdominal manipulation, and trauma to the chest wall are capable of initiating bronchoconstriction and increased Broncho secretion. Allergy is also responsible for atelectasis via the bronchospasm (spasm of thebronchial or bronchiolar musculature and production of an exudate that occludes the lumen.

No narration of the lung is usually due to complete obstruction of the conducting airway withresorption of all dismal air or to instability and collapse of the terminal air spaces, Oftenassociated with inadequate surfactant as in hyaline membrane disease or shock, lung. The extent of the nonaeration or collapse may vary from entire lung to involvement of only verydistal air spaces in localized or diffuse obstruction.

PATHOLOGY

The atelectasis areas, are airless, congested, deep red, have a firm consistency, and depressed below the neighemoglobinring healthy or emphysematous lung. When there is extensive; atelectasis ofone or more lobes, there is usually compensatory emphysema of the air-bearing lung.

CLINICAL FINDINGS

The clinical features depend on the extent and distribution of the atelectasis. And its cause indeed. A small area of the atelectasis will be asymptomatic. Patients may present with persistent cough and fever. When a large area of the lung becomes atelectatic, and especially when it does so suddenly, there is dyspnea with rapid shallow breaths, tachycardia, and often cyanosis. in the obstruction is removed, »the symptoms disappear suddenly. Even atelectasis of the entire lobe may not be responsible for changes in the. Percussion notes, due to compensatory emphysema of the adjacent lung tissue. Physical examination may reveal tachypnea, rales or wheezing, or a localized decrease in breath sounds. ln pts. With chronic: atelectasis, the volume loss In the affected area, may be so complete that no localized dullness to percussion or decreasedbreath sounds can be detected on physical examination of breath And voice sounds are decreased orabsent over extensive atelectasis areas if there is

an infection; elsewhere in the lung, there may be temperature elevations tuberculin test is done, with associated leukocytosis if there is an infection inolder pts. With significant atelectasis, or it may be possible to measure a decrease in lung volumesby pulmonary function testing. Most patients with significant atelectasis, particularly those with reactive airway disease such as asthma, will also have decreased maximal expiratory flow rates on pulmonary function and testing.
A chest X-ray may show diffuse patchy, lobar, or linear infiltrates, signs of unilateral or more localized volume loss (unilateral _diaphragmatic elevation, mediastinal shift, hilar elevation, or elevated or lowered fissure lines.) or areas of compensatory hyperinflation. When the atelectasisareas are small, there is difficulty in differentiating them from the pneumonic consolidations, those areas which Involve several lobules of a lobe; can be identified by the contraction of the area. When one or more lobes are atelectatic, the X-ray picture is that off massive collapse.

Bronchoscopy examination will reveal a collapsed main bronchus when the obstruction is at thetracheobronchial junction and may also disclose the nature of the obstruction.

TREATMENT

The bronchoscopic examination is indicated when an isolated area of atelectasis persists for several days and immediately if it is the result of the foreign body if there is Reason to believe that it isdue to any relievable bronchial obstruction. Frequent changes in the child 's position and deep breathing are beneficial. Vigorous: treatment of the underlying disorder is started, and vigorous chest percussion and postural drainage combined with bronchodilator administration are inhaled. Oral or both). The pulmonary physiotherapy should be directed toward the affected If a localizedlobar or segmental atelectasis persists for 1-2 months diteoptimal medical therapy, bronchoscopic examination and therapy is indicated -Various- types of positive pressure mechanical breathing devices may aid in re-expanding the involved pulmonary, segment.

Oxygen therapy is indie a ted when -there is- dyspnea. Morphine or Atro nine are contraindicated. Lobectomy is indicated only after failure to. Expand the lung with at least. 1-years of optimal therapy. There is no evidence that intermittent positive. Pressure breathing iseffective long-term therapy for atelectasis due to large airway obstruction. Children with right middle lobe atelectasis should be evaluated for asthma and, if appropriate,treated with chronic bronchodilator therapy.

MASSIVE PULMONARY ATELECTASIS

Massive collapse of one or both lungs is most often a postoperative complication but occasionally results from other causes such as trauma, asthma, pneumonia, tension pneumothorax,The aspiration of foreign material, either a solid object large enough to obstruct a main stem bronchus or liquids such as water or blood, or paralyses- such as that in diphtheria or poliomyelitis. Massive atelectasis is usually produced by a combination of factors- immobilization or decreased use of the diaphragm and the respiratory muscles, obstruction of the bronchial tree, and the abolition of the cough reflex. In postoperative cases, the onset is within 24 hours after the operation but may not occur for several days. There is dyspnea, cyanosis, and tachycardia. The child is extremely anxious, there is likely to be prostration, and the older patient complains of pain in. the chest. The temperature is up to104F. The physical signs are characteristic: the chest appears flat on the affected side, where there is also decreased respiratory excursion, dullness to percussion, and feeble or absent breath and voice sounds.
Lower lobes are more frequently involved than upper ones.

The heart and mediastinum are displaced toward the affected side. X-ray shows the collapsed lung, the elevation of the diaphragm, narrowing of the intercostal spaces and displacement of the mediastinal structures and heart towards the affected side. Bilateral massive collapse is usually rapidly; fatal, though bronchoscopy aspiration procedure and artificial respiratory may be lifesaving. When there is bilateral atelectasis, bronchoscopy aspiration should be performed immediately. When there is only unilateral atelectasis, the child should be placed on the unaffected side. Forced coughing or crying; while the child is lying on the unaffected side and positive pressure ventilation may alsobe. Helpful. If these measures are not helpful, bronchoscopy aspiration should be performed.
Relapses are frequent, and the child should be kept under constant observation.

PNEUMOTHORAX

Pneumothorax pneumomediastinum, pneumopericardium, pulmonary interstitial emphysema Acute pulmonary interstitial and mediastina emphysema (air block) and pneumothorax are characterized by an extraneous collection of the in the. Interstitial-tissues of the lungs, the mediastinum, and their facial extensions interfere with normal circulatory and respiratory functions. Especially in newborn infants, pulmonary interstitial emphysema usually precedes the other manifestations of air leak, such as pneumomediastinum pneumopericardium, pneumoperitoneum, subcutaneous emphysema, and pulmonary pseudo cyst. Pneumothorax is not common, in childhood except in the neonatal period where it occurs in 1 - 2%(incidence is higher in the premature infants), where it may be related to factors incident to birth, and be associated with interstitial emphysema and pneumomediastinum. Pneumothorax may be spontaneous, but most often, it is associated with birth trauma, positive pressure ventilation, or continuous positive airway pressure in newborn infants or in others. In staphylococcal pneumonia and- infancy, the incidence of pneumothorax is relatively high.Aside from the accidental introduction of air into the pleural cavity during thoracentesis, pneumomediastinum is uncommon in childhood. Pneumonia may occur—is because of pneumothorax, especially when in association with empyema; it may also follow pulmonary abscess, gangrene, infract, rupture of a cyst, or an emphysematous bleb (as in asthma), foreign bodies in the lung, and external thoracic trauma or surgical procedures.

In older children, it may occur with trauma-restrictive or obstructive lung disease, asthma, cystic fibrosis, or pneumonia, Broncho pleural fistula, or rupture of audio cysts, may complicate tracheotomy in them when it is associated with mediastina emphysema. Accidental or operative trauma, overinflation of the lungs, with alveolar rupture during resous citation, acute or chronic infection, atelectasis, or congenital anomalies may lead to rupture of the alveoli, with the release of the air into the perivascular sheaths. The air then diffuses along the artificial channels, with the formation of mediastinal emphysema. With further increase of pressure, the air is forced into the pleural space, causing; pneumothorax, and it may even extend into the subcutaneous tissues. Pneumothorax may be associated with, serious effusion (hydropneumothorax) or a purulent effusion (pyopneumothorax). In pneumothorax the lung collapses towards the hi plus, unless prevented! by adhesions. Bilateral pneumothorax is rare. Large accumulation of extra pulmonaryair can cause significant interference with normal venous return, thus decreasing cardiac output and blood pressure, can cause secondary atelectasis, shunting and hypoventilation -Some patients may have recurrent pneumothorax; about 20% of cases of spontaneous pneumothorax will recur,mostly within 1 year Patients with

2-3 recurrences of pneumothorax in the same hemi thorax, especially with no apparent underlying disease, need pleural stripping to remove the pleural apace.

X-rays of the chest obtained with barium swallow in various views to permit evaluation of all 4 cardiac chambers both great arteries., and pulmonary vasculature to determine the magnitude of pulmonary flow. Cardiac catheterization with visual contrast studies is the only definite way by which the complete hemodynamic, functional, and anatomic picture of the patients abnormality can be obtained. It gives information regarding oxygen saturation and pressure changes in the various heart chambers, and great vessels; systemic and pulmonary blood flowsand resistances; localization of, direction, and quantitation of shunts; and changes in cardiac and pulmonary function. Obstructive or regurgitating lesions can be identified.

Angiocardiography in two planes provides a clear picture of the cardiac anatomy. Other diagnostic measures as vectorcardiography, phonocardiography, and exercise testing may helpin diagnostic and assessment efforts. Echocardiography is important as an aid in planning themore definitive invasive procedures. Some use radioactive tracer techniques. Recognition of CHD in the neonate depends upon the early detection of cyanosis, cardiac murmurs, and cardiac failure. Cardiac murmurs in neonate do not necessarily mean severe cardiac disease, their presence deserves careful evaluation, however. The absence, of a cardiac murmur does not exclude heart disease-indeed absence of murmurs in presence of cardiac failure or cyanosis in the newborn period is indicative of a severe cardiac abnormality.

- The primary presentation of CHD in the neonatal period-presenting as cyanosis, TGA, tetralogy, pulmonary atresia pulmonary stenosis with intact ventricular septum tricuspid atresia, complex obstructive syndromes (Pulmonary nary obstruction) as: dextrocardia, asplenic syndrome, or polysplenia syndrome; Ebstein's anomaly of the tricuspid valve,and total anomalous pulverous return with obstruction.

- presenting as CCF, PDA, VSD, double outlet right ventricle, single ventricle, persistent truncus arteriosus, TGA with VSD, aortic atresia, coarctation of aorta syndrome, hyperplastic left heart syndrome, total anomalous pulmonary venous return, arteriovenous; fistula, and endocardia fibroelastosis.
- Presenting as cardiac murmurs. PDA, VSD, persistent atrioventricular canal, aortic stenosis, pulmonary stenosis, single ventricle double outlet right ventricle, atrioventricular valvularregurgitation arteriovenous, fistula -presenting as arrhythmias, supraventricular tachyarrhythmia, and complete congenital heartblock.

Ventricular Septal Defects (VSD)

VSD is the most common congenital cardiac defect accounting for 1/4 of all patients with CHD. Defect may occur anywhere in the septum but most commonly in in the membranous septum below the crista supraventricular is close to aortic valve in the outflow area of the left ventricle. The size ofdefect is more important than its site and the commonest type is a small one about 0.5 cm in diameter. Defects may less commonly be larger in other locations and in muscular parts of the septum also. Defects commonly involve the outflow area of the ventricle, and defects they are in the inflow portion of the septum are muscular and may be single or multiple. The commonest one is a single isolated lesion.

HEMODYNAMICS

This depends on the size of the defect, and the response of the pulmonary vasculature. With a small de feet, cardiac chambers and pulmonary vessels are normal. When large significant L-

Pshunting and pulmonary. Hypertension occurs, leading to RVH and LVH and dilatation, and enlargement of the left atrium. The pulmonary artery is large. The fetal circulation is not jeopardized even with a large communication between the ventricles because the high pulmonary vascular resistance of the fetus limits the left-to-right shunting. After birth, the magnitude of the L- P shunt is determined by the size of the defect and the ratio of systemic to pulmonary vascular resistance. Left to right shunting occurs as pulmonary vascular resistance falls. (this may take several weeks). Therefore, torrential pulmonary flows are not usual in neonate, and death with overt COF is also not usual in isolated VSD in the first month. Since the fall of pulmonary vase resistance is rapid in premature, with, a large defect, COF manifests earlier.

In the older child, the defect does not permit large L-P shunting and rt ventricular and pulmonaryarterial pressures are normal ordinarily, but since the magnitude of the shunt is inversely related tothe pulmonary vascular resistance, a marked increase in pulmonary vase resistance will limit the magnitude of L-R shunting and may result in a bidirectional shunt, or a predominately R~L (reversed) shunting. Thus, Kisenmengers syndrome is where pulmonary hypertension with reversedshunt through the VSD occurs. Increased pulmonary vascular resistance may be due to hypertrophy of the media of the small muscular pulmonary arterioles (During infancy, the media of the small pulmonaryarteries and arterioles are thick, which may represent retention of the normal fetal pulmonary vasculature »or a Response to pulmonary hypertension).

In the presence of a L-R shunt the right ventricular output is supplemented by blood shunted across the defect so that pulmonary arterial blood flow increase, increasing the return of pulmonary venousblood to the left atrium and ventricle. The resultant left ventricular diastolic overload producesa larger stroke volume and left vent hypertrophy with dilatation.

Increased pulmonary flow contributes to increased pressure (hyperkinetic pulmonary hypertension), but other factors also may be important for pulmonary hypertension since the closure of the shunt is not always followed by the immediate reduction of pulmonary arterial pressure.

Clinical features: The features of VSD depend on the hemodynamics which in turn is determinedby size of the defect and the state of pulmonary vasculature. Patients with small or moderate left to right shunting usually have no cardiovascular symptoms butmay have a h/o frequent reap infections in infancy and early childhood.

With small defects: There is small L-R shunting, and pulmonary arterial pressure is normal. The patients are asymptomatic, there are no lifts, heaves, thrills, or shocks. The lesions are only found on routine examination. The first sound at the apex is normal, and the 2nd sound at the pulmonary area is split (physiologically). The typical finding is a loud, rash, or blowing left parasternal pansystolic murmur, heard best over the lower left sternal border. An associated thrill may be present. There are no diastolic murmurs. The murmur may be present at birth or may appear weeks after birth. In a few cases the murmur ends well before the 2nd sound because there occurs closure of defect during late systole. This atypical murmur become pan systolic after administration of phenylephrine. The long systolic murmur (hallmark of VSD) may be inaudibleduring first few weeks in neonates because the pulmonary vascular resistance remains elevated in neonates with VSD which limits the left-right shunting. In premature the baby- the murmur isaudible early since the pulmonary vascular resistance falls early. The murmur is best heard at the left sternal border in the 3rd and 4th space, but slight radiation to entire precordial occurs., and to back.

Moderate defects with moderate L-R shunting, Some

moderate defects behave as mild lesionsand some as large one's Moderate defects may result in large left to right shunts, and mild to moderate increases in pulmonary arterial pressures and resistance. During infancy, the symptoms are tachypnea, dyspnea, feeding difficulties, slew physical development, and recurrent pulmonary infections with or without CCF. The cardiac failure usually responds to medical therapy. There isslight predominance of precordial, and sternum systolic thrill is palpable at the lower left sternal border between the 3rd and 4th space. The 2nd sound at the pulmonary and apical area is most often normal and split but may be single. Murmurs in moderate defects-A harsh pan systolic murmur, which is loud and harsh, heard best atthe lower sternal border in the 3-4th space area, has a wide distribution over the precordium andmay be heard at back (but loudest at the lower left sternal area). The increased pulmonary blood flow produces a systolic ejection murmur heard best at the uppersternal border.

The increased pulmonary venous, return leads to à large flow across the mitral valve which generates the rumbling mid-diastolic murmur, best heard at the apex. This murmur indicates that the flowacross the mitral valve is large, and that pulmonary: systemic blood flow ratio is at least 2:1.
The small and some moderate defects frequently close, by 2 years of age spontaneously, but the closure, may be delayed until later childhood. Improvement after 1-2 years is usual with moderatedefects, due to relative _or absolute decrease in size of the defect.

Patients with large defects is sick in early infancy, with recurrent respiratory infections, includingbouts of pneumonitis, growth retardation, feeding difficulties, profuse perspiration, episodes of CCF, dyspnea, exercise intolerance, and fatigue. Episodes of COF develop between 1-6 months only. PC cyanosis, in the absence of raised pulmonary pressure, is not seen, but a dusky plethora may be noted during infections and crying. The anterior portion of the cheat gets protruded (especially left precordium and sternum)-there is cardiomegaly with a palpable parasternal lift and apical thrust, common systolic thrills, the usual murmur as in moderate defects, but thesound of Pulmonary valve closure is louder, and the 2nd sound is narrowly split or single (with accentuated pulmonary component). If the apical diastolic murmur is present, it indicates a significant L-R shunt (as the blood returns to the left side of the heart via the mitral valve) Large defects cause the excessive pulmonary left side of the heart via the mitral valve). Large defects cause excessivepulmonary flow and thus pulmonary hypertension When the defect is extra-large progressive increases, in shunting occurs as the pulmonary bleed- vascular resistance continues to fall. Thelarge pulmonary blood flow places an increased diastolic load on the left ventricle, which eventually fails, followed by right ventricular failure. In these patients COF occurs by 6-12 weeks only. In severe cases (and some moderate ones with pulmonary blood flow more than 2 times the systemic blood flow the 3rd sound in the mitral area is frequently heard, usually before the mid-diastolic murmur., due to the rapid inflow of large amounts of blood in the early-stage diastolic phase from the left atrium to the left ventricle across the normal mitral area.

If the shunt across the defect is limited by a significant elevation of pulmonary arterial pressure, the symptoms may appear to be less severe, but physical underdevelopment and easy fatigabilityare usual. Mild cyanosis due to concomitant R-L shunt may be observed during intercurrent pulmonary infections. There is a bulge of precordial and sternum, moderate cardiomegaly with aprominent left parasternal lift, a pulmonary ejection click is frequent and initiates a systolic ejection murmur; the 2nd sound is narrowly split, with a booming pulmonary component. An early diastolic murmur (od pulmonary valve incompetence) is somctimes heard. Thus, the essentials: of diagnosis in VSD are small or moderate shunts, without pulmonary hypertension-an asymptomatic child having thetypical murmur, without any accentuation of P2.

Large L-R shunts present with CCF, easy fatigue ability, hyperactive heart with biventricularenlargement, the typical murmur, with accentuation of P2, and diastolic murmurs at the apex.
Insignificant L-R shunt or bidirectional shunts present as mild cyanosis, quiet pericardium withright ventricular lift, palpable P2, and short ejection systolic murmur along the left sternal border.

X-RAYS:

1. In mild defects, rays are usually normal, but there may be minimal cardiomegaly and slight increase in the vasculature of pulmonary vessels
2. Moderate size defects. Show moderate cardiomegaly with some prominence of both ventricles and the left atrium. The shadow of the main pulmonary artery may be prominent, pulmonary over circulation is usual.
3. With large defects gross cardiomegaly is usual, within prominence of both ventricles, the leftatrium, and pulmonary artery. The ascending aorta and aortic knob are relatively small.
4. In cases where, due to elevated pulmonary arterial resistance, shunting is limited, there is moderate cardiomegaly, some prominence of both a right and left ventricular shadows.

Prominence and increased pulsations of the pulmonary artery trunk and its primary divisions contrast with the narrow peripheral branches of the pulmonary arterial tree. In cases with advanced pulmonary vascular disease, theheart is smaller, the main pulmonary artery bulges, and pulmonary blood flow is reduced.

ECG.

ECG estimates the size of the VSD and the type of pulmonary vasculature Response to it.

- In small defects, ECG is normal usually (but there may be isolated left or combined VH)
- Moderate and large defects with normal pulmonary arterial pressures usually show LVH (prominent Q and R waves).
- With larger defects with pulmonary hypertension, there is combined hypertrophy as RHV, and RHV. Pulmonary hypertension may be due to increased flow or increased resistance, or both.
- With pulmonary hypertension from, pulmonary vascular obstruction, there is pure RVH. Thus, in Eisenmenger's complex we have severe RVH and marked rt axis deviation. When left atrium isenlarged, peaked, or notched waves may be seen.

CARDIAC CATHETERIZATION

Cardiac catheterization quantitates the effects of VSD on pulmonary and systemic circulation and adds to diagnose any undetected clinical abnormalities that may be associated with VSD. The blood from the right ventricle has a higher 02 concentration, than, from the right atrium, the differences of pressure in heart chambers, and main arterial trunks are noted.

Pulmonary pressure may be normal or equal to systemic. Small defects, have normal right ventricular and pulmonary artery pressures, while as in larger defects, these pressures are elevated and may approach systemic level. The catheter may pass from the right into the left side of heart via the defect. Angiocardiography reveals the septal defect with passage of contrast medium from theright into left ventricle via the defect. Thus, left ventriculography established the location and number of defects. The indisputable evidence of VSD is passage of catheter from right to left ventricle via the septaldefect.

PROGNOSIS AND COURSE

-About 50% of the VSDs close spontaneously; these are usually small defects, and close within the first few months of life. It is unusual for moderate to large feets to close spontaneously –but they may decrease in size or close. If the patient survives the first 1-2 years, the patient improves symptomatically. Larger defects have closed spontaneously in the 2nd-3rd decades.

Asymptomatic patients with hearts normal in size on X-ray and without pulmonary hypertensionhave shunts of less than 2:1 on cardiac and catheterization, and their defect shrinks slowly, and eventually, get smaller. These have small defects that need no surgery. Thus, many children regain asymptomatic without evidence of an increase in heart size, pulmonary arterial pressure, or resistance.

Even if the patient is asymptomatic from a small defect, there is the risk of SABE; it occurs in less than 1% of cases of VSD. A small but significant number of patients get recurrent respiratory infections and CCF. Infants with large defects develop COF during infancy and, if not treated, die. These pts. may heed surgery during infancy because of the intractable CCF, or surgery before 2 years of age because of the progression of pulmonary hypertension, or surgery between 2-5 years of age as an elective procedure. During childhood and adolescence, patients who survive the first 2 years of life do well, during early adulthood, may develop the irreversible pulmonary vascular obstructive disease.

Some are born with pulmonary hypertension that does not regress and thus are rendered inoperable, others develop inoperable pulmonary hype tension progressively over years. It is apparent that most cases of irreversible pulmonary hypertension can be prevented by surgical repair of the defect before 2 years of age. Pulmonary hypertension, in most of cases, does not progress during childhood but in some cases may increase during childhood, or more particularly in adolescenceand adulthood. A small number develop pulmonary stenosis, which protects the pulmonary circulation in these patients the clinical picture changes from that of VSD with large L-R shunt to that of a VSD with pulmonary stenosis.

Treatment

-Patients who develop COF should know be treated vigorously, and. those who respond well shouldcontinue digitalis until surgical correction is tin defect is done. It is often possible to discontinue digitalis after age 2. But if the patient does not respond to vigorous- anti-failure treatment, or shows signs of developing progressive pulmonary hypertension, surgeryis done without delay.

- As a protection against SABE, the integrity of the primary and secondary teeth should be carefully maintained, and the child should receive a large dose of penicillin to cover dental extraction, tonsillectomy, and adenoidectomy. Intercurrent infections should be treated vigorously.
- Surgery is mostly done electively between the 2-5 years of age; the ideal Candidate being a symptomatic pts, who has a moderate pulmonary hypertension and a large L-R shunt. (In these patients thesurgical mortality risk is about 5%). Patients who has pulmonary systolic pressures, approaching those of systemic level, but have no R-L shunt or but have large L-R shunts are still the candidates, butthe mortality is higher.

The candidates for surgery are those with cardiomegaly, poor growth, poor exercise tolerance, orother clinical abnormalities who have cardiac catheterization findings of the significant shunt (2:1 or greater) and without significant pulmonary hypertension (greater than 10 units of resistance).

In general patients with mean pulmonary artery pressures equal to systemic pressures, who are not responsive to 02 administration, with no left to right shunt or bidirectional shunt, and pulmonaryresistance to be greater than 10 units or pulses resistance ratio more than 0.7, are considered inoperable generally. There are others who have pulmonary hypertension of lesser degree, but operative risk is higher. Operative mortality without pulmonary hypertension is only while as it is 25# in those with upper limits of operability. Thus, patients with significant R-L shunts and small L-R shunts are inoperable.

Infants: with large VSD, torrential pulmonary blood flow through-the, pulmonary hypertension grease and uncontrollable COF present with problems, but digitalis and diuretics, treatment of intermittent infections, especially pneumonitis, and anemia may improve the clinical course significantly when emergency operation is needed for intractable COF before 2 years., pulmonaryarterial banding helps in decreasing pulmonary blood flow., relieving CCF, and decreases frequency of recurrent pneumonitis. In latter years, the pulmonary artery is demanded and VSD closed.

In asymptomatic pts, who have a normal heart, normal ECG, and normal pressures at catheterization in lesser circulation, small defects that cause no cardiac burden (where Qp/Qs is less than 1.5-2). To prevent pulmonary hypertension, from becoming inoperable early surgical interventionshould be done in patients who have increased pulmonary resistance.

<u>VSD with AI</u>: VSD is complicated by prolapse of the aortic valve and aortic insufficiency. The features of VSD are found, and superadded features of AI, as a diastolic murmur and wide pulse pressure and the patient is confused with PDA. The patient may range from asymptomatic one with trivialaortic regurgitation and small L-R shunt to one with florid incompetence, CCF, angina pectoris, and massive

cardiomegaly who urgently will require surgical closure of the defect and relief of the aortic incompetence

<u>VSD with Lt vent-Rt atrial shunt</u>
VSD associated with an abnormal septal leaflet of the tricuspid valve leads to the ejection of left ventricular blood into the right atrium via the defect during systole giving rise to findings of VSD or ostium primula defect. As a reflection of high atrial pressure, there is a large systolic venous pulsation in the neck. Cardiac catheterization by showing an L-R shunt at the atrial level may lead to misdiagnosis of ASD. Left ventriculography rapidly leads bopacification of atrium. Treatment is closure of VSD.

VSD with the origin of both great vessels from the Rt ventricle
Since both aorta and pulmonary artery arise from the left ventricle, the only outlet to the left ventricle is a VSD. Clinically it is like uncomplicated VSD with a large L-R shunt and in majority pulmonary hypertension is present. ECG is that of ostium premium defect, right ventriculography shows the origin of aorta, and echocardiography shows discontinuity of mitraland aortic valves.

<u>VSD with PDA</u>

In some cases, the signs, of VSD predominate and the murmur of PDÀ is inaudible. In others the signs of PDA predominate hut a systolic murmur and thrill are often present along the lowersternal border. Cardiac, catheterization reveal the left to right at the ventricular level, and the catheter passes from pulmonary artery to aorta via the ductus. Both defects are closed at the sametime.

<u>Multiple ventricular septal defects</u>
"Rarely multiple defects involve the septum, and generally these patients present in infancy with signsof large L-R

shunts and pulmonary hypertension; multiple defects are established by ventriculography only.

USD with ASD

In. patients with VSD with ostium secondum, VSD dominates the clinical picture, and the clinical picture is that of moderate or large VSD. Cardiac Catheterization shows L-R shunts at both atrial and ventricular levels.

VSD with coarctation

The signs of coarctation of aorta are clear, while the signs of VSD are confused with collaterals,associated with coarctation.

VSD with left SVC

Clinically not detectable, is established by catheterization when catheter the persistent leftsuperior vena cava from the coronary sinus. Both persistent SVC and PDA pose problems, of bleeding at the time of operation, if undetected. Otherwise, persistent SVC does not itself need treatment.

VSD with endocardial sclerosis

In pts. with VSD jet of blood shunting across the defect to the opposite right ventricular wall leading to thickened white patches in the endocardium of the right ventricle; endocardia sclerosismay occur in left atrium and left ventricle in VSD are infrequent.

VSD with heart block

Heart block is rare in VSD pts, but systolic murmurs are not unusual in patients with complete heart block and are caused by turbulence of blood associated with the large stroke volume. Patients with VSD and complete heart block should be suspected of having corrected transposition of thegreat vessels.

ATRIAL SEPTA DEFECT (ASD)

ASD accounts for 10-12% of cases of CHD in children but is the commonest condition in adults.Atrial septal defects are of 3 types:

OSTIUM SCANDIUM DEFECT:

Almost 90% cases of ASD fall in this group, and females are affected twice more commonly. It isa defect in the fossa ovalis caused by maldevelopment of the septum second. This is situated in the midportion of the interatrial septum. The atrioventricular valves are normal, but a common associated finding is partial anomalous, venous drainage from the right lung. The defects may be multiple. In symptomatic children the openings may be more than 2cm in diameter. Large defect may extend inferiorly towards the inferior vena cava and ostium of the coronary sinus and superiorly toward the superior vena cava, or posteriorly.

Hemodynamics: There is a considerable shunting of oxygenated blood from the L to R side andthis blood is added to the normal venous: return to the R atrium and is pumped to the lungs. Thepulmonary blood flow becomes 2-4 times of the systemic flow. The actual factor of importance that leads to shunting is the greater distensibility of the right side of heart (atrium, ventricle), the low pulmonary resistance, and the fact that the R-atrial pressure is slightly higher than the right L-atrium. In the infants, right ventricle is thick and less compliant which limits the L-R shunting –and therefore there is paucity of the symptoms and signs in infants. As the infant gets older, the R-ventricle becomes thinner and, the L-R shunting increases. The large workload of the R-heart leads to R-sided hypertrophy and dilatation of the pulmonary artery.

With the large pulmonary blood flow, pulmonary arterial pressure is normal (or only slightly raised) during childhood, but pulmonary hypertension and increased pulmonary vascular resistance increasesafter the 3rd decade of life; at this time L-R shunting decreases and finally R-L shunting will develop. Thus, in ASD, RVH and pulmonary dilatation occurs while as left ventricle and aorta are smaller than usual due to less amount of blood carried by them. Progressive dilatation of the R- ventricle may lead to heart failure. Cyanosis in ASD is either associated with COF or Eisenmenger's syndrome.

CLINICAL FEATURES

The patients is usually symptomatic when it is discovered during routine examination. With larger defects, the older child may complain of recurrent episodes of pneumonitis — frequently complicated by segmental pulmonary collapse, mild fatigue, exercise intolerance, and dyspnea on effort. Thus, some may develop easy fatigability whereas others mayremain absolutely symptom free during childhood. COF rarely develops in infants and young children and thus, most children with ASD do not have cardiovascular symptoms. But an occasional child may present with florid COF often unresponsive to drugs thus necessitating early surgery. Physical development of the children is usually normal but may be retarded.

Arterial pulses are normal, and equal throughout, venous pressure is normal unless there is associated tricuspid insufficiency or heart failure. The heart is of variable size and may be grossly enlarged or normal.

There is a systolic lift (heaving impulse) felt along the left sternal border, and it even can bepalpated up to the midclavicular line; it is due to systolic contraction of the dilated R- ventricular (there is a hyperdynamic R-ventricular heave). There are no thrills, but in thin chests, when a murmur is loud, the thrill may be present A loud first heart sound precedes the murmur; sometimes, a pulmonary ejection sound may accompany it). The 2nd heart sound is widely split and fixed in all phases of respiratory in the majority of patients atthe pulmonary area (at the upper left sternal edge). Wide splitting of the 2nd sound is due to prolongation of R-ventricular systole because of large stroke volume -which can 't be reduced, as in the normal, on expiration. Without the widely split 2nd, a sound diagnosis of ASD is questionable. Pulmonary valve closure is accentuated.

Typical murmur-a soft systolic murmur (ejection type), blowing, seldom accompanied by a thrill. Best heard over the upper left sternal border, radiating into the upper lung fields, best heard at the left y upper sternal border in the 2nd space, caused by the torrential flow of bloodacross the valve into the pulmonary artery.

There is a tremendous flow across the tricuspid valve, which leads: to a mid-diastolic murmur best heard at the lower left sternal border and apex_ (low tricuspid murmur). (caused by tremendous flow during the diastole). The presence of this murmur suggests a high flow P:S blood flow ratio over 2:1. The diastolicmurmur of pulmonary incompetence may be heard (rare). A murmur of relative pulmonary artery stenosis-may be heard in. infants.
-Associated abnormalities which may be found on. Physical examination includes pigeon chestkyphoscoliosis and high-arched palate. Lutembachers syndrome is ASD with congenital or Rhmitral stenosis.

X-RAY
Varying degrees of cardiac enlargement are usually slight due to the prominence of the right ventricleand atrium. The cardiothoracic ratio is greater than 0.5. The pulmonary artery is large, the pulmonary vascularity greatly increased, while the left ventricle and aorta are small. On fluoroscopy, increased pulsations may be noted in the hilar region (hilar

dance).

ECG

There is right axis deviation and RVH (the so-called incomplete Rt bundle branch block) ^these findings must be present for the diagnosis of uncomplicated secondium defect. Occasionally one may find tall P waves, prolonged PR interval, atrial fibrillation and complete heart block, Wolff-Parkinson-White syndrome, and complete bundle branch block. Or the ECG may be normal. There is no evidence of atrial enlargement, which is a very valuable -ve finding.

CARDIAC CATHETERIZATION

A more than 7% increase in the oxygen content of the right atrium as compared with superior vena cava and inferior vena cava samples is highly suggestive of the diagnosis. Pulmonary artery pressure is usually normal. Higher oxygen concentration in the right atrium may also be found in anomalous pulmonary venous, return to the right atrium, with VSD with tricuspid insufficiency, with ventricular-septal defects with left ventricular, right atrial shunts, and- with aortic-right atrial communications, as the ruptured sinus of Valsalva. Selective angiocardiography differentiates these. Angiocardiography in the left atrium confirms the ASD when the contrast medium passes into the right atrium. Pulmonary arteriography excludes anomalously draining pulmonary veins. In a minority of patients mixing of blood is incomplete in theright atrium so that the principal site of the shunt appears to be at the ventricular level. The pulmonary arteriolar resistance is usually normal. The shunt is usually high, as high as lit/min/sq. meter ofbody surface.

Echocardiography shows the paradoxical motion of the ventral septal wall, moving in the same direction rather than the direction opposite to that of the free left ventricular wall and dilatedright vent cavity with increased tricuspid valve excursion.

Course: Secundum septal defects, are usually well tolerated during childhood, so that in most cases. Symptoms will appear in the 3rd decade or later. Life may be normally passed,except increased frequency of respiratory infections. Cardiac failure pulmonary vascular obstructive disease, become more common after the 3rd decade. Pulmonary hypertension, atrial dysrhythmias, tricuspid incompetence, and heart failure may occasionally occur in infants and children. Bacterial endocarditis is so rare that its occurrence suggests presence of an associated CVS anomaly. Presence of symptoms, Or absence, and progressive cardiomegaly guide the prognosis. Secundum defect is usually isolated defect but may be associated with partial anomalous pulmonary venous return pulmonary valve stenosis, VSD, pulmonary arterial branch stenosis and persistent left SVC.

Treatment: A secundum defect in which P:S blood flow ratio is greater than 2:1 is closed generally. The mortality rate of the operation is less than 1% and is advised in all cases (even theasymptomatic cases) prior to entry into the school (the surgical mortality is higher in adults). Direct vision, open heart surgery is done using extra-corporeal circulation. Surgical mortality in adults is increased by pulmonary hypertension, cardiac; failure, tricuspid incompetence oratrial arrhythmias, surgery is best done between 4-7 years, just before entry to school.
The results are more gratifying in children with large shunts; symptoms disappear rapidly, andfrequently physical development is enhanced, heart size may become normal, but persistent cardiomegaly is not unusual after surgery, and many arrhythmias of atria (atrial tachycardia, flutter, fibrillation) may occur.

ENDOCARDIAL CUSHION DEFECTS

It is an anomaly resulting from the incomplete fusion of

endocardia cushions. (Endocardia cushions form the lower portion of the atrial septum, the membranous portion of the ventricular septum, and the septal leaflets of the tricuspid and mitral valves. These defects may be completeor incomplete. The complete form is the Persistent common atrioventricular canal, while the incomplete form is mostly osmium primum defect, the persistent common atrioventricular canals are a rare disorder but are 20 times more common in Downs children. The anomaly consists of a high Veda low ASD of osmium premium variety (thatis continuous with the VSD) cleft in the septal leaflet of the tricuspid valve, and in the anterior leaflet, of the mitral valve (leading to regurgitation). Thus all 4 cardiac chambers are in communication.

Thus, this lesion has, in addition to interatrial and interventricular defers, an atrioventricular valvecommon to both ventricles, consisting of an anterior and a posterior leaflet related to the ventricular septum and a lateral leaflet in each ventricle. The incomplete form of endocardia cushion defect can manifest as one of these, but the commonest is osmium primum defect; transitional varieties may occur as osmium primum defect with clefts in the anterior and septal tricuspid valve leaf lets, less commonly osmium primum with normal atrioventricular valves. In others atrial septum is normal, but VSD simulates that found in the common atrioventricular canal.

The most common partial form of endocardia cushion defect is the osmium primum defect with a cleft in the mitral valve. Thus, an osmium primum defect is situated in the lower portion of the atrial septum, overlying the mitral and tricuspid valves; the tricuspid valve is usually normal,but (there may be some thickening of the septal leaflets), but most have a cleft in the anterior Leaflet of the mitral valve.

Hemodynamics: In the Common atrioventricular canal, the L-R shunt is trans atrial as well as trans ventricular (large shunt), tricuspid and mitral regurgitation, and marked pulmonary hypertension, and commonly increased pulmonary vascular resistance. With increased pulmonary vascular resistance, the shunts get bidirectional at both atrial and ventricular levels. Usually, R-L shuntingis small and seldom causes unsaturation in the absence of increased vascular resistance, but with significant shunting, clinical cyanosis may develop; in the isolated ostium primum defect, there isL-R shunting primarily across the atrial defect with mitral regurgitation, the shunt is usually moderate or large, and degree of mitral incompetence mild to moderate, and pulmonary arterial pressures are usually normal or only moderately increased.

CLINICAL FEATURES:

Ostium premium When isolated presents as ostium secondum; many children are asymptoticand discovered on routine examination only. In them, shunts are moderate, and incompetence trivial. In them, correct diagnosis is based on apical systolic murmur and classic ECG. With larger shunts and significant incompetence, there is growth failure, dyspnea, fatigue,recurrent respiratory infections, and cardiac failure that may occur early in life.

With mitral valve insufficiency, the heart is hyperactive precordial bulge present —both right and left ventricular impulses can be palpated at the left sternal border and apex-a hyper dynamic parasternal right ventricular lift, and a left ventricular heave suggesting significant mitral incompetence. The heart is moderately enlarged. A systolic thrill may be present at the left lowersternal border and apex. On auscultation, the first heart sound is normal; the 2nd sound is widely split and fixed, the pulmonary component loud, a pulmonary ejection systolic murmur (somctimcs prcceded by a click) that radiates to the upper lung; a rumbling mid-

diastolic murmur at the lover left sternal edge (all these are signs of L-R shunt); to these may be added signs of mitral incompetence-a harsh, apical pan systolic murmur, heard at the left lower sternal border and apex with radiation to the left axilla(this murmur may even be short and musical).
In common atrioventricular canal-patients are severely affected, and COF often develops in infancy. Recurrent bouts of infection are common in infancy. Therefore, contrary to the above, severecardiac failure, repeated Respiratory infections, and failure to thrive are common and seen early.

The findings are often consistent with a large VSD; an undernourished and small infant with signs of cardiac failure; sternum bulging anteriorly from a markedly enlarged heart the heart hyperactive and both right and left impulses are palpable; a systolic thrill may be palpated at the lower left sternal border;2nd sound is split with accentuated pulmonary component; first sound normal or accentuated, and followed by the Haran, widely distributed pan systolic murmur (transmitted to the entire pericardium, out best heard at the lowboy left sternal border); 2nd sound is widely split because pulmonary blood flow is torrential; if severe pulmonary hypertension develops, the splitting is not wide, but pulmonary valve closure is loud. A mid-diastolic murmur of low Frequency (low pitched) is audible at the lower left sternal border, and at the apex. A pulmonary cystoleic ejection murmur is produced by the large pulmonary flow.

When severe pulmonary vascular obstruction is present, there is evidence of dominant right ventricularenlargement. A shock of the 2nd sound can be palpated in the pulmonary area. No thrill is present. The sin 2nd sound is markedly accentuated but single; a short systolic murmur (nonspecific) is heard at the lower sternal border. There is no diastolic murmur (flow murmur). Cyanosis may be seen with significant R-L shunts.

X-RAY

X-RAY in ostium primum is like that in ostium secondum, if isolated, but with significant mitral regurgitation, there is cardiomegaly; with L ventricle-R atrium shunting, the right atrium may be enlarged. In complete form, there is the enlargement of all 4 chambers of the heart; pulmonary vascular markings are increased due to over circulation in the lung, and the main pulmonary arteryis enlarged; in patients with pulmonary vascular obstruction, only the pulmonary artery segment and its branches are prominent, and the peripheral markings are decreased. Hilar dance is not unusual on fluoroscopy. The aorta is normal or small.

ECG

ECG may show large P waves suggesting atrial enlargement; prolongation of the PR interval is common; right ventricular volume overload with an incomplete right bundle branch block patternor RVH is present; there is left axis deviation in all cases of endocardia cushion defect (occasionally extreme right axis deviation) signs of biventricular hypertrophy; with mitral regurgitation, LVH occurs. Cardiac catheterization: in estium primum defect shows L-R shunting at the atria level as in ostium secondum defect; and a step up in oxygen saturation at both right atrial and ventricular levels, greatly increased pulmonary blood flow, in the complete defect. Selective angiography (Left ventriculography) a characteristic Goose-Neck deformity, is seen in the complete form, the distortion of the outflow of the left ventricle. Crystal echocardiography and contrast c echocardiography are highly useful in differentiating the subgroups of endocardia cushion defects.

COURSE:

Course and prognosis depend on the magnitude of the L-R shunt, the degree of pulmonary vascular resistance, and the severity of mitral incompetence. Death during infancy is common with complete defect, many patients with ostium primum defects is asymptomatic or have only minor non-progressive symptoms until they reach the 3-4th decade because of the associated anomalies as mitral regurgitation, more severe symptoms may present with ostium primum than with secondum defects. Complete defect usually develops cardiac failure during early infancy, and in untreated cases, death may occur before months of age, and in older children progressive pulmonary vascular obstructive disease is common and may occur for 3 years of age.

TREATMENT

In incomplete form. Surgical repair(5-8years) surgical repair is done, it is technically more difficult than in secondum defects, because of the associated anomalies and because of the proximity of the specialized conduction system. Mortality rate is low, 2-5% mortality rate is higher 15-25% with complete variety therefore these cases are treated better medically i.e., for COF etc. otherwise complete correction is advised in the first year of life, before the irreversible pulmonary hypertension develops.

FORAMEN OVALE

At birth or soon after the foramen, the ovale closes in 80%of hearts. The closure is permanent. In others, a slit-like opening persists an isolated, patent foramen ovale is of no clinical significance if the right atrial pressure is increased, as secondary to pulmonary stenosis or pulmonary hypartensicnvenous Wood may be shunted from the right to left atrium aero sac, the frames and result in cyanosis. Because of the anatomic structure at the valve of a patent foramenovale, blood cannot be shunted from the left atrium to the right atrium. An isolated patent foramen ovale does meet need for any treatment

SIUMS VENUS DEFECT

These defects are situated in the upper part of the atrial septum in close relation to the entry of the superior vena cava. One or more pulmonary veins, usually from the right lung, drain anomalously into the superior vena cava. Sometimes the superior vena saves straddles the defect sothat some systemic venous blood enters the left atrium. The abnormal hemodynamics are like those of secundum ASD, consisting primarily of a volume overload at the right ventricle. Clinical picture. ECG and X-ray are like those of secundum ASD. In the chest X-ray bulge of the superior V.C shadow may suggest the diagnosis, but anomalous pulmonary veins are not recognized on routine chest x-ray. Anatomic correction requires the insertion of a patch to ensure the entry of anomalous: veins into the left Atrium.

PATENT DUCTUS ARTERIOSUS

Functional closure of the duct, which takes a large part of the pulmonary arterial blood into the aorta in the fetus) normally occurs aeon after birth., but if the ductus remains patent, aortic blood, in.shunted into the pulmonary artery. PDA in a common anomaly and is very common in mothers who had rubella during the first trimester of pregnancy; the incidence in higher at high altitudes,above 10 thousand feet, is twice as more common in females, and PDA is more common In premature babies. It is peculiar among the CHEMOGLOBINs that it frequently occurs as an isolated anomaly, but associated lesions can be coarctation and VSD (thus all the 3 can be commonly associated. In some, associated anomalies it in the lesion of PDA that keeps the child alive, as in pulmonary atresia. The size of the communication is variable and. may be small to large. The aortic end of the ducting is usually distal to the left subclavian artery and the pulmonary artery is entered at the bifurcation.

HEMODYNAMICS

Since the aortic pressure is much higher than the pulmonary artery pressure, therefore the bleedwill enter from the aorta to the pulmonary artery, both during the systole and diastole. The degree of the shun depends on the size of the ductus end and the pressure gradient between the aortaand the pulmonary artery. In extreme cases, 1-/2-2/3 **cases** of the left ventricular output may be shunted through the ductus, and the oxygenated blood recirculates through the pulmonary circulation. In most cases, the pressures in the pulmonary artery, right ventricle, and right atrium are normal, but the pulmonary arterial and. right ventricular may be elevated. In large shunting, there is engorgement of the lung, hypertrophia of the left ventricle, and dilatation of the left atrium since the blood is continuously shunted through the duct us, there in a continuous murmur. Occasionally pulmonary hypertension develops. The total blood volume in increased and returned to normal limits after the surgical closure of the ductus.

CLINICAL FEATURES

The clinical features depend on the size of the shunt and the degree of pulmonary hypertension. There are usually no symptoms as the shunt is small; when the shunt is of moderate size, symptoms vary from poor feeding, slow weight gain and tachypnea (in infants), and fatigue and effort dyspnea in older children. Symptoms may appear at any age .and may include slowly progressive exceptional dyspnea followed by left Vent failure or franc CCF. With moderate shunts, symptoms may increase up to the 2nd to 3rd month but by 1 yr due to compensatory ventricular hypertrophy. improvement is seen Large defects are invariably symptomatic in infancy with the features of left ventricular failure Retardation of physical growth may be the manifestation. Rarer symptoms are precordial pain due to complicating neurecirculatery asthenia) and hoarseness from the involvement of the adjacent recurrently

SIGMA

Peripheral arterial pulses are full, and with a moderate sized shunt, the pulses are bounding; dynamically, PDA is an arteriovenous shunt of considerable extent, signs of and large pulsepressure are produced, including water-hammer pulseipicous arterial, pulsations in the neck (Corrigons).

In babies, the finding bounding pulses is often a useful the pointer to the correct diagnosis. BP recording shows a wide pulse pressure; pulse pressure is greater than; half of the systolic pressure. The law of diastolic pressure says further fall during exertion. The' heart size is usually normal and precordial activity normal, but with mode rate shunting, the precordial is hyper dynamic; the apical impulse is normal, or a left ventricular tap may be present due to LVH systolic thrill is often palpable-at: the upper left sternal border; the thrill is usually systolic butoften extends into diastole, and in some cases, are palpable throughout the whole cardiac cycle system-diastolic)

The first sound is normal, and the 2nd heart sound is narrowly split very rarely with maximal shunts2nd sound, gets paradoxically split-the 2nd sound closes on inspiration and splits on expiration.The paradoxical splitting is due to the maximal overload of the left ventricle and the prolonged lection of the blood from this chamber Murmur. The classic murmur is a systo-diastolic murmur, loud in intensity very rough machinery, continuous humming top millwheel or rolling thunder in quality, begins soon after thefirst sound, reaches maximum intensity at the end of the systole (at the 2nd heart sound) becomes a crescendo murmur during the late diastole waning to disappear before the first sound sound-The murmur may be localized to the 2nd left space but fairly well, over the lung fields anteriorly but poorly over the lung fields, posteriorly, thus, radiates down the left sternal border, or to the left clavicle. The murmur is harsh and does not have the blowing quality of the acquired lesions.

In infants, the murmurs may be typical, being prominent in systole, the diastolic component being short or indefinite in few patients with pulmonary hypertension may have only a systolic murmur. Rarely the murmur confined to the diastole only, which is due to pulmonary valvular insufficiency. In patients with a large L-S shunting, a low-pitched mitral diastolic murmur may be audible and is dueto the large blood flow across the mitral valve. With small shunts there is no CCF, and with large shunts, there is a CCF. X-ray; with small lesions, there is no abnormality with moderate and large shunts. Varying degrees of cardiomegaly are evidently affecting the left atrium and left ventricle. The pulmonary artery and main pulmonary artery branches are prominent. The cardiacsize depends on the degree of the L-R shunt. The aortic knob is prominent and pulsates vigorously. Vascularity of the lungs is increased. ECG, in most cases this, is normal with large shunts. There is left atrial and left ventricular hypertrophy. RVH may also be present Biventricular hypertrophy is especially seen when there is palm hypertension due to increased blood flow. In those with pulmonary vascular obstruction pure right VH is seen but in uncomplicated cases of PDA. LVH is seen and not RVH only. The waves are sometimes deep and indicate left diastolic ventricular overload. In the young infant a pattern of LVH and strainmay be seen.

In ordinary cases clinical features with X-ray and ECG are sufficient for diagnosis but in some cases special studies may be needed. Echo cardiograph measures left atrial hypertrophy which isan important clue to the presence of COF especially useful in premature with PDA and **CCF.**
Cardiac catheterization. In complicated cases with associated defects or PDA in infancy hemodynamics tests should be done. Confirmation of clinical diagnosis' may be obtained by demonstration of a 3-5% rise of the oxygen content of blood

from the pulmonary artery over that obtained from the right ventricle or by direct probing of ductus catheter entering the descendingaorta from the pulmonary artery. Aortography by injection of contrast medium into the ascending aorta shows opacification of the pulmonary artery from the aorta via the duct. The shunt is visualized.

COURSE AND PROGNOSIS

Many patients with PDA is asymptomatic, but the lesion is not benign; patients with small to moderateshunts usually do quite well even without surgery, but in the 3rd-4th decade of life, symptoms of easy fatigability, dyspnea on exertion and exercise intolerance usually develops because ofte development of pulmonary hypertension or CCF. Patients may live a normal life span without anycardiac embarrassment. Spontaneous closure may occur during infancy. The fare first year, especially in the prematures, but such a thing; occurs only extremely rare beyond the first year; since SABE is a potential complication, surgical ligation is recommended if the lesion persists beyond the first yr.

PDA reduces life expectancy; many patients succumbs to COF which may be preceded by attacks of left ventricular failure most common in the 3rd decade but may occur at any age; it is controlledby drugs, but patient should be operated on as soon as the condition permits SABE is the most commoncomplication in late childhood but may occur at any age. Pulmonary emboli are common -when the ductus is involved, systemic emboli occur. Once controlled by drugs. Surgery should be done optimal time for surgical treatment is 3 months after the cure of the infective process. Rarer complications are aneurysmal dilatation of the pulmonary artery or the ductus, calcification of the ductus, non-infective thrombus, thrombosis of tine ductus with embolization, paradoxical emboli and acquired rhotic heart disease and Eisenmenger's complex.

TREATMENT

All patients with PDÄ (except those with increased pulmonary vascular obstruction are ligated electively at years of age. Patients with large shunts and pulmonary hypertension may be ligated sooner (even before the age of less than l year) to prevent the development of progressive pulmonary vascular obstruction. Some advice elective surgery for simple PDA at 1 year only. Once COF is present or SABE has occurred surgery should be done as soon as these conditions have been medically controlled. COF occurs in infancy same applies. Some stretch the ligation of the asymptomatic case to 3-10 years. Operative mortality is less than 1%, and the upper limit of the surgical repair in the asymptomatic patient is 35 years since, in older people, the regional vessels are more rigid or associated with degenerative changes, and the cardiac reserve is reduced in them. Pulmonary hypertension is not a contraindication to operation if the shunt is from the aorta to the pulmonary artery and notreversed. Division with suture if feasible is better than simple ligation.

After surgery symptoms of frank or incipient cardiac failure rapidly disappear and if the patient was physically stunted there is usually an improvement in physical development within a year or two. The pulse and blood pressure return to normal, and the machinery murmur is replaced by twonormal heart sounds. In a few patients a systolic murmur over the pulmonary area may persist. The murmur may be the result of turbulence in a persistently dilated pulmonary artery, or rarely an unsuspected associated VSD or ASD. X-ray signs of cardiomegaly and pulmonary overcirculation also disappear and ECG becomes normal. If preoperatively pulmonary hypertension was present, it also recedes.

Patients with nonreactive pulmonary vascular obstruction

who have a resistance greater than 10 unitsand a pulmonary/systemic resistance ratio of more than 0.7 should not be operated upon since they are made worse by the closure of the ductus (ductus in them serves as an escape route limiting the degree of pulmonary hypertension.

PDA in INFANCY

Aside from the usual symptoms, an isolated PDA may occasionally produce symptoms of severe COF or left-sided heart failure during the first 2 years of life; these symptoms are frequently precipitatedby respiratory infections. Again, the presence or absence of the diastolic component of murmur depends on the pressure relations between the aorta, and the pulmonary artery-If secondary pulmonary hypertension develops lops, there is no flow of blood during diastole, and only a systolic murmur is present. If the pulmonary arterial pressure is normal, the typical machinery murmur may present early, even in infants a few weeks of age. ln addition, the pulse pressure is the wide band the heart is moderate to grossly enlarged, the main chambers involved are the left ventricle and atrium. X-ray shows the enlargement of the chambers and reveals prominent pulmonary arteries and increased aortic pulse actions. ECG may be normal or show evidence Of left ventricular dominanceor biventricular hypertrophy. Surgical intervention produces marked relief of symptoms. Surgical therapy is indicated in all symptomatic patients irrespective of age and has been successfully performed invery young infants

PDA IN PREMATURE BABIES

PDA is present in 10-15% of premature babies, those weighing less than 1500g, which is due to a precipitous fall in pulmonary vascular resistance at birth, due to a diminished amount of smoothmuscle in the pulmonary arteries of premature infants. Many of these babies are asymptomatic and need no specific therapy. The peripheral pulses are jerky, and the majority have the typical continuous murmur; sometimes, the murmur is audible only in systole, with mid or late systolic accentuation-the ductus closes spontaneously, usually within 12 weeks. In others, the shunt acrossthe duct is moderate or large and is complicated by cardiomegaly, pulmonary oedema, and heart failure; many respond, to digitalis and diuretics, with subsequent spontaneous closure, but in some the response to therapy is inadequate, and surgical obliteration of the duct is necessary to controlcardiac failure

A premature during or after clinical course of RDS may have significant associated PDA.that is paradoxically difficult to detect-clinically but is often threatening in magnitude. A soft nonspecific murmur (systolic) or no murmur is more common than the classic continuous.

Murmur. The peripheral pulses and more are often bounding, but typically are not characteristic for some days, after the onset of a large L-R shunt. An early sign indicating the presence of a significant **L-R** shunt with concomitant **COF** is increasing dependence on oxygenand respiratory support. In addition, increasing X-ray cardiomegaly and pulmonary edemaincreasing echocardiography evidence of a L-R shunt differentiate it clinically and laboratory from bronchopulmonary dysplasia.

Generally adequate assisted ventilation and correction of anemia improves the signs produced bythe PDA. Prolonged assisted ventilation with high Oxygen concentrations may result into bronchopulmonary dysplasia. The clinical picture of this syndrome may be aggravated by a large flow across a PDA and surgical obliteration may be necessary.

DIFFERENTIAL DIAGNOSIS

There are some conditions which produce systolic and

diastolic murmurs in thepulmonary area without cyanosis:

1. Venous hum
2. Aorticopulmonary septal defect
3. Ruptured sinus of Valsalva into the right side of the heart or pulmonary artery
4. Coronary arteriovenous fistulas.

In these 4 conditions, the dynamics are those of an arteriovenous fistula with a machinery murmur and a wide pulse pressure. Sometimes the murmur is not maximal in the pulmonary areahut is heard along the lower left sternal border.

1. Truncus arteriosus with torrential pulmonary flow may be extremely difficult to differentiatefrom PDA especially in infancy.
2. Pulmonary branch stenosis is associated with systolic and diastolic murmurs, but the pulsepressure is normal.
3. Arteriovenous fistulas of medium sized intrathoracic vessels as internal mammary producessigns of PDA.
4. VSD with aortic insufficiency and combined rheumatic aortic and mitral insufficiency may beconfused with PDA because the combination of murmurs produced by these lesions superficiallyresemble those of PDA diagnosis is by careful auscultation and absence of pulmonary over circulation.

AORTICOPULMONARY WINDOW (septal defect):

There is a communication between the ascending aorta, and main pulmonary artery the defect islocated just above the aortic valve, resulting from the incomplete septation of the bulbous cordisInto the ascending aorta and main pulmonary artery. Presence of pulmonary and aortic **valves** and an interventricular septum differentiates it from truncus arteriosus.

Symptoms will depend on the size of the defect, and symptoms of a large V.SD or a. large PDA. There are recurrent pulmonary infections. COF and occasionally minimal cyanosis. In the absence of pulmonary hypertension., physical signs are that of a large PDA, wide pulse pressure, cardiomegaly and a variety of cardiac murmurs-the murmurs may be systolic and diastolic, or continuous Clinically the only clue may be that the murmur is somewhat a typicaland situated lower and more medial than with. PDA Patients in early infancy present with tachypnea. X-ray shows moderate to gross cardiomegaly depending on the size of the defect The pulmonary artery is prominent and pulmonary vascularity prominent.

ECG shows usually shows a typical picture of a large PDA, and there may be left, right orbiventricular hypertrophy.

Cardiac catheterization shows systemic pressure in the pulmonary artery and Rt ventricle and alarge L-R shunt at the pulmonary artery level. The course of the catheter may be diagnostic. In PDA, the catheter enters the pulmonary artery and passes across the ductus into the descending aorta, while as in the aorta pulmonary septal defect, the catheter enters the ascending aorta from the pulmonary artery. Selective angiography with infection of the contrast medium into the ascending aorta can demonstrate the lesion accurately. In most cases, the defect is in theintracardiac portion of the aorta, thus needing cardiopulmonary bypass for the surgical closure, preferably before the age of 3 years death may occur from COF during infancy, or infection (pneumonia.) during childhood, or from pulmonary vascular obstructive disease, or cardiac failure with early treatment, prognosis is improved.

Fistula of the Coronary artery:

A congenital fistula between the coronary artery and vein or a coronary artery may empty directly into the heart usually the right ventricle). In both cases, there is a machinery murmurwhich is more diffuse, and signs are like PDA. In the coronary arteriovenous fistula, oxygenated blood enters the coronary veins, which in turn empty into the coronary sinus; the right atrial blood has a higher Oxygen content than samples from the vena cava. When a coronary artery directly empties into the right ventricle, there is. L-R shunt at the ventricular level which can be anatomically demonstrated by injection of contrast medium into, the ascending aorta. Fistula should he surgically treated fistula of the coronary artery enters the differential diagnosis of PDA.

Ruptured Sinus of VALSALVA:

One of the Valsalva's sinuses of the aorta weakened by congenital or acquired disease may lead to aneurysmal formation and rupture into the right atrium or ventricle; clinically, it is like PDA except that the machinery murmur may be in the unusual site. Cardiac catheterization showsthe L-R shunt at the atrial ventricular level, and aortography with injection of contrast mediuminto the ascending aorta demonstrates the site of aneurysm and rupture Treatment is surgical.

PULMONARY VALVE STENOSIS

Pulmonary stenosis may exist as an isolated abnormality or with defects in the atrial or ventricularsepta. In all instances, the origin of the aorta is normal. Normally the aortic root differentiates itfrom tetralogy of Fallot, in which the aorta is dextrose. Pulmonary stenosis with normal aortic root can be classified as simple pulmonary stenosis; valvular, infundibular, and combined valvular and infundibular.

Pulmonary stenosis with an arteriovenous shunt; as PS with VSD (acyanotic Fallot), PS with ASD, PS with PDA- Pulmonary stenosis with a venoarterial shunt; PS with VSD (like tetralogy of Fallothemodynamically), PS with reversed interatrial shunt through PFO or ASD.

SIMPLE VALVULAR P.S- with INTACT SEPTUM and NORMAL AORTIC ROOT

In 80% of cases of isolated pulmonary stenosis existing as an Isolated lesion, 80% of cases have valve stenosis, where the valve cusps have fused into a dome-shaped membrane with a small central oreccentric opening. The ventricular and atrial septa are normal. The pulmonary artery beyond the stenosis is often enlarged. The hole may be 2 mm-1cm in diameter. Occasionally there may be the fusion of 2 cusps only producing a bicuspid pulmonary valve. In severe cases, secondary infundibular stenosis. The pulmonary valve ring is usually small. There is marked post-stenotic dilatation of the main pulmonaryartery and the left pulmonary artery. Patent foramen ovale is common.

Pulmonary stenosis obstructs the flow of blood from the right ventricle to the pulmonary artery; the pressure load **patient** the right ventricle is increased during systole to push blood through the hole in the valve. Pressures may be much greater than the systemic, the increased work of the ventricle leading to severe RVH. and eventually right ventricular failure. This contrasts with tetralogy of Fallot where because of the communication between the ventricles, the maximal pressure that the right ventricle may develop is equal to systemic pressure and not more than systemic pressure, and heart failure is extremely uncommon. Arterial oxygen tension saturation is normal, and in severe cases: the cardiac output- is low and fixed.

In severe stenosis, in the presence of a patent foramen ovale, there may be R-L shunt of variable magnitude causing cyanosis. The presence of cyanosis, in pulmonary stenosis indicates a relatively severe degree of valvular obstruction.

CLINICAL FEATURES

With mild to moderate stenosis, there are usually no

symptoms; thus, the majority of patients are completely asymptomatic throughout infancy, childhood, and adolescence. There isno cyanosis in mild cases. It is with a more severe lesion, develop cyanosis, and COF very early, even, in the neonatal period.

In moderately severe cases, there is progressively increasing cyanosis, easy fatiguability, effort dyspnea, and exercise intolerance may be reduced to walking a few yards. Cyanotic spells characterized by a sudden onset of a marked increase in cyanosis and dyspnea are much less common than in tetraology and squatting is very uncommon. Substernal pain and rarely effort syncope may occur in severe cases. Patients with mild to moderate stenosis are acyanotic, but patients with severe or critical stenosis showscentral cyanosis. Patients are well built and well-nourished and often have round, bloated, or moonshaped facies and widely spaced eyes.

Pulmonary stenosis with a dysplastic valve is found commonly in. Noonan's syndrome With stenosis of a mild degree, the venous pressure and pulse are normal, the heart is not enlarged-theapical impulse is normal, and the rt ventricle is not palpable. A loud pulmonary systolic ejectionmurmur, frequently accompanied by a thrill, is audible maximally over the pulmonary area. The murmur is usually preceded by a pulmonary ejection sound. The murmur is often present at birth and invariably during; the first month of life. The 2nd sound is split, with a delayed pulmonary element of normal intensity.

In stenosis of a moderate degree, the physical signs are the same but exaggerated. The venouspressure may be slightly elevated with an intrinsic wave. -

Their precordium is prominent, a right ventricular sternal lift (heaving impulse of the rt ventricle)is palpable; a systolic thrill is palpable in the pulmonary area and frequently in the suprasternal, notch the first sound is normal, but the 2nd sound, in mild stenosis, is normally split, and then the pulmonary component is normal in intensity, hut in moderate stenosis, it is more widely split, and the pulmonary component is softer (of diminished intensity) and delayed. In patients with mild and moderate stenosis, a prominent pulmonary type of ejection click is heard best at the 2nd left space; this click varies with respiration and becomes more prominent during expiration than inspiration. The systolic ejection murmur is accentuated in later systole. The click follows the first sound.

In severe degrees of stenosis, peripheral cyanosis is present, due to small cardiac output, compensatory vasoconstriction and To surgical blood flow through the skin. Arterial oxygen saturation is normal. The venous pressure is elevated due to a large presystolic A-wave (in older children), which is sometimes transmitted to the liver as a presystolic pulsation Occasionally, a large jugular wave is seen due to functional tricuspid incompetence. The heart is greatly enlarged, with à conspicuous sternal and parasternal lift, which extends to the midclavicular line (right ventricular lift). A loud systolic ejection murmur, frequently accompanied by a thrill, is audible, maximally in the pulmonary area, but radiates widely over the whole pericardium, into the neck, over both lung fields and into the back (upper lung fields posteriorly). The murmur is a rough stenotic type and has a late systolic accentuation. The 2nd heart sound is single, and hence the pulmonary component is not audible (or is la very late and soft). A right atrial presystolic gallop is usually heard in the presence of a large venous A-wave.

Thus, the essentials in the right ventricular lift; systolic ejection click at the pulmonary area inmild to moderate cases, widely split **2**nd sound with very soft pulmonary component, obstructive systolic murmur at the pulmonary area. There is no diastolic murmur, clubbing with severe cases, and hepatomegaly

X-ray

Maybe present with in most cases, which are asymptomatic. Also, the heart size is normal, and the only finding on X-ray is posted stenotic dilatation of the pulmonary artery; otherwise, a chest X-ray is normal- In moderate to severe cases, the heart is enlarged mainly the right ventricleand in severe cases, right atrium also. The heart shows gross enlargement in cases of CCF. There may be no post stenotic dilatation. The pulmonary vascularity is decreased, especially inpatients who are cyanotic.

ECG

In mild cases, it is normal or may reveal minimum right ventricular hypertrophy, with moderate to severe lesions, there is evidence of right ventricular hypertrophy with more severe cases, there are also tall, spiked P waves (P Pulmonarynale) right ventricular strain pattern in rt precordial leads (T wave inversion). In the most severe cases, right atrial hypertrophy is seen, and axis deviation is also seen.

Cardiac catheterization demonstrates an abrupt change in pressure across the pulmonary valve with low pulmonary artery pressure but much-raised pressure in the right ventricle which may be higher than systemic pressure in severe cases. There is no increase in oxygen saturation on the right side of the heart. In the most severe cases, there is an R-L shunt at the atrial level (via the PFO) - The gradient across the pulmonary valve is 10-200mm, depending on the severity of the obstruction. In severe cases, right atrial pressure is elevated with a prominent A-wave. Angiocardiography is an injection of contrast medium into the right ventricle shows the thickening of the pulmonary valve and the very narrow opening of the pulmonary valve a Jet of medium from the right ventricle into the pulmonary artery seen as a narrowing of the right ventricular outflow tract during ventricular systole followed by a widening this area.

COURSE AND PROGNOSIS

Children with mild stenosis can lead a normal life without specific treatment; many cases of moderate obstruction are similar, but their progress should be re-evaluated at frequent intervals) Progression of obstruction to right ventricular outflow' is indicated by a change in the systolic murmur with the development of late systolic accentuation. Generally, there is a good correlation between the width of the splitting of the 2nd sound and peak right ventricular pressure in so the duration of the split in milliseconds approximates the peak. pressure in mmHg. (If the duration of the split is 80 sec, the right ventricular systolic pressure is 80 mm Hg). Progressive ECG changes of right ventricular hypertrophy also indicate an increasing obstruction to right ventricular outflow.

Patients with mild stenosis live a normal life and have a normal span of life. Those with moderatestenosis are initially normal but later show symptoms of easy fatigability and dyspnea on exertion, which may be progressive. Those with severe stenosis develop severe cyanosis and: COF in early life, and the infant will die if not treated surgically.

TREATMENT.

Mild cases and many moderate cases do not need any treatment, and should be encouraged to lead normal lives, but dental and ENT surgery must be covered by antibiotic prophylaxis. Patients in whom right ventricular pressure is more than 75 mm Hg or in whom the pressure gradient across the pulmonary valve is more than 50 mm Hg, should be treated surgically. Patients who has symptoms or cyanosis are treated immediately by surgery. All patients with severe isolated pulmonary stenosis require surgery (Pulmonary valvotomy). In the majority of cases, it gives good results; the gradient across the pulmonary valve is abolished, but a pulmonary diastolic murmur may be heard and is due to surgically created pulmonary valve incompetence. It has no clinical significance. The operative mortality is 1-10% depending on the age and the condition of the pt.

Part II: Pulmonary Issues

INFUNDIBULAR PULMONARY STENOSIS (without VSD)

Infundibular stenosis is due to failure of involution of the bulbous cordis leading to a muscular or fibrous obstruction in the outflow tract of the right ventricle. The site of the obstruction may be close to the pulmonary valve or well above it, and an infundibular chamber is present between the right ventricular cavity and the pulmonary valve. When there is combined valvular and infundibula stenosis (i.e. the pulmonary valve is abnormal, the infundibular stenosis may be due to hypertrophy of the right ventricular outflow tract secondary to pulmonary valvular stenosis pure infundibular stenosis is rare the hemodynamics and clinical manifestations are similar to those described above, but there are some exceptions- the systolic thrill and murmur are frequently maximal in. the 3rd and 4th space on the left side, but radiates widely (it is Maximal. In 2nd space in the valvular stenosis) also the murmur is long. The ejection click Is absent. On X-ray post stenotic dilatation of the pulmonary artery may be present but is not usual with an Infundibular chamber and valvular pulmonary stenosis, 2 pressure gradients are noted during cardiac catheterization (between the right ventricular and infundibular chamber and between pulmonary artery and the infundibular chamber).

Angiocardiography is confirmatory, demonstrating the site of the infundibular stenosis, presence of an infundibular chamber, and associated abnormalities of the pulmonary valve. Since the clinical picture of isolated infundibular stenosis closely mimics that of acyanotic tetralogy of Fallot, therefore it is essential to prove the intactness of the ventricular septum. The clinical course is like simple valvular stenosis. Pulmonary valvuloplasty is done in severe cases where there is associated pulmonary stenosis.

PULMONARY STENOSIS WITH ARTERIOVENOUS SHUNT:

Valvular or infundibular pulmonary stenosis may be associated with a L-R shunt across an atrial ASD, VSD or PDA. The clinical picture depends on the degree of stenosis and magnitude of the L-R shunting.

1. With ASD: If the stenosis is dominant, and the shunt small, the clinical picture is as simple valvular stenosis. If the stenosis is slight and shunting large, the features are of ASD, but the murmurs are harsh and accompanied by a. thrill. Diagnosis is by cardiac catheterization, demonstrating a shunt at the atrial 1evel, and the pulmonary stenosis is shown by the presence of a. pressure gradient across the valve. Selective angle cardiography also shows the presence of pulmonary stenosis, and indicator dilution studies confirm the **L-R** shunt across the ASD.
2. With VSD: If VSD is dominant and pulmonary stenosis slight, the clinical picture is that of VSD, while the pulmonary stenosis is not recognized except by pressure gradient during catheterization. If the VSD is small but the stenosis at the Pulmonaryni level is dominant, again: the combination is difficult to diagnose. Rarely in patients VSD, progressive ventricular hypertrophy may lead to the development of infundibular pulmonary stenosis, which obscures the presence of the septal defect. The small shunt across the VSD may not be recognized even at the cardiac catheterization. Selective left ventriculography proves whether the ventricular septus is intact.
3. With PDA: In addition to the signs of pulmonary stenosis, a machinery murmur is heard over the pulmonary area. This

combination of anomalies is suspected when there are signs of PDA with.RVH.Pulmonary atresia is excluded by the absence of cyanosis and the presence of poststenotic dilatation of the pulmonary artery.

These anomalies are treated by direct vision surgery; the defect in the atrial ventricular septum is closed, and pulmonary stenosis is relieved by pulmonary valvuloplasty or infundibular resection. If PDA is present it is divided during the same procedure. Surgery is recommended only for severe or progressive cases.
With the successful operation, the shunt is obliterated, and the gradient across the valve is reduced orabolished. -

PULMONARY STENOSIS WITH VENTROATRIAL SHUNT

Patients with moderate to severe valvular or infundibular pulmonary stenosis have right ventricular systolic: hypertension in addition the right atrium, has difficulty in emptying during right ventricular diastole which occurs, during right atrial. systole)., the right atrial pressure also rises which results in reversal of shunt(R-L) access the ASD and in cyanosis; Same is true with a patent foramen ovale Pulmonary stenosis with ASD or PFÖ is Trilogy of Fallot. Cyanosis may be present at birth or appear later (frequently during adolescence) and is accompanied by clubbing of digits and polycythemia. JVP is increased with an intrinsic A-wave. Other findings: are of severe pulmonary stenosis-The R-L shunt produces arterial oxygen saturation. Treatment is surgical in. all. Valvotomy plus closure of ASD). When pulmonary stenosis presents with, reversal of shunt, via a VSD, it is like Tetraology of Fallot.

DISTAL PULMONARY STENOSIS'

PERIPHERAL PULMONARY BRANCH STENOSIS

Constriction coarctations), which may be mild and localized or multiple and extensive, may affect the branches of the pulmonary artery in the periphery of the lung. This condition is frequentlyassociated with other CHD lesions such as pulmonary valvular stenosis, tetralogy of Fallot, PDA, VSD, ASD, and supravalvular aortic stenosis but may be found as an. Isolated lesionis, more common in congenital rubelia syndrome. Supravalvular aortic stenosis with pulmonary arterial branch stenosis has been observed in patients with idiopathic hypercalcemia. of infancy.

If the constriction is small, there is little effect on the pulmonary circulation. With multiple severeconstrictions, there is an increase in the pressure in the right ventricle, and pulmonary artery proximal to the site of obstruction-When the lesions are isolated, diagnosis is suggested by unusual murmurs: heard over both lung fields both, anteriorly and posteriorly. These murmurs are usually midsystolic (but may be systolic, diastolic, or continuous). Transient pulmonary branch stenosis murmurs of infancy are innocent. Frequently the physical signs are dominated bythe associated anomaly Of tetralogy) If the stenosis is seven, there is ECG evidence of RVH and right atrial hypertrophy. In severe lesions, there is cardiomegaly and prominence of the main pulmonary artery. Usually the pulmonary vasculature is normal, but in some cases, intrapulmonary vascular shadows are seen (which. on. arteriography is seen- to be the areas of post stenotic dilatation). Severe resobstructions of the main pulmonary artery and its primary branches should be respected. The most common cause of this condition is congenital rubella (in which PDA. may be less common) followed by hypercalcemia syndrome and Ullrich-Noonan syndrome.

SUPRAVALVULAR PULMONARY STENOSIS

There is coarctation of the body of the main pulmonary artery or of the bifurcation of the main pulmonary artery; the clinical picture is identical to that of valvular pulmonary stenosis, but the murmur is maximal in the first left space at the sternal border and in the suprasternal natch; there is no ejection, click; the 2nd sound is narrowly split, but the pulmonary component is quite loud, as a result of the closure of the pulmonary valve under high pressure. The murmur radiates well itothe neck and over the lung fields.

ABSENCE OF A PULMONARY ARTERY

This may be an isolated lesion, or may come in association with other lesions. Occasionally itis seen in patients with Tetralogy.

PULMONARY VALVULAR INSUFFICIENCY

Pulmonary valve insufficiency is seen in cardiovascular diseases associated with severe pulmonary hypertension or may follow surgery done for right ventricular outflow obstruction (pulmonary valvotomy and infundibular resection) or rarely may be an isolated lesion when it is mild and symptomatic. There is a diastolic murmur at the upper left sternal border, which simulates, in quality, the murmur of aortic incompetence, but the murmur starts later, has a low pitch, and may increase in intensity during inspiration. Chest X-ray shows prominent main pulmonary artery and the ECG is normal or shows minimal RVH. Cardiac catheterization confirms the diagnosis shows a low pulmonary arterial diastolic pressure). Selective arteriography demonstrates the incompetent valve. Generally isolated pulmonary valvular incompetence is well, tolerated and requires no treatment except prophylaxis against bacterial endocarditis.

The absence of a pulmonary valve is usually associated with other defects especially tetralogy of Fallot and VSD. The pulmonary arteries become markedly dilated and compress the bronchi, resulting in. recurrent episodes of wheezing, pulmonary collapse, and pneumonitis. Florid pulmonary incompetence is not tolerated, and death may occur during infancy from bronchial compression and heart failure. Valvular grafting can be done, but gross dilatation of pulmonary arteries remains.

CONGENITAL AORTIC'STENOSIS

Congenital aortic stenosis occurs more commonly in males (3:1). Anatomically, it is divided into 4types:

- -Most of the cases (75%) are valvular; there is stenosis of the valve itself.
- If this critical stenosis presents in infancy, the lesion is usually in the form of a unicuspidal diaphragm structure without well-defined commissures, whereas preschool and school children present with bicuspid valve, while young adolescents present with a. tricuspid (but partially fused) leaflets.
- The fusionof the cusps produces a. dome-shaped valve with an eccentric opening.
- Occasionally the valve ring is hypoplastic

Rarely there may be other sites where the stenosis affects. Stenosis may be sub-valvular, with a discrete membranous or fibrous obstruction that forms a diaphragm with a central hole obstructing the left ventricular outflow tract (20% case In others, the lesion is supravalvular-; there isconstriction of the ascending aorta just above the coronary arteries. Supravalvular aortic stenosis may be associated with pulmonary arterial branch stenosis and may present with a family history, with a typical elf like facies full face broad forehead, flattened bridge, long upper lip, and rounded cheeks), growth retardation, mental retardation, and idiopathic hypercalcemia of infancy (Supravalvular syndrome). In idiopathic hypertrophic subaortic stenosis (IHSS). Thereis a marked hypertrophy of the entire ventricle, including the ventricle and the outflow tract with the contraction of the ventricle, the hypertrophic portion of the septum, together with the mitral valve, causes obstruction of the left ventricular outflow.

HEMODYNAMICS

Obstruction to the outflow from the left ventricle, causes the left ventricle to work harder to empty the- itself, and to maintain an adequate pressure and flow, into the systemic circulation, leading to the left ventricular hypertrophy, which in turn needs more oxygen With, severe stenosis, oxygen requirements may be more than, what the coronaries can supply, and insuch cases coronary insufficiency also occurs. In critical stenosis, left ventricle may fail (Usually left ventricle tolerates increased pressure load for longer periods before developing failure at coronary insufficiency). Physiologically as is a condition., where there is a. systolic pressure gradient of more than.10 mm between the left ventricle and the aorta., and anatomically, it is the obstruction to the outflow tract of the left ventricle.

CLINICAL FEATURES

As, except in infants in whom the lesion is severe and who may develop CCF, is generally asymptomatic. Mostly they have no cardiovascular symptoms, their physical development is good, and the abnormality is detected on routine examination. These patients (except the severe ones) may do. well up to 3rd to 5th decade, but some may have mild exercise intolerance or easy fatigability. With severe obstruction patients develop ,within the first decade, fatigue and effort intolerance, and a small percentage, show dizziness, angina pectoris, syncope, or episodes of pulmonary edema due to left ventricular failure (indicatingcritical stenosis.' Presence of precordial pain and syncope indicate severe functional impairment.

Sudden death may occur in all forms but is most, common with IHSS.

Though isolated valvular stenosis rarely produces symptoms in infancy, severe COF may
occur, and Response poorly to drugs and surgery is needed. Physical signs mostly depend on the type of the lesion-
In most cases (Valvular stenosis), the patients are well-developed and well-nourished. The pulses are normal and equal throughout (but if the lesion is. severe and the gradient is more than80 mm, the pulses are small in volume, with a slow upstroke, and are anacrotic). There is a. left ventricular thrust at the apex (due to hypertrophied left ventricle) in some cases, but in most cases, the heart is normal in size, and the apical impulse is normal. A. systolic thrill is palpable at the left sternal border,2nd right space close to the sternum, the suprasternal notch, and over both carotid arteries.is palpable in moderate lesion. In milder disease only the right carotid manifests the thrill.

AUSCULATION

The first heart sound is normal; prominent systolic ejection clicks, or ejection sound (aortic type) is best heard at the apex, but is audible all along the left sternal border, at the 2nd; right intercostal space, and at the apex. This ejection, dick is separated- from the first soundby a short but appreciable interval. lt does not vary' with respiratory. The 2nd sound is normally split, but the aortic component is diminished or of good intensity.

The murmur is a coarse rasping, medium to high-pitched, systolic (ejection type) murmur, heard maximally in. the aortic area, radiating to the neck and down to the left sternal border and towards the apex radiates- weekly to the suprasternal notch and along the carotids), and is accompanied by the thrill.

In discrete membranous subvalvular stenosis, the physical signs are the same, but the ejection click is absent and the thrill and murmur are more intense at the left sternal border in the 3rd and4th space than at the aortic area. The concomitant aortic insufficiency is common in children after 5 years and leads to an aortic-blowing systolic murmur.

In the asymmetric septal hypertrophy, the murmur is ejection in quality and heard from the left sternal border towards the apex. An apical mid-diastolic rumbling murmur may be heard due to the normal mitral valve, or the murmur of mitral insufficiency may be heard. There may be an atrial 4th sound also. There is no ejection click and the arterial pulse has a rapid up stoke and frequently a bisferiens quality. In the supravalvular stenosis, unlike other types, there is the abnormal facies (full face, broad forehead with hypertelorism, flattened bridge of the nose, short and upturned nose, prominent upper lip, and rounded cheeks), subnormal mentality, and associated hyperkalemia in some cases. The thrill and murmur uncharacteristically heard over the suprasternal notch and over the carotids, but are well transmitted over the aortic area and nearthe amid left sternal border. A difference in pulses and blood pressure between the right and left arm may be found, with those on the right side being more prominent. The aortic component of the 2nd sound may be accentuated. X-ray. In most of cases the heart is not enlarged, but mild to moderate cardiomegaly due to left ventricular hypertrophy may be seen. In valvular, and less commonly subvalvular, there is poststenotic dilatation of aorta (ascending aorta). Ascending aorta is normal in supravalvular and IHSS lesions. Infants with COF show severe cardiomegaly. Though the ascending aorta is frequently prominent in valvular aortic stenosis, the aortic knob is normal.

Valvular calcification may be seen. ECG Correlates with the severity of obstruction. Patients weigh mild stenosis and thus a small gradient across the aortic valve show normal ECG. Patients with severe lesions obstruction show LVH and left ventricular strain but may be normal even with severe stenosis (such children have abnormal vector cardiogram). A progressive increase in left ventricular hypertrophy on serial ECG indicates significant obstruction. A strain pattern (with ST or Twave changes) suggests a severe functional impairment. For proper evaluation of the severity of the lesion, cardiac catheterization is done Progressive increase in LVH, or appearance of a strain pattern points to the need for eat surgery. Left cardiac catheterization, using retrograde catheterization, shows difference of pressure across the aortic valve (gradient between the aortic pressure and left ventricular pressure). If the gradient between the left ventricle and aorta is less than 50 mm, it is a mild lesion, if it is more than 70 mm, it is severe. And if in between these two limits, it is moderate stenosis. Withdrawal of the catheter across the left ventricular outflow tract and aortic valve localize the lesion Patients with severe AS may be asymptomatic and have normal chest X-rays, and normal ECGs, but serial. Catheterization is the only dependable guide to the severity of the lesion. In case of a. valvular stenosis, an asymptomatic patient with a resting gradient of more than 70 mmHg is thought to need surgery. If the gradient is less but the patient is symptomatic again surgery is needed. Cineangiocardiography (a cardiac imaging technique using cine imaging to visualize heart and blood vessels) helps to localize the lesion and outlines the anatomy of the valve Echocardiography is used in initial evaluation and follow-up of IHSS.

Course and prognosis in most cases, the prognosis is good, but there is a high incidence of sudden death in children (5%), most common with IHSS. Sudden death is frequently precipitated by severe physical exertion. In such patients there is frequently gross left ventricular hypertrophy. The prognosis is also affected by the associated anomalies as VSD, ASD, coarctation, and pulmonary stenos Infants with AS, who die from CCF, frequently have endocardia sclerosis of the left ventricle and left atrium and of the mitral valve.

Surgery is needed in patients who are symptomatic (irrespective of the gradient), patients with ECG evidence of gross LVH, and pressure gradients of more than 20 mm. Open heart surgery using cardiopulmonary bypasses are needed. Valvular stenosis is treated by valvotomy, but some mayneed valve replacement. Discrete sub aortic stenosis is reseed results of surgery in subvalvular stenosis are better than in valvular where the results are not satisfactory on may produce or aggravate aortic insufficiency which is a worse lesion than the original disease for which the surgery was done. In supravalvular lesion stenosis can be relieved if the area of obstruction is discrete and not associated with a hypo plastic aorta. If the gradient is abolished or reduced, angina dizziness, syncope, or effort intolerance and ECG improvement with alleviation of signs of LVH are seen. When time gradient is more than 50 mm, at rest, the calculated aortic valve orifice is less than 0.7 sq. cmm/sq meter of body surface, significant ST segment depression is evident during and immediately after graded exercise. Even after successful surgery, obstructionmay recur after 5-1.5 years(frequently). Patients with AS should not be allowed to participation active competitor support, but otherwise should lead unrestricted normal levels. IHSS is treated medically with beta-adrenergic blockers as propranolol. Patients should be re-evaluated on an annualbasis and operated if progression is seen. Penicillin prophylaxis for dental, oral and ENT Surgery should be given

CONGENITAL MITRAL STENOSIS

A rare anomaly, in which valve leaflets are thickened and fused to produce a diaphragm-like or funnel-like structure with a central opening. Chrodae tenenae (the ligaments located within the small intestine that support the movement and function of the organ) are shortened and deformed. The lesion may be isolated or associated with the lesions especially PDA, aortic stenosis and coarctation of the aorta. Most patients: develop symptoms early in life (within the first 2 years); the infant is underdeveloped, has obvious dyspnea, and frequently has cyanosis or pallor. Episodes of pulmonary edema and COF æcommon. The heart is enlarged, due to dilatation and hypertrophy of the right ventricle and left atrium is a regular sinus rhythm. First heart sound is loud, the pulmonary part of the 2nd sound is loud, and 2nd sound is split (Both sounds are loud). Ab opening snap of the mitral valve may bepresent. Mostly there is a presystolic crescent murmur heard at the apex others have described a rumbling diastolic murmur followed by a loud first heart sound, but mostly systolic murmurs are found). Rarely no murmur is heard at all. X-ray shows left atrial and right ventricular enlargement and pulmonary congestion. ECG shows right axis deviation, RVH, bi atrial enlargement (and normal, bifid, or siked P Waves). Cardiac catheterization reveals increase in right ventricular, pulmonary arterial and wedge pressures, and associated anomalies if present. Echocardiography reveals the abnormal valve structure and shows reduced excursion. Angiocardiography may show delayed emptying of teleft atrium. The prognosis is poor, and most children succumb within first 2 years of life. Only an occasional patient is saved by surgery.

CONGENITAL MITRAL INSUFFICIENCY

Again, a rare disorder, which may be found as isolated, but usually is found associated with other congenital heart Lesions, as PDA, coarctationof the aorta, VSD, corrected transposition of the great arteries, anomalous origin of left coronary from the pulmonary artery, endocardia, endocardia fusion defects, and Mar fans syndrome.

Mitral incompetence is an integral part of many endocardia cushion defects and frequently is associated with congestive cardiomyopathy. The mitral valve angulus is usually dilated, chordaetendinae a short and may insert anomalously. The valve Leaflets are deformed, and endocardia sclerosis of varying degrees is present. In significant mitral incompetence, the left atrium enlarges to accommodate the regurgitate flow; the left ventricle hypertrophies and dilates, further increasing the degree of mitral incompetence. Increased pulmonary venous pressure results in ultimate right ventricular and atrial hypertrophy and dilatation mild lesions produce no symptoms, the only sign is the murmur. But since uncomplicated congenital mitral incompetence is rare, and in most patients significant regurgitation occurs., symptoms occur at an early age. These symptoms are poor physical development, frequent respiratory infections, fatigue on exertion, and episodes of pulmonary edema or CCF. There is cardiomegaly, and the typical apical pan systolic murmur an associated apical mid- diastolic murmur or late diastolic rumbling murmur is frequent. In presence of pulmonary hypertension, the pulmonary component of the 2nd hear sound is accentuated. ECG shows bifidP Waves, usually signs of LVH, and sometimes signs of RVH. X-ray shows an enlargement of the left atrium (which at times is aneurysmal the ventricle is prominent, time aorta is small, and the pulmonary vascularity increased. Left ventricular angiography outlines the left atrium by contrast medium that regurgitates across the mitral valve. Cardiac catheterization shows an elevated left atrial pressure, and at times pulmonary hypertension. Occasionally there is a dilatation of the valve ring only with a normal valve otherwise) but mostly chordae tendinae are also malformed, and that leads to regurgitation. Treatment is by valvuloplasty, which results in striking improvement in symptom and heart size. In children beyond 3-4 years, it may be difficult to exclude rheumatic fever as the cause of mitral insufficiency.

(Late systolic mitral regurgitation is a syndrome resulting from an abnormal mechanism that allows billowing of the mitral leaflets especially the posterior one into the left atrium toward the end ofsystole. It may be congenital and associated with other anomalies mainly ASD secundum or mayfollow rheumatic or viral myocarditis which leads $0 papillary muscle dysfunction. Mostly affects girls which are generally asymptomatic but may get incapacitating left precordial stabbing pain lasting for hours to days, there is a late apical systolic murmur preceded by a click Notreatment is needed during the childhood, but SABE may occur.

PULMONARY VENOUS HYPERTENSION

Many lesions can lead to pulmonary venous hypertension followed by pulmonary arterial hypertension and then COF (as congenital MS, MI, some varieties of total anomalous pulmonaryvenous return, left atrial myxomas, and less frequently cortriatrium, individual pulmonary venous stenosis and supravalvular steno sing of the ring of the left atrium There is irritability, recurrent pulmonary infections, and CCF. Physical signs are dominated by the presence of pulmonary hypertension. ECG shows RVH with spiked p waves. X-ray shows cardiomegaly, prominent pulmonary veins, prominent right ventricle, prominent right atrium, and prominent pulmonary arteries. The left atrium is nor mal in size or only slightly enlarged.

Cardiac catheterization excludes the presence of a shunt and demonstrates, pull onaryhypertension with an elevated pulmonary arterial wedge pressure. Selective arterial angiocardiography may delineate the anatomic lesion.

COR ATRIATUM

An extremely rare anomaly, where there is stenosis of the common pulmonary vein, and the pulmonary veins enter a separate chamber rather than pass directly into the left atrium: the chamber communicates with the left atrium through an opening of variable size. Physiologicallyit is like mitral stenosis, and the clinical picture depends on the size of the opening. If the opening is very small, symptoms may appear in very early life. But if large patients may remain asymptomatic for a long time, cardiac catheterization shows a high pulmonary venous pressure and a low left atrial pressure. Angiocardiography shows 2 Left atrial chambers. Echocardiography may show a hard shadow in the left atrium, Surgical repair is successful later, and surgical mortality is very high in your infants.

TETRALOGY OF FALLOT

Tetralogies od Fallot is the commonest cyanotic heart disease and consists of 4 components, 2 ofwhich comprise the basic defects (pulmonary valvular or infundibula stenosis + a large high VSD); the right ventricle is hypertrophied, and in 25% cases right aortic arch is present. The 4 components therefore are

1. Ventricular septal defect (VSD) is usually large, located in the membranous part of the septum just below the aortic valve, and related to the posterior and Right aortic cusps. The VSD is quite large and in some cases, may be in the muscular area.

2. Obstruction to the right ventricular outflow tract. The stenosis is usually infundibula (75%), or at both valvular and infundibula Levels (25%), and only rarely at the valvular level alone. The pulmonary arterial trunk is also smaller than usual. Hypertrophy of the crista supraventricular is, contributes to the infundibula stenosis and results in the formation of an infundibula chamber ofvariable size and contour. The pulmonary valve may have a small ring and be loci cuspids.

3. The aorta is juxtaposed and overrides because a. varying proportion of its origin is from the right ventricle; thus, overriding is present because the position of the VSD in

relation to a dilated and dextranase aorta The cortex arches to the right in 20-25% cases and ASD is seen in 1.5% cases. Hemodynamics thereis a right ventricular outflow VSD leading to an R-L shunt at the ventricular level, and thus, the unsaturation of blood. The degree of the desaturation and the extent of cyanosis depends on the size of the shunt, which in turn depends on the resistance to the right ventricular outflow, the size of the VSD, and the systemic radicular resistance. Thus, the greater the obstruction, the larger the VSD, and the lower the systemic vascular resistance, the greater is teR-L shunt. Though the patient may be deeply cyanotic, the amount of pressure the right ventricle is able to develop is limited to that of the aorta (systemic pressure), and right ventricular pressure can exceed the pink left ventricular pressure, and right ventricle is usually quite able to maintain this level of pressure without developing heart failure.

The diastolic and systolic pressures in both ventricles are similar. The pulmonary blood flow is restricted by the pulmonary outlet obstruction but may be supplemented by bronchial collateral.]

CLINICAL FEATURES:

1) Cyanosis-Cyanosis may be present at birth or may not be present inthe immediate post-neonatal period due to the persistence of PDA.; if the ductus remains Open, sufficient blood passes through the lungs to prevent cyanosis even with atresia of the rightventricular outflow tract). As the ductus constricts later, the cyanosis becomes apparent gradually, in the case of the children getting an infection, suddenly. Cyanosis usually becomes apparent, with crying, during the first 6 months of life. But a child with maximal right ventricular obstruction may present with deep cyanosis right at birth. The cyanosis is usually progressive and is most prominent in the mucous membranes of lips and mouth, and finger- and toe-nai ls (but the entire skin may have a dusky bluish color). The csclerae are gray, and the blood vessels at

the periphery of the eyes are engorged (simulating mild conjunctivitis). The blood vessels of the retina are large and dark. The mucosae of the pharynx are purple, and the tongue is deep blue and often large and fissured, inert papaillae. The gums are frequently inflamed and bleed easily from light pressure,

2) Progressive cyanosis leads to retardation of growth and development, clubbing of the fingers and toes generally by 1-2 years of age.
3) Easy fatiguability and dyspnea on exertion are seen. Infants, and toddlers will play actively for a short time and then sit or lie down. Older children also will stop walking or playing for rest. Characteristically a child who can walkwill assume a squatting position for the relief of dyspnea due to physical effort. Assuming squatting position after exercise or playing leads to decreased venous return and increased systematic arterial resistance, the ease of which would tend to decrease the R-L shunt and increase the pulmonary blood flow. This re increased oxygen saturation so that the child can resume physical activity within a few minutes.
4) Some infants and children exhibit sudden episodes of hyper cyanosis associated with irritability, pallor, hyperventilation, and flaccidity, terminating in loss of Consciousness5) Growth and development are retarded; the stature and nutritional status are below: the average,and the muscles and SC tissue flabby and soft Puberty is delayed. Therefore, the children are small and underdeveloped.

CARDIOVASCULAR EXAMINATION

Cyanosis may be from clinically undetectable to due cyanosis at rest. Clubbing is seen Pulse is usually normal, venous, and arterial pulses are normal. The left anterior hemithorax bulges forwards. The precordium is quiet. There is a taping apical impulse (right ventricular lift or tap). A prominentsystolic thrill is present in 1. /2 cases, along the left sternal border in the 3rd and 4th spaces, or at the lower or mid sternal borders.

The first heart sound is normal. The 2nd sound is single (produced by closure of the aortic valve) and loud. If the closure of the pulmonary valve is audible, it is delayed and diminished, occasionally, there is an ejection click at the apex, that is, aortic in origin. Murmur is a loud, harsh, either ejection or pansystolic, most intense at the left sternal border in the 3rd interspace, but is transmitted widely, radiating over the anterior and posterior lung fields. In cases of pulmonary atresia or at the height of an anoxic spell, there may be no murmur. In some cases, the systolic murmur is followed by diastolic murmurs leading to a continuous murmur, which may be heard anywhere in the chest, anteriorly or posteriorly, and is due to enlarged bronchial collaterals vessels or rarely persistence of a PDA, and frequently occurs in pulmonary atrescia/X-ray of chest: May sometimes be absolutely normal and typically,there is a normal or small heart, with a large right ventricle and uplifted. Cœur en sabot (French for "clog-shaped heart" or "boot-shaped heart"); thus in the anteroposterior view we see a narrow base, concavity of the left border(in the area normally occupied by a pulmonary artery); the main pulmonary segment being small and concave. The rounded apical shadow situated high above the diaphragm is produced by the right ventricle chiefly and looks like a sheep's nose; the entire cardiac silhouette resembles a wooden boot. In lateral view, the anterior clear space may or may not be encroached upon by the enlarged right ventricle in many patients the right ventricle displaces the leftventricle posteriorly so that the posterior border of the heart may overlap the spine in the left anterior oblique view.

All these features suggest RVH, but ECG is the more sensitive index of RVH. The aorta is large, and in 20-25% of cases, the aorta arches to the right instead of to the left (which is visible in an anteroposterior view or may be confirmed by the displacement of a barium-filled esophagus to the left). In the left oblique view, a right aortic arch may indent the esophagus. The Hilary areas of the lung are clear and do not pulsate due to diminished pulmonaryblood flow. For the same reason, the lung fields are clear (poorly vascularized). The heart size isnormal usually. Variations from the typical picture include post-stenotic dilatation of the pulmonary artery (associated with valvular pulmonary stenosis); the pulmonary vascularity may be made prominent by a reticular network of collateral bronchial circulation radiating from the hilus of the lungs localized infundibula stenosis an infundibula chamber may produce a bulge at the upper left cardiac border in the frontal protection, which is distinguished from the pulmonary artery because it remains prominent in the right anterior oblique view ECG: Right ventricular hypertrophy and right axis deviation are demonstrated early without the evidence of right ventricular dominance, the diagnosis is not likely, and it is found in the right precordial chest leads where the configuration the QRS complex. The P wave is typically normal, which is a common occurrence and significant. It may be tall and peaked or sometimes: in 1/3 cases, withevidence of slight right a trial hypertrophy. VA is always seen but right ventricular strain patterns are if diagnosis is in doubt, other tests are done. Cardiac catheterization and angiocardiography are essential to elucidate the anatomical abnormalities, and to exclude other defects which may mimic the tetralogy of Fallot (especially double outlet right ventricle with pulmonary stenosis, and arterial transposition with pulmonary stenosis). Cardiac catheterization indicates absence of a significant L-R shunt, and arterial desaturation of varying degree. The presence of an R-L shuntat the ventricular key is shown. The right ventricular pressure is at the systemic level, and the pressure contour in the right ventricle is almost identical to that of the left ventricle. The pulmonary arterial pressure is very low. The degree of arterial unsaturation is depending on the magnitude of the R-L shunt and at rest, is 75-85% usually. There is a sudden fall of pressure as the catheter enters from the right ventricle into the infundibula chamber or pulmonary artery. Thesystolic pressure in both the ventricles is 80-11.0 mm while as the pulmonary artery pressure is only 5-1 mm... The selective right ventriculography outlines the heavily trabeculated right ventricle by contrast medium: it, in addition to outlining the right ventricle, will show the length, size, width, contour, etc. of the infundibula stenos, will outline the infundibula chamber, and outlines the pulmonary artery, pulmonary valve, out flow tract of the right ventricle, and the size and location of the VSD, as the contrast medium passes from the right into the left ventricle via the VSD. The pulmonary valve may be normal, but frequently the leaflets are thickened, and the valve ring is small. Nearly simultaneous opacification of the aorta and pulmonary artery is usual. The size of the pulmonary trunk varies, but in severe cases it is small or hypo plastic The infundibula stenosis varies in length, wisdom, and distensibility. The VSD is usually very large and is situated below. The large aorta is. Well opacified the aorta is seen to arch to the right in 25% of cases. Complications 7) cerebral thrombosis and brain infarction-cerebral thrombosis, usually in the ins and Dural sinuses, and occasionally in the cerebral arteries are more common in the presence of extreme polycythemia and may be precipitated by dehydration.They occur more frequently in patients under the age of 2 years of great importance is the fact that 1/3 of these patients with cerebrovascular accidents has Fe deficiency anemia; these infants with microcytic hypochromic anemia may have hemoglobin and hematocrit in the normal range so that microscopic examination of the blood smear and measurement of cell indices are essential, Braininfraction is not uncommon, and the cause varies with child's age to some extent. In the first 2 years of life, the major cause is anoxia, resulting from the marked arterial blood desaturation and the relative iron deficiency anemia that exists in many of these pts. Children with a hematocrit under 55% may be the development of an anemic., anoxic infarction, but this is much less common over age 2 years when Fe deficiency is less of a problem. Therefore, all the children should be followed with a hemoglobin, hematocrit, RBC count, and if there is any indication of iron. deficiency they should be given iron. (orally). In older children, infarction is due to ischemia, making the surgical increasing of pulmonary blood flow essential. When the hematocrit increases by more than 75%, the viscosity of the Toilood (Toilood stands for "task, occasion, invitation, location, object, and outcome, ownership, and deadline." It is a mnemonic device used in the medical field to guide healthcare professionals in efficiently organizing and prioritizing tasks and activities related to patient care. By considering these aspects, healthcare providers can ensure that all necessary tasks are completed, and patient care is effectively managed within the given timeframe) markedly increases, and the possibility of thrombotic infarction develops. In these cases, therapy will involve ensuring proper hydration, particularly for patients in a coma. For patients with very high levels of polycythemia, phlebotomy and volume replacement with fresh frozen plasma should be considered. Physical therapy to the affected extremities should be instituted early.

Heparin is of no use since it does not affect the viscosity of the blood and cannot prevent extension of the basis and is dangerous in hemorrhagic cerebral infarction. 2) Brain abscess is rarer thanbrain infarction. Children over 2 years of age with tetralogy who develop CNS, especially brain damage, should be considered to have brain absces6 until proved otherwise. Brain abscess is seen to develop in areas of previous. microscopic-sized infractions. Because of the R-I shunt, bacteria that usually are filtered out by the lungs can pass into the systemic circulation and henceto the area of infraction in the brain. Common presenting symptoms are those of an expanding intracranial mass and there is usually also a respiratory infection. 1-2 weeks prior to the onset of neurologic symptoms. The illness typically begins slowly, with a low-grade fever. There may be tenderness in the area of the skull, and blood tests may show elevated levels of erythrocyte sedimentation rate (ESR) and total leukocyte count (TLC). In others the symptoms may start suddenly with headache, nausea, vomiting, epileptiform seizures, and localized neurologic signs depending on the site of and size of the abscess, and the presence of increased intracranial tension. Echograms, brain scans, and cerebral angiography help in identification of the site of theabscess. Treatment consists of massive doses of antibiotics, but usually, surgical removal of abscess is needed. Bacterial endocarditis is rare in operated patients but common in children who have had a palliative shunt operation during infancy. Penicillin prophylaxis is essential in all surgical procedures in which the patient may develop bacteremia, dental surgery, and ENT Surgery. Although rare, individuals with mild lesions may experience cyanosis and initial symptoms of chronic obstructive fluid (COF). In infants, COF can be triggered by iron deficiency anemia.

ASSOCIATED CVS ANOMOLIES

Associated anomalies with CVS are commonly seen but can be challenging to diagnose clinically. In infancy, patent foramen ovale (PFO) and patent ductus arteriosus (PDA) are frequently observed. It is essential to identify the drainage of persistent left superior vena cava (SVC) into the coronary sinus before surgery, as systemic venous return occlusion is necessary prior to craniotomy. Intracardiac catheterization is used to recognize secundum type atrial septal defects (ASD). Radical surgery should include closure of atrial septal defects, including PFO, as high venous pressure after surgery can cause cyanosis through right-to-left shunting. When the pulmonary valve is absent, a specific syndrome manifests characterized by mild or absent cyanosis, enlarged and hyperdynamic heart, and loud murmurs. Wheezing and recurrent pneumonitis from bronchial compression can occur due to aneurysmal dilatation of the pulmonary artery. Approximately 25% of tetralogy of Fallot cases exhibit stenosis in a pulmonary artery branch, which can be diagnosed through selective pulmonary arteriography or right ventricular angiocardiography. Surgery is performed to alleviate significant stenosis in major pulmonary arteries. If there are differences in X-ray appearance of the pulmonary vasculature on the two sides, the absence of a pulmonary artery may be suspected. Usually, the left pulmonary artery is absent, resulting in increased vascularity in the right lung. This condition may be accompanied by hypoplasia of the left lung. Distinguishing between absence of the left pulmonary artery and severe stenosis with occlusion can sometimes be challenging. Other associated anomalies include relative hypoplasia of the left heart, aortic or subaortic stenosis, bicuspid aortic valve, aberrant coronary artery, and anomalies of the aortic arch.

COURSE

Most infants experience increasing cyanosis during the first 6 months of life. Some may have hypercyanotic spells that can be fatal, but the majority of infants grow out of this condition without any serious problems. However, untreated patients have limitations in their activities, and as they get older, the cyanosis and symptoms become more severe. By the end of the second decade, death may occur. Cerebrovascular accidents, cerebral abscesses, and subacute bacterial endocarditis (SABE) contribute to the poor prognosis of untreated patients.

The treatment for this condition involves several approaches. Firstly, general measures include protecting against SABE and brain abscess through the use of antibiotics during dental and ENT surgeries. Monitoring the hematocrit and hemoglobin levels is critical to detect anemia and polycythemia, both of which can worsen hypoxemia and increase the risk of cerebral vascular accidents. Prompt treatment of hypovolemia and dehydration is necessary to avoid concentrated blood and possible cerebral infarction. Paroxysmal cyanotic attacks may be triggered by relative iron deficiency in infancy, and iron therapy can decrease their frequency and improve overall well-being. Maintaining hematocrit levels between 55-65% is considered safe. Sedation with medications like promethazine or oral propranolol can also be used to reduce the frequency and severity of dyspneic spells.

In terms of surgical interventions, palliative anastomotic procedures are recommended for severely symptomatic infants in whom complete correction is difficult. Different types of anastomotic procedures include the Blalock-Tausig operation, Potts operation, and Waterston operation. These procedures aim to improve symptoms and exercise tolerance by creating connections between blood vessels. Palliative therapy with shunt procedures carries a 2% risk of mortality and should only be performed on severely affected patients under one year old. Postoperative complications may include chylothorax, Horner's syndrome, and cardiac failure.

Total correction surgery is another option and involves opening the right ventricle, closing the ventricular septal defect, and removing the obstruction in the right ventricular outflow tract. This can be done in patients with near-normal size pulmonary arteries and pulmonary valve rings. Total correction surgery leads to significant improvements in cyanosis, growth, development, and symptoms. However, there is a risk of sudden unexpected death due to arrhythmias, particularly complete heart block. The surgical risk for total correction is around 10% and may be higher in cases with significant deformity of the right ventricular outflow tract and in adolescents and adults.

PROGNOSIS

Infants with the most severe farm are deeply cyanotic at birth, and generally, those who are cyanotic at birth usually die before their first birthday. Anoxic spells may occur during the neonatal period, and death may occur during a severe anoxic spell. Many patients who survives the first year of life seem to improve, which may be due to the development of systemic to pulmonary collateral vessels. Although anoxic spells may decrease in severity, these patients remain deeply cyanotic and markedly limited in their activity and seldom survive 2nd decade without surgery. Those who develop cyanosis during the first year of life may live till 2nd to 3rd decade, but unless successfully operated on, they lead the life of invalids. Infants with moderate obstruction to right ventricular outflow do well, and cyanosis, though present in early life, is not severe but may progress in severity, and cyanotic spells may occur. They do well during childhood but progressively deteriorate during the 2nd and 3rd decades, and death occurs during the 3rc decade from cerebrovascular accidents, brain abscess, SABE, anoxia, or pulmonary hemorrhage. Patients with the mildest form of the disease is called to have acyanotic tetralogy. The degree of obstruction is extremely mild, and the R-L shunt very small (very frequently there is, a L-R shunt Cyanosis in these cases develops during childhood, but as the age increases, the obstruction increases, and combined with the increased activity, results in progression of cyanosis. Many of them live normal lives, but dyspnea on exertion becomes increasingly troublesome, and life expectancy is decreased, death usually occurs by the 3rd to 4th decade.

PAROXYSMAL DYSPNEIC ATTACKS (Hypoxie, hypercyanotic, or blue spells)

Infants with tetralogy of Fallot often experience sudden episodes of paroxysmal dyspnea, accompanied by marked cyanosis. While this condition can rarely occur in other types of cyanotic congenital heart disease, it primarily affects infants within the first two years of life. During these episodes, the infant may exhibit a sudden onset of cyanosis, difficulty breathing, restlessness, and gasping for air. Their cry may weaken, and some infants may exhibit signs of precordial pain by clutching or scratching their chest. The intensity of the ejection systolic murmur associated with tetralogy of Fallot temporarily disappears or decreases during these spells. These episodes can last anywhere from a few minutes to a few hours and can occasionally be fatal. Changes in consciousness can vary from restlessness and irritability to syncope. After shorter episodes, the infant may experience generalized weakness and sleepiness, while more severe episodes can result in unconsciousness and, in rare cases, convulsions and partial paralysis. These spells can occur spontaneously, but they may also be triggered by activities such as feeding, crying, bowel movements, or infections, or be exacerbated by iron deficiency anemia. While these episodes can begin in the neonatal period, they commonly continue until the child reaches preschool age. It is uncommon for these episodes to occur for the first time after the age of two. Cyanotic spells in infants with tetralogy of Fallot occur due to a sudden decrease in pulmonary blood flow, increased right-to-left shunting, and systemic hypoxemia. However, the exact mechanism that triggers this sequence of events is not fully understood. Typical examinations reveal spasms in the infundibulum of the right ventricle. The systolic murmur disappears or weakens, arterial oxygen saturation decreases, and arterial pressure in the pulmonary artery reduces. Other explanations for these symptoms include inadequate systemic venous return, reduced systemic vascular resistance, and a vicious cycle of arterial hypoxemia caused by increased respiratory rate (hyperpnea). It is believed that hyperpnea may precipitate an attack by increasing systemic venous return.

In the presence of fixed or decreased pulmonary blood flow, there is an increased right to left shunt, resulting in arterial hypoxia, metabolic acidosis, and increased CO_2. This further stimulates the respiratory mechanism to maintain continuing anemia, which may predispose to cyanotic spells. These spells are characterized by sudden onset dyspnea, increased cyanosis, and can progress to loss of consciousness, convulsions, and even death. The intensity of the murmur may be reduced or completely disappear. Laboratory data includes hypoxemia, acidosis, diminished pulmonary flow on X-ray, and increased voltage of P waves on ECG. Treatment options depend on the severity and may include positional changes, oxygen therapy, medications such as morphine or propranolol, blood transfusion, and palliative surgeries.

Double-outlet right ventricle is a rare anomaly where both major arteries arise from the right ventricle. The aorta is completely transposed while the pulmonary artery remains in a relatively normal position. This results in a large VSD being necessary for blood to be ejected from the left ventricle. The location of the defect can vary, with different symptoms and degrees of cyanosis. Pulmonary stenosis can further increase cyanosis. Echocardiography, cardiac catheterization, and angiocardiography are used to diagnose this condition. Treatment options include palliative surgery to increase pulmonary blood flow and corrective surgery to establish aorta-left ventricle continuity.

In cases of double outlet right ventricle with pulmonary stenosis, palliative surgery involving shunts between systemic and pulmonary circulation is performed. For those without pulmonary stenosis and in cardiac failure, pulmonary artery banding may be done. Corrective surgery to establish aorta-left ventricle continuity can be challenging.

PULMONARY ATRESIA

Pulmonary atresia with VSD is a severe form of tetralogy of Fallot in which blood cannot flow from the right ventricle into the pulmonary artery due to the atretic or absent pulmonary valve. The pulmonary trunk is also underdeveloped. In this condition, the entire output of the ventricle is ejected into the aorta via the VSD. In order for normal function to be maintained, there must be an additional communication and pathway for blood to enter the lungs, typically through the PDA or bronchial circulation. The extent of pulmonary blood flow depends on the size of the ductus or collateral channels. If these pathways are large, patients may fare well, even better than severe cases of tetralogy of Fallot. However, if the pulmonary blood flow is minimal, severe oxygen deprivation can occur early in life, potentially leading to sudden death if the PDA closes after birth.

The clinical features of pulmonary atresia with VSD are similar to those of tetralogy of Fallot, but cyanosis appears within a few days after birth, whereas in tetralogy of Fallot it usually appears later in the first year. The systolic murmur is often absent or soft, and there may be an ejection click after the first heart sound. The second heart sound is moderately loud, and continuous murmurs from the PDA or bronchial circulation may be heard throughout the chest. The heart may appear enlarged on X-ray, and the bronchial collateral flow pattern may be visible. Right ventriculography can reveal opacification of the large aorta from the VSD and the pathway of pulmonary blood flow from the aorta. If dependency on the PDA is established, infusion of prostaglandin E1 can be used to dilate the PDA and stabilize the patient until surgery.

Severe cyanotic spells and increasing hematocrit levels are common during infancy, indicating a need for surgical systemic-pulmonary arterial anastomosis. Later corrective surgery can be attempted if the pulmonary arteries are of adequate size. Many patients with this condition have malformations of the primary divisions of the pulmonary arteries, such as hypoplasia or stenosis, or even absence of a pulmonary artery, accompanied by large bronchial collaterals. These malformations typically require surgical correction. The ideal correction involves bypassing the obstructed right ventricular outflow and closing the VSD. In some cases, total obstruction of the right ventricular outflow may occur after a systemic-pulmonary anastomosis for tetralogy of Fallot, necessitating further corrective surgery.

In cases where the ventricular septum is intact, there is usually associated hypoplasia of the right ventricle, which is thick-walled and lined with thick endocardium. The tricuspid valve orifice is often small. However, in some patients, the right ventricle may be normal or large, and the tricuspid valve may be functionally incompetent. Intermediate forms between these two extremes can also occur. The main pulmonary arteries are almost always patent. In order for normal function to be achieved, there must be an intertribal communication and another pathway for blood to enter the lungs, typically through a PDA or bronchial circulation. Since there is no egress from the right ventricle, blood from the right atrium is shunted into the left atrium via the foramen ovale or ASD, mixes with pulmonary venous blood, and is pumped into the aorta by the left ventricle. Pulmonary flow occurs through the PDA and bronchial vessels.

The pulmonary circulation is primarily maintained by the PDA, although it is usually insufficient to maintain adequate pulmonary blood flow. Therefore, whether a patient with pulmonary atresia with VSD survives depends on the patency of the ductus, and death can occur within a few days of birth if it constricts and closes. As the ductus closes, hypoxia becomes more severe, leading to death. Cyanosis and tachypnea are usually present at birth or appear soon after birth, although if the ductus is widely patent, cyanosis may not be intense. Some patients may be initially normal at birth and develop cyanosis in early infancy.

Progressive deepening of cyanosis is accompanied by severe dyspnea, and metabolic acidosis develops as cyanosis increases. Cardiac failure can occur early, especially in the presence of tricuspid incompetence and right ventricular dilatation. Cardiomegaly is often observed. The second heart sound becomes single, and there may be no murmur in the presence of a competent tricuspid valve. However, a blowing systolic murmur may be heard at the pulmonary valve area or under the left clavicle due to the associated PDA, or continuous murmurs may be heard anywhere indicating good pulmonary blood flow through the ducts. If tricuspid regurgitation develops, as seen in cases where the right ventricle is normal or dilated (type 2), a loud, pan-systolic murmur is heard at the lower sternal border. The liver may exhibit pulsations. ECG findings include tall spiked P waves (indicative of left atrial enlargement) and evidence of left ventricular hypertrophy with left-axis deviation. With a hypoplastic and small right ventricle, there may also be evidence of right ventricular hypertrophy, and the axis may be in the normal plane or deviated to the right. X-rays typically show a markedly enlarged heart with reduced pulmonary circulation. In cases with significant tricuspid insufficiency, there may be massive right atrial enlargement, and the cardiac silhouette may fill the entire chest. Cardiac catheterization shows high pressure in the right atrium, often higher than systemic pressure, and demonstrates R-L shunting.

Angiocardiography reveals the size of the ventricular cavity, the atretic pulmonary valve, tricuspid regurgitation, and the successive filling of the right atrium, left atrium, left ventricle, aorta, large ducts, and pulmonary arteries. Right ventriculography shows the hypoplastic right ventricle and may reveal large sinusoids that fill with contrast medium, draining in a retrograde manner into the coronary arterial system. Echocardiography confirms the absence of the pulmonary valve and can show varying degrees of hypoplasia of the right ventricular cavity.

Treatment for pulmonary atresia with VSD aims to increase pulmonary blood flow and manage heart failure. As soon as the diagnosis is made, a balloon atrial septostomy is performed to create an adequate flow in both directions, followed immediately by surgery. The surgical procedure involves pulmonary valvotomy, followed by a systemic-to-pulmonary artery anastomosis. A Blalock-Taussig procedure may also be performed to improve blood flow to the lungs. Since the majority of patients have hypoplastic right ventricles, the initial procedure may involve creating a systemic-to-pulmonary artery anastomosis and a large ASD using balloon septostomy, followed by pulmonary valvotomy in the hope that the right ventricular cavity will grow. However, surgery carries a high risk, particularly in neonates with hypoplastic ventricles. If the tricuspid valve, right ventricle, and pulmonary valve ring are nearly normal, valvotomy can relieve the obstruction. Infusion of prostaglandin E1 can help maintain patency of the ductus until surgery is performed. In type 1 patients, the dimensions of the right ventricle significantly increase after the initial procedure.

TRICUSPID ATRESIA

Tricuspid atresia is a rare condition where the tricuspid valve is completely missing, resulting in no normal connection between the right atrium and right ventricle. The right ventricle is smaller than usual. Systemic blood that normally enters the right atrium is redirected through a patent foramen ovale (PFO) or atrial septal defect (ASD) into the left atrium, where it mixes with pulmonary blood. This mixed blood then enters the left ventricle. Most of this mixed blood goes into the aorta, while some is shunted through a ventricular septal defect (VSD) into the hypoplastic right ventricle and then into the pulmonary artery. The right ventricle may be underdeveloped or narrow in shape. In some cases, the pulmonary artery and pulmonary valve may also be underdeveloped or completely blocked, in which case the pulmonary blood supply is maintained by a patent ductus arteriosus (PDA). Generally, there is a small VSD and hypoplastic pulmonary arteries. If the septum between the ventricles is intact, pulmonary atresia is usually present, with the pulmonary artery being a normal size and the VSD being large. There are two types of tricuspid atresia: with and without transposition of the great arteries. In 70% of cases, the great arteries are in their normal positions, while in 30% there is transposition.

1. When there is tricuspid atresia but no transposition(majority), we may have no VSD, hypoplasia, or atresia of the pulmonary artery: PDA. Small VSD; pulmonary stenosis, hypoplastic pulmonary artery large VSD; no pulmonary stenosis normal sized pulmonary artery
2. When there is associated transposition: with VSD and pulmonary stenosis with VSD, but no pulmonary stenosis. As a result of lack of direct communication between the right atrium and right ventricle, the development of the ventricle depends on the presence of an L-R shunt at the ventricular level. Therefore, severe hypoplasia of the right ventricle is seen in those forms in which there is no ventricular septal defect or in which the VSD is very small. When pulmonary stenosis is present with tricuspid atresia and arterial transposition, the hemodynamics and clinicalpicture simulate those of tricuspid atresia with normally related great arteries. Clinical_features: In the great majority of cases, symptoms are present at birth or develop very early in infancy. - Cyanosis is present at birth, except in cases where pulmonary blood flow is great. When pulmonary blood is compromised at cyanosis, polycythemia, easy fatigability, exceptional dyspnea, and anoxic hyper cyanotic attacks occur early in infancy. Growth and development are very poor, and there is Hurled fatigability at feeds, tachypnea, dyspnea, and evidence of right heart failure. Cyanosis in intensity depends on the amount of pulmonary blood flow, and in infants with pulmonary atresia or severe pulmonary stenosis, cyanosis is deep. Hypoxic spells occur in infants below 6 months of age.

Cardiac failure may be present if pulmonary blood flow is large. After (thus left heart failure is seen in patients with a marked increase in pulmonary flow sepatients with large VSD, no pulmonary stenosis, and the normal sized pulmonary artery; and in case of transposedarteries, with VSD but no pulmonary

After infancy, clubbing is common, but squatting is not as common as in tetralogy. Thus, the older child will have clubbing, cyanosis, effort dyspnea, squatting, and growth retardation. If the interatrial communication is small, right atrial hypertension results in a prominent jugular A-waveand presystolic pulsation of the enlarged liver.

A slight bulge on the right side of the sternum may be seen-The heart may or may not be enlargedwith a heaving left ventricular apical impulse. The first heart sound is single and loud, and the heart sound is single (only aortic component due to the absence of pulmonary component). The usual murmur is a harsh, blowing systolic murmur (pansies to lie or ejection), best beard! At the lover left sternal border Pan and systolic murmur is from VSD). The murmur may be absent in very small infants. In the precise, absence of a significant murmur in a cyanotic baby should suggest a cause other than Fallots with pulmonary atresia associated, the harsh blowing systolic murmur is present.
X-ray Heart is normal sized or may be slightly enlarged; the main pulmonary segment or- is usually small or absent there is deficiency of the shadow of Pulmonarynar aretery; pulmonary vascular markings are decreased (pulmonary under circulation. The cardiac contour is variable. In the PA view the right border may be straight or rounded due to the large right atrium (the size of the right atrium varies, depending on the size of the communication at the atrial level). In the left anterior oblique view, the posterior border of the heart overlaps the spine because of the large left ventricle. The anterior border may be normally receded from

the sternum or be displaced forward by the large left ventricle. The apex is high in PA veiw. In many cases, cardiac silhouette is like teratology. When pulmonary blood flow is increased, gross cardiomegaly with a large main pulmonary artery and plethoric pulmonary vaseular is seen. With left atrial enlargement, the heart may have a square appearance.

ECG:

ECG is a much more sensitive index of the state of the ventricles; the axis deviation, left ventricular hypertrophy, and abnormal P waves are usual (tall and peaked P waves indicating rightatrial hypertrophy). The size of the P waves depends on the right atrial pressure, which in turn depends on the wave the size of the interatrial communication (the taller the P wave, the smaller the communication.

Left ventricular preponderance or hypertrophy is seen in some cases. In the right precordial leads, the normally prominent R wave is replaced by a complex; the left precodrial leads show a qR complex followed by a normal or insetted T wave. In an obviously cyanotic Infant with an X-ray picture as above, left axis deviation, left ventricular hypertrophy and right atrial enlargement almost established the diagnosis of tricuspid atresia. Right vetrlcular forces are absent or decreased.

CARDIAC CATHETERIZATION

Revelas a. right to left shunt at the atrial level; there is an elevated rightatrial pressure with prominent a wave; it is impossible to enter the right ventricle from the rightatrium. If the catheter is advanced through the inferior vena cava and right atrium, it usually passes across the aerial defect into the left side of the heart.

ANGIOCARDIOGRAPHY

When an injection is made into the right atrium, it shows a lack, of communication between the right atrium and right ventricle; the absence of flow from the right atrium to the right ventricle results in infilling defect between the right atrium and left ventricle) the contrast medium passes from the right atrium into the left atrium, and thus the left ventricle and aorta. The tiny right ventricle may be opacified if there is a VSD); otherwise, the pulmonary arteries are filled via. a PDA. Selective left ventriculography may be done to detect the presence of associated transposition of arteries and pulmonary stenosis.

TREATMENT

Treatment is palliative and is aimed at creating a large interatrial communication; to relieve the right atrial hypertension and to increase the pulmonary blood flow (done by balloon atrial septostomy of RashKind type at the time of cardiac catheterization or the Blaock-rienlon operation and systemic pulmonary arterial anastomosis preferably Waterston type. The results arenot as gratifying as with- tetralogy. Good results may be obtained from end-to-end anastomosis ofthe superior vena cava to the right pulmonary artery (Glenn 's operation) the operation failure isincreased by left ventricular failure and failure tedrecegnise a small interatrial communication. Systemic to pulmonaryenary anastemesis should only be done in patients in whom pulmonary blood flow is markedly decreased and in whom cyanosis is severe. When pulmonary blood, flow is excessive cardiac failure should be treated by digitalis and diuretics followed by pulmonary artery binding may Be done. Recently a valve-hearing conduit has been introduced from the right atrium directly into the pulmonary artery (Eentan procedure) while closing the ASD. Prognosis depends on the balance between the pulmonary blood flow, which should be optimal, permitting adequate oxygenation of tissues without producing intractable CCF; in untreated cases, it is dealt with securely within the first 6 months; only a minority survive without palliative surgery, and they have non-restrictive inter-atrial communication and adequate pulmonary blood flow. The immediate, as well as long term prognosis are poor, and most patients will not survive beyond 15 years since presently, it is an uncorrectable lesion.

COMPLETE TRANSPOSITION OF GREAT ARTERIES

Complete transposition. of the great arteries is the 2nd most common cyanotic disorder and more common in males 3:1and is due to embryologic abnormality in the spiral decision of the truncus arteriosus, The aorta arises from the right ventricle and the pulmonary artery from the left Ventricle, Systemic veins return to right atrium; and pulmonary veins to left atrium,,Therefore the blood from the right side of the aorta passes to the aorta and pulmonary blood flow is returned to the lungs. These two independent circuits cannot sustain life unless there is an associated compensatory shunt as foramen pvale, PDA, ASD, or VSD. This condition is commonest cause of death in infants under 1 yr having CHD. Many patients has family h/o diabetes mellitus. The aorta lies anterior superior and to the right, whereas the pulmonary artery lies posterior inferior and to the left (Less commonly, the aorta may be directly in front of the pulmonary artery or maybe anterior but left to it, or both may be side to side). In most cases, associated cardiac abnormalities are present, including VSB, ASD, pulmonary stenosis, and PDA. Obstructive changes within the pulmonary arteriolar bed are common in patients past infancy. Generally, the right coronary artery arises from the aorta above the posterior sinus of Valsalva and the left above the left sinus while as in normal infants, the rt coronary artery arises above the right sinus and the left abovethe left sinus in 50% of cases have a VSD. Therefore, the transposition is classified as transposition with the intact ventricular septum, where it may be with pulmonary stenosis, valvular or subvalvular, or bdhor without it, transposition with VSD; where it may be with pulmonary stenosis, with pulmonary vascular obstruction, or without pulmonary vascular obstruction and thus normal pulmonary vascular resistance.

The mem hemodynamics depends on the reaction of the pulmonary arterial and veno circulationsand on the presence of the associated defects. Neonates with a virtually intact ventricular septum show an increase in the pulmonary arterial and venous pressures gross arterial oxygen desaturation, Marked increase of pulmonary vascular resistance may be present early but is generally found in older children and with a large VSD. In pts, with intact ventricular septum, arterial blood mixin occurs at the atrial and ductal level, but in most of these cases, the communications are small, and the ductus closes shortly after birth. These patients are, therefore, severely cyanotic, and COF occurs rapidly due to a marked increase in cardiac output. Patients with a VSD show a greater or lesser degree of cyanosis depending upon the ratio of the pulmonary to systemic blood flow patients with VSD and pulmonary stenosis are usually severely cyanotic because of the limited flow to the lungs. Patients with VSD and pulmonary vascular obstruction, there is a moderate degree of cyanosis. Patients with VSD and normal pulmonary resistance show the least cyanosis but develop COF very early from enormous pulmonary blood flow.

Therefore, the clinical features in transposition include cyanosis, CCF, dyspnea, tachypnea, which dominate the picture, but the method of presentation depends on the associated defects. Cyanosis is present at birth or appears shortly after birth or within the first week of life (occasionally does notdedpuntil later). Patients with the intact ventricular septum, and those who have VSD with, Pulmonaryinc stenosis are most deeply cyanotic, whileas those with VSD but normal vascular resistance in the lungs is least cyanotic. Many of the neonates are quite large, some weighing 4 kg at birth. Retardation of growth and development after the neornatal period are common. The cyanosis is progressive and present at rest. Polycythemia, and arterial unsaturation, are usual in older infants. Occasionally moderate cyanosis appears late in. patients who have torrential pulmonary blood flow. In some pts, legs are less cyanotic than rest of the body, as arterialized blood flows via the PDA from the pulmonary artery to the descending aorta. Differential cyanosis is seen only if there isassociated preductal aortic coarctation. Hyper cyanotic blue spells are rare. COF occurs in patients with intact septum and those with large VSD and normal pulmonary vascular resistance. COF develops not only because of the high cardiac output but also because of the poor oxygenation ofthe myocardium and the presence of systemic pressure in both ventricles. COF develops within 2-4 weeks usually. Patients with VSD and pulmonary stenosis (it is clinically identical to tetralogy) there isno CCF, but they have severe anoxic spells in early life; if they survive the first yr retarded growth is common, and cyanosis becomes progressively more severe, but intellectual development is unaffected. Although these infants are large at birth, growth, and development is. retarded, so that by 6months to 1yr they are usually below the 3rd percentile in. both height as well as weight. Cyanosis is marked. Clubbing is present after 1 yr of age. Cardiomegaly may be present, usually with, hyperactive precordium, and righ ventricular lift especially after the first month; but heart may benormal-sized in. the neonate. The first heart sound is loud and. sharp: the second is also loud and single (or very narrowly split). Soft unimpressive systolic murmurs may be heard. Signs of pulmonary hypertension will incilde-a systolic ejection click, a booming second heart sound, short systolic, ejection murmur, and sometimes anearly diastolic murmur of pulmonary incompetence.

X-RAY:

X-ray reveals a progressive cardiomegaly, increased pulmonary vasculature, and a narrow cardiacbase in PA view. The characteristic findings are lacking in the newborn infant but may be absentin any age period. Progressive generalised cardiomegaly develops rapidly and is much more striking if pulmonary blood flow is excessive. With absent pulmonary stenosis there is marked pulmonary overvascularization bilaterally. The narrow cardiac base in the frontal projection is due to superimposition of the shadows of aorta and pulmonary artery; it may be obscured by a large thymic shadow. At birth and within first 7-10 days thereafter, the chest may be essentially normal, but the heart is always enlarged after the first month. The right ventricle is more markedly enlarged than the left. When pulmonary vascular obstruction is present, there is only mild to moderate cardiomegaly, and pulmonary vessels are prominent at the hila but are narrow peripherally. Classically the heart has an egg-on-side shape with a narrow supracardiac mediastinal shadow that widens out in the oblique and lateral view.

ECG:

As the right ventricle is pumping blood into the aorta against systemic resistance, there is right ventricular hypertrophy, and since later pulmonary vascular changes haveset in, a pattern of combined ventricular hypertrophy may be seen.ECG in infancy reveals the usual amount of right ventricular predominance and hypertrophy expected for age. Thus, ECG may show right axial deviation, RVH, and frequently pulmonary; but ECG is least helpful, especially during early infancy, when right ventricular hypertrophy is normal. Echocardiography helps to establish the transposed location of the vessels, if it is demonstrated that the great anterior vessels is in front or to the right of the posterior vessel. With cardiac catheterization, the pulmonary artery is entered from the left ventricle and the aorta from the right ventricle. Pressures in the right ventricle are equal to the aortic pressure, and the leftventricular pressure is usually lower than the right ventricular pressure.

Angiocardiography (right ventriculography) opacifies the aorta, and in the lateral projection, the aorta is seen lying anterior to the pulmonary artery, and aortic valve cusps; are higher than normal; As soon as thesurgeon identifies the nature of the lesion; Rashkind septostomy is done. Without an intact ventricular septum, patient survives only if there is a large ASD, and with VSD, the best survival rate is seen in those who have mild to moderate pulmonary stenosis. A large PDA portends a bad prognosis. The majority of patients die within a month without surgical intervention.

ISOLATED (SIMPLE) TRANSPOSITION

In these pts, the ventricular septum is intact, and mixing of the circulation occurs from the bidirectional shunting across the foramen ovale. Cyanosis and tachypnea appear within the first weeks of life and generally within the first days. If the foramen ovale is patulous, significant mixing may occur so the recognition of cyanosis is difficult and may be delayed for weeks but the presence of cyanosis and tachypnea in a neonate of normal weight should be taken as isolated transposition, which constitutes a medical emergency. In the first few days of life, the physical examination may be normal except for hepatomegaly since murmurs are absent in the majority, and cardiomegaly is unusual in the neontal period. _i'wo distinct components of the 2nd heart sound help to exclude the diagnosis of hypoplastic heart syndrome. Chest X-ray may be normalor may show cardiomegaly, a narrow cardiac waist, and increased pulmonary arterial and venous circulation. If cyanosis is in doubt, confirmation of tne desaturation may be obtained from pO2 determination of arterial blood; in these pts, the arterial pO2 is low, and doesnot rise significantlyafter the patient breathes 80-100% of oxygen. The heart may have the typical appearance of an egg ona string.If there is pulmonary stenosis, pulmonary vasculature may be decreased. Cardiac catheterization shows right ventricular hypertension. The catheter enters the aorta directly from the right ventricle; the atrial communication ASD or PFO may be delineated; the blood in the pulmonary artery has a. higher oxygen concentration than in the aorta here is marked systemic unsaturathon. A pressure gradient exists between the atria, and the left atrial pressure exceeds the right one. Right ventriculography demonstrates the origin of the anterior placed aorta from the right ventricle, shows the Intactess of the right ventricle excludes association of the PDA, the aortic valve is cehalad to the pulmonary valve, the origin of the coronary arteries is also showwn. Left ventriculography shows that the pulmonary artery- arises exclusively from the posterior ventricle and that the septum is intact. It is established that both ventricles are normal.

Some patients with isolated transposition have adequate mixing of blood across the interatrial septumand may only present at the age of 2-4 weeks or occasionally even at the age of few months; in addition to intense cyahosis and hypoxemia, there is marked cardiomegaly; ECG shows right ventricular or biventricular hypertrophy and chest X-ray the typical progressive cardiomegaly, andsignificant increase in pulmonary vascularity due to the prominence of both arterial and venous shadows. The narrow cardiac base is due to superimposed shadows of the two arteries; and prognosis is bad.

TREATMENT

The prognosis of the hypoxic neonate is extremely poor, and without treatment,1/2 will die in the first week of life. Particular attention must be paid to maintaining normal body temperature since hypothermia intensifies the signs of metabolic acidosis which frequently occurs from hypoxemia. Early recognition of the disease, the prevention of hypothermia, and the rapid correction of acidosis and hypoglycemia, which may occur in these patients is essential. As soon as the diagnosis is made, balloon atrial septostomy (Rashkind) is done immediately enlarging the atrial communication by repeatedly pulling a dye-filled balloon acrossthe foramen ovale, tearing the septum. After an adequate septostomy, mixing of the blood occurs at the atrial level, the high pressure in the left atrium and pulmonary veins is restored to normal, signifleant elevation of arterial oxygen saturation occurs, and tachypnea is relivedbecause of reduction of pulmonary venous pressure.

Cardiac catheterization is done in the neonatal period for diagnostic and therapeutic purposes; then repeated at 4-6 months with catheterization of the pulmonary artery to assess the progression of pulmonary vascular obstruction, determination of the presence of left ventricular outflow obstruction, and repeat Rashkind septostomy if needed? Then repeated at 8-10 months if surgery has not been done. Some pts, following the septostomy, may have a recurrence of cyanosis due either to inadequate shunting of blood at the atrial level or to the development of sub-valvular pulmonary stenosis. These patients have polycythemia, effort intolerance, irritability,poor weight gain,and are liable to develop cerebrovascular accidents. After significant pulmonary stenosis is excluded, either blbon septostomy is repeated, or surgical atrial septostomy is done, if the is under 6 months of age. Intra-atrial surgical correction (Mustard operation) is done in older babies.

Intra-atrial correction should not be postponed beyond the age of 1 yr, even if the cyanosis is only moderate. Symptomatic improvement after the Mustard operation is dramatic, with the disappearance of cyanosis, and a marked increase in effort intolerance, but carefully follow-up for many years is essential, for the following complication may arise after the operation arrhythmias are common and primarily atrial in origin; they consist mostly of bradytachyeardiae arrhjhtmias due to the sick sinus syndrome, atrial tachycardia with block, atrial flutter, and conjunctional rhythm-in some complete heart block occurring Sometimes, arrhythmias may occurafter Blalock-Hanlon operation (atrial seprostom: and thus precede the Mustard cooperation.

Recurrences of cyanosis may occur as a rupture of the atrial baffle created during theoperation and bidirectional atrial shunting. superior or inferior cava syndrome or pulmonary vascular (venous) obstruction may result fromthe obstruction of these veins entering the atria by the atrial baffle. tricuspid incompetence may occur with an increase in the left atrial pressure, pulmonary edema, adCCF.

TRANSPOSITION WITH VSD

If the defect is small, the clinical picture and treatment are as of isolated transposition, but a long systolic murmur is audible along the left sternal edge because of the flow across the VSD. A significant number of defects close spontaneously (depriving the patient of the necessary mixing). When the defect is large, significant mixing of the blood occurs, and the clinical picture is dominated by CCF. The onset of cyanosis is subtle and delayed and varies in intensity. Usually, cyanosis develops within the first month but occasionally may be delayed for months. If the presence of cyanosis is dubious, a low arterial p02 and its failure to rise when the patient breathes 80- 100% oxygen resolves the problem. Hypoxemia is associated with polycythemia. Heart is enlarged; the murmur is pansystolic; ECG shows prominent P waves, right ventricular or biventricular hypertrophy; usually right axis deviation (but may be normal, or even, to the left); chest X-ray shows marked cardiomegaly, a narrow, cardiac waist, and extreme pulmonary plethora;

cardiac catheterization confirms the diagnosis, with angiocardiography. Right and left ventriculography to indicate the transposition and site and size of VSD. At the time of catheterization, ballooon septostomy is done to decompress the right-atrium left atrium even though adequate mixing occurs at the ventricular level. Elective pulmonary banding is done sincepulmonary vascular resistance develops rapidly in these ppts. These patients also need digitalis and diuretics. The operation later consists of pulmonary artery debanding, closure of the VSD, and Mustard operation. The operative risk is increased if there is associated development of sub-pulmonary stenosis. The prognosis in these patients is poor, the majority dying within the first yearbecause of CCF, hypoxemia, and pulmonary hypertension. Those who survive infancy without surgery, are essentially dealt with as Eisenmngers syndrome due to a large VSD.

TRANSPOSITION WITH A LARGE PDA

In the neonatal period; a large. PDA may be beneficial, hut later on it is not an asset and persistent patency beyond the first weeks of life aggravates the situa tion, since the dominant flowacross the duct is from aorta to pulmonary artery, further increasing the pulmonary blood flow the clinical picture is dominated by COF and cyanosis may not be obvious. After effective palliation with balloon septostomy, many of these babies remain in uncontrollable CCF, and require surgical closure of the duct. Presence of PDA accelerates rising pulmonary vascular resistance, and its spontaneous closure may disastrously disrupatient the delicate balance of mixing.

TRANS-POSITION WITH PULMONARY STENOSIS

This condition mimics; tetralogy of Fallot. The site of obstruction is valvular or subvalvular, and there may be an associated hypoplastic pulmonary arterial trunk a VSD may or may not be present. Subvalvular obstruction may have resulted from atrial septostomy or pulmonary arterial banding Symptoms may start soon after birth or may start in late infancy; manifesting by cyanosis, hypercyanotic spells, decreased exercise tolerance, and poor physical development; COF is not common during infancy but may result later. On examination, physical signs mimic tetralogy, but the cyanosis is more intense, and the heart is enlarged-pulmonary vasculature may be normal or reduced, and in cases where pulmonary stenosis is not severe is increased instead. ECG shows right axial deviation, RVH sometimes, spiked tall P waves. Cardiac catheterization shows that the pulmonary venous pressure is low, and its oxygen saturation exceeds that of the aorta selective rt. It ventriculography demonstrates the abnormal origin of the arteriesan in addition to VSD and pulmonary stenosis.

Treatment is difficult; Mustard operation is not always practicable and has high risk, if the subvalvular obstruction is long and narrow and if the main pulmonary artery is hypoplastic;. Inmost cases, Rastelli operation an aortic homograft from, left ventricle to pulmonary arteries is more ideally done. Systemic-pulmonary arterial anastomosis is done in patients who are cyanotic hutare not in failure.

TRANSPOSITION WITH TRICUSPID ATRESIA

When transposition of great arteries accompanies tricuspid atresia and pulmonary stenosis, the syndrome mimics tricuspid atresia, but if pulmonary stenosis is absent, then pulmonary low excessive cyanosis is mild and seldom conspicuous. Tachypnea feeding difficulties, poor weight gain, recurrent respiratory infections and COF are usual-increased venous pulsations that may lead topresystolic pulsations of a large liver and a prominent A-wave in the jugular venous pulse. Thereis marked cardiac enlargement, systolic and ejection murmurs, and the 2nd heart sound is

loud and single. ECG usually shows prominent P waves, left axis deviation, and LVH.
X-ray shows cardiomegaly and increases pulmonary vascularity.
Diagnosis is confirmed by selective left ventriculography, delineating a large left ventricle, small right ventricle arterial transposition and relative size of the pulmonary artery and aorta. Generally, the prognosis is poor especially when the aorta is hypoplastic, and the pulmonary artery flowis torrential. Surgical palliation is given by pulmonary artery banding.

TRANSPOSITION OF THE AORTA AND OVERRIDING PULMONARY ARTERY- (TAUSSIG BING SYNDROME)

In this malformation, the aorta rises from the right ventricle, and the pulmonary artery (which is large) overrides the ventricular septum. A VSD is always present. The clinical picture is dominated) by the presence of severe pulmonary hypertension. Cyanosis is present from birth, and tachypnea, frequent Respiratory infections, decrease exercise tolerance, and poor physical development are usual. In the infant, heart is enlarged, but later, the pulmonary vascular disease reduces pulmonary blood flow, and the heart is normal sized in the older children. Auscultatory findings include an early ejection click, a mid-systolic ejection murmur, a hooming 2nd heart sound, and sometimes an early diastolic murmur of pulmonary valve incompetence (all features of pulmonary hypertension). The systolic murmur is longer and louder if pulmonary blood flow is torrential. Pulmonary stenosis is rarely present.
ECG shows RVH with prominent P waves since, during infancy, there is a large pulmonaryflow. LVH is also seen in them.
Chest X-ray shows cardiomegaly and increased pulmonary vascular obstruction during infancy As pulmonary vascular obstruction develops, the heart size decreases, the major branches of thepulmonary artery become prominent, and

there is attentuation of the vascular pattern in the outer lung fields.
Cardiac catheterization reveals right ventricular hypertension and pulmonary hypertension, and the pulmonary arterial oxygen saturation exceeds that of theaorta. Selective right ventriculography shows the abnormal anatomy of the aorta and pulmonary artery. The mustard operation may be useful (interatrial venous
and if there is no pulmonary vase obstruction and closing of VSD.

EISENMENGER SYNDROME

Eisenmenger's syndrome is the combination of pulmonary hypertension with reversed or bidirectional shunt through a VSD, ASD or PDA or other communications between the aorta andlesser circulation. The principal physiological abnormality is thus elevation of the pulmonary vascular resistance. In the normal infants and soon after birth, pulmonary vascular resistance is high. Within a few weeks, the structure of the pulmonary arteriole's changes to that of the adult with a thin wall and large lumen, and the pulmonary vascular resistance falls to the adult levels. In this syndrome, this resistance remains abnormally high. This abnormal resistance is present from the very birth. In some cases of a large VSD, the resistance may fall somewhat, only to rise again in later childhoodor adult life.

Symptoms are usually present in the first year of life, in patients with VSD; these include dyspnea feeding difficulties, fatigue, failure to gain weight, and recurrent pneumonia. As the child grows older, dyspnea on effort is obvious, when VSD and ASD are present. Cyanosis may be present early and gets progressively worse when the child approaches puberty, it is associated with clubbing and polycythemia; and there are squatting, angina pectoris, hemoptysis, and episodes of syncope. If there is a PDA, venous blood from the pulmonary aryery is shunted down the descending aorta and results in differential cyanopsia (blue lower limbs and pink upper limbs JVP is raised when COF or functional tricuspid insufficiency is present. Heart size is variable, normal in VSD, and large with ASD. There is a conspicuous left parasternal (right ventricular) heave, with palpable pulmonary arterial pulsations sometimes. A systolic murmur preceded by a pulmonary ejection, click. The 2nd heart sound is loud and. booming; and is closely split or single in many cases of VSD but widely split with ASD. Functional incompetence of the pulmonary valve resulting; in a blowing diastolic murmur down the left sternal border (Graham Steel mu ring) is common and assisted with a normal peripheral arterial pulse.

X-ray shows a heart that may be normal to greatly enlarged; the larger hearts are seen with ASDand the smaller ones with VSD and PDA, but there is a large overlap. The pulmonary artery is enlarged; the pulmonary vessels are enlarged in the hilar areas and diminish in calibre in the periphery's branches. The right atrium and right ventricle are prominent. ECG shows RVH, occasionally associated with incomplete right bundle branch block. The Pwaves are tall and spiked. Sometimes there are signs of biventricular hypertrophy. Cardiac catheterization shows a bidirectional shunt generally; the catheter may traverse the defect with a PDA or ASD. The sÿstolic pressures are usually equal in the systemic and pulmonarycirculations, and pulmonary vascular resistance is raised.
Indicator dilution curves demonstrate the bidirectional shunts or the unidirectional right to leftshunts.
Selective angiocardiography locates the site of the shunt. With PDA, the contrast medium entersthe descending aorta from the pulmonary artery. The presence of this syndrome contraindicatesthe surgical closure of the defect Pulmonary hypertension with increased pulmonary blood flow but without a R-L shunt isnot Eisenmengers syndrome, and surgery may be lifesaving in them.

Treatment of Eisenmenger's syndrome is primarily symptomatic, and older children with significant polycythemia may be improved by cautious, repeated small venesections.

SINGLE VENTRICLE (COMMON VENTRICLE)

Both atria open into the common ventricle via two separate AV valves. From this common ventricle, both aorta and the pulmonary artery arise. The single ventricle, in most cases, has the morphologic characteristics of a left ventricle. This complicated defect is always associated withother cardiac anomalies. A rudimentary rt ventricular outflow chamber without a rt ventricular sinus, separated from the single ventricle by a muscular ridge and communicating with it via a bulboventricular foramen, other associated anomalies may be present, as transposition of the arteries, dextrocardia or other cardiac mamalposition, aortic outflow obstruction with or without coarctation, ASD, common atrioventricular canal, etc. The more common is the single ventricle associated with arterial transposition and a rudimentary outlet chamber from- which the aorta arises or a single ventriclewith pulmonary stenosis.

The hemodynamics and clinical picture depend extremely on the associated anomalies and thus is variable. Single ventricle may mimic a large VSD, transposition of the arteries (with VSD) tetralogy, tricuspid atresia, and persistent truncus arteriosus Patients usually present soon after birth. If the single ventricle presents with pulmonary stenosis, there is cyanosis from infancy, which increases in intensity during childhood when clubbing and polycythemia also appear. Dyspnea and fatigue are present, and blue spells may occur.

There is cardiomegaly, a left parasternal lift systolic thrill, a loud pansystolic murmur, and ejection click, and a single and loud 2nd heart sound.

When a single ventricle is associated with a rudimentary systemic outflow tract, pulmonary bloodflow is torrential. These patients have tachypnea, dyspnea, poor physical development, recurrent pulmonary infections, and CCF. Cyanosis is mild cardiomegaly marked -left parasternal lift palpable systolic ejection murmur not intense, 2nd; sound loud and closely split-a _3rd heartsound is heard which may be followed by a short mid-diastolic murmur. The development ofpulmonary vascular resistance- the disease may restrict pulmonary blood flow so that cyanosis increases and heart size decreases so that signs of cardiac failure appear to improve.

ECG is not specific usually, right axis deviation is present (but left axis deviation may be present); P waves are normal, spiked or bifidjprecordial lead past era will show Right ventricularhypertrophy, combined hypertrophy, or sometimes left ventricular hypertrophy. X-ray shows cardiomegaly. The rudimentary systemic outflow chamber may produce a bulge on the upper left border of the cardiac cell Houtte in the PA projection. In the absence of pulmonary stenosis, pulmonary vascular nature is increased, with the prominence of the major branches of the pulmonary artery. With the development of the obstructive pulmonary vascular disease, attenuate ion of the size of the peripheral pulmonary arteries occurs. With, pulmonary stenosis, pulmonary vasculature is decreased.

Echocardiography demonstrates a large ventricular atrio-ventricular valve leaflet that moves fr anteriorly; ventricular septal echoes are absent. Selective ventriculography will demonstrate the single ventricle and the position and relation of the pulmonary artery and aorta-Presence of pulmonary stenosis or a rudimentary outflow chamber is identified. Many patients with single ventricle dies during the neonatal period, and more than 1/2 die in the first year many succumb during infancy from COF and superimposed pulmonary infection those who survive till adolescence later die of pulmonary hypertension. Those with pulmonary stenosis have a better prognosis; if there is a pulmonary stenosis, systemic-pulmonary arterial anastomoses can result in improvement. Similarly, an anastomosis of the SVC to the right pulmonary artery in them can be beneficial. In those with a large pulmonary flow and cardiac failure pulmonary artery, banding is done.

EBSTEIN DISEASE

Epstein's anomaly can be variable-the most typical lesion is where posterior and medial leaflets ofthe tricuspid valve are displaced downwards into the right ventricle and get attached to the ventricle wall near the apex, while the anterior cusp of the valve retains some attachment to thevalve ring some redundancy of the valve cusps affects all the cusps. Right ventricle is divided into two chambers by the abnormal valve-the first chamber Is continuous with the cavity of right atrium (materialized portion), and the 2nd consists of a thin-walled ventricle. The right atrium is huge. Tricuspid incompetence may also be present. The degree of right ventricular Impairment depends on the amount of materialized ventricle, the size of the remaining ventricular body, and howintimately the valve tissue is adherent to the ventricular wall. The effective output from the right side of the heart is decreased because of the small size of the functioning right ventricle and possible obstruction produced by the large, sai1-like anterior tricuspid leaflet (Similar hemodynamics is produced by thinning of the right ventricular wall due to hypoplasia of the myocardia = Uhls anomaly).

The degree of symptoms depends on the degree of displacement of the tricuspid valve. In many pts, the only complaint is fatigue, and some may remain asymptomatic for many years. In halfof the pts, the initial symptoms occur in infancy, when they may also show growth retardation. Others present with cyanosis (which depend on the Integrity of the atrial septum; if foramen ovale is patent or there is an ASD, there is right to left shunting leading to cyanosis and polycythemia); other features are effort dyspnea, fatigue, and CCF. Cyanosis can appear at any age but is intense only In some pts. With associated tricuspid insufficiency JVP is raised. Cardiac Arrhythmias are common, especially numerous attacks of supraventricular tachycardia or numerousextra-systoles.

On palpation the precordium is quiet, the cardiac impulse is diffuse; a systolic thrill may be present; the systolic murmur of pulmonary stenosis or tricuspid regurgitation may be present the 2nd heart sound is soft, and the systolic murmur is audible over most of the left anterior chest. Gallop rhythm is common, and triple or quadruple rhythm may be heard. A high-pitched, scratchy, diastolic murmur is commonly heard at the left sternal border-this murmur is superficial and may mimic a friction rub(pericardial). A series of systolic ejection clicks, and an opening snap of the tricuspid valve may also be audible is enlarged. Though some may remain asymptomatic up to adult life, others may present with cyanosis in the neonatal period along with cardiomegaly and long systolic murmurs; in such pts, mortality is higher due to hypoxemia and cardiac failure. Rapid improvement may occur in some due to a decrease in pulmonary vasc resistance.

ECG shows a first-degree heart block, with a right ventricular conduction disturbance and tall and broad P waves due to right atrial enlargement. Complete rigi bundle branch block and Wollf Parkinson White syndrome patterns are common. X-ray shows cardiomegaly with right atrial (and sometimes right ventricular) enlargement. Fluoroscopy shows cardiomegaly with diminished pulsatile activity, resembling a large pericardial effusion. The intrapulmonary vasculature may be normal decreased, and the aorta is small. Cardiac catheterization shows an elevated right atrial pressure with a prominent V wave. In the absence of an associated anomaly ventricular pressure is not usually increased. The right atrium is enlarged, and R-L shunt is determined if absent. Intracardiac ECG in the right ventricle artialised right ventricle (the right ventricle between the atrioventricular junction and the abnormal attachment of the valvecusps forming a common chamber with the right atrium) and right atrium produces typical diagnostic findings. These studies may lead to cardiac arrythmias and even rupture of the atrium.

Right ventriculography show displacement of the tricuspid valve (seen as a radiolucent notch or crescent to the left of the spine); tricuspid regurgitation may be present, and the right atrium is markedly enlarged. Treatment is symptomatic for most of the pts. Medical treatment is directed towards the control ofthe COF and supraventricular dysrhythmias. Surgical treatment is not needed during childhood, but in deeply cyanotic pt, Glenn, anastomosis between the SVC and Rt pulmonary artery leads to improvement. Replacement of the abnormal tricuspid valve with a prosthesis has- been performed. Prolonged strenuous exercise should be avoided. In severe untreated cases, death may occur during infancy, most commonly from cardiac failure, hypoxia, and supraventricular tachycardia. Life expectancy in untreated patients is 30-40 years.

HYPOPLASTIC LEFT' HEART SYNDROME.

It includes varying degrees of hypoplasia- of the left ventricle due to severe valvular or vascular obstructive lesions of the left side of the heart; the lesion may include severe stenosis atresia or hypoplasia of mitral or aortic valve or both the valves, and there may be obstructive lesions of the aortic arch. The anomalies thus include underdevelopment of the left atrium and leftventricle stenosis or atresia of the valves on the left side of the heart and hypoplasia of the ascending aorta.

Associated anomalies may be VSD, ASD, and endocardial fibroelastosis. There is a severe obstruction to the filling or emptying of the left ventricle. Therefore, the quantity of blood that fills this ventricle is very small, resulting in hypoplasia of this chamber. Following birth also, there is marked impairment of circulation because of the very small size of the left ventricle and the obstructing lesions. The left ventricle is small, but its wall may toe if left ventricular outflow obstruction is associated with mitral stenosis. If mitral atresia and aortic atresia coexist, the left ventricular cavity is minute. The left ventricle is virtually nonfunctional, and the right ventricle maintains both pulmonary and systemic circulation pulmonary blood passesthrough an ASD or VSD from the left to the right side of the heart where intermixing occurs. If the ventricular septum is the intact whole of the right ventricular outflow is ejected into the pulmonary arteries the systemic circulation is maintained via a PDA. With a VSD and a. small patent aortic orifice, right ventricular blood enters the left small ventricle and ascending aorta as well as pulmonary artery. Anomalies may be so severe as to preclude adequate cardiac output. Because ofthe obstruction of arterial flow, high pressure develops in the left atrium, pulmonary venous system, and pulmonary artery, placing a marked burden on the right ventricle. The major hemodynamic abnormalities are inadequate maintenance of systemic circulation and pulmonary venous hypertension.

CLINICAL FEATURES

Symptoms appear early in life, often within the first 1-2 hours of birth, though somepatients present a few days later Signs of heart failure appear during early weeks, with dyspnea and hepatomegaly. All peripheral pulses are weak and sometimes impalpable a grayish-blue color ofthe skin is soon apparent, and cyanosis may or may not be present within the first 48 hours. Cyanosis is generalized. If the aortic valve has a small opening or there is a hypoplasia of the aortic arch, there is differential cyanosis. (In these pts, oxygenated blood from the left ventricle enters the ascending aorta and innominate artery resulting in a normal color in the right arm and right side of the head and neck, in contrast to the cyanosis in the rest of the body.) The results of pulmonary obstructionare tachypnea, respiratory distress, and pallor. The infant usually exhibits mar respiratory distress and tachypnea. Heart is enlarged with a palpable right ventricular parasternal lift. In many cases there are no murmurs, but in some are short and mid-systolic murmurs. Heart failure develops very early.

X-RAY

X-ray shows cardiomegaly after a few days with pulmonary venous congestion. Chest x-rays arenormal at birth; usually, but rapid and progressive cardiomegaly occur, early in aortic atresia ECG shows right axis deviation, RVH, and Right atrial hypertrophy (P waves prominent). When in earlier cases, ECG shows RVH, it-is normal, and if the patient survives, RVH and RAH supervene. There is the absence of left ventricular forces, and an absence of q wave in V6.

Echocardiogram is diagnostic and eliminates the need for catheterization and an echocardiography. It shows the absence of the normal mitral valve echo, an absent or small aortic root, a small posterior (left) ventricle, a large anterior ventricle, and an easily identifiable tricuspid valve. If done, cardiac catheterization reveals the right heart and left atrial pressures with low descending aortic pressure. Angiocardiography shows a contrast medium flowing from the right ventricle to thepulmonary artery, through a PDA, and into the ascending aorta. Aortography reveals a hypoplastic aorta and coronary arterial system. Infants usually die during the first week or at the most within first month. Patient with aortic atresia-develop COF early (usually within the first week), and death occurs early in this group. Patients withmitral atresia who have large ASD or VSD may live longer (Some have lived beyond the first decade) Patients with involvement of the aortic arch die within the first month. Treatment is essentially symptomatic and medical in severe forms. In less severe forms, some surgical palliation may be possible.

TRUNCUS ARTERIOSUS

In this condition, only one single- huge arterial trunk arises from the ventricular portion of the heart and supplies the pulmonary, systemic, and coronary blood supply. The cause is the complete lack of formation of ridges that divide the fetal truncus arteries into the aorta and pulmonary artery. Since a portion of the ventricular septum is contributed by this spiral septum, there is a necessary VSD in all (a high VSD). The number of the semilunar valve Varies from 2-6. The valvemay be competent incompetent or stenotic. The classification depends on the origin of the pulmonary artery-mostly there is to be a pulmonary artery that arises from the base of the trunk just above the semilunar valves and runs parallel to the ascending aorta (In the majority, pulmonary arteries arise proximal to the innominate artery). In some, two pulmonary arteries arise side by side from the posterior aspect of the truncus; in others, these arise from either side of the truncus. In some, there isno pulmonary artery and no ductus arteriosus. The pulmonary circulation is maintained by bronchial collaterals arising from the descending thoracic aorta. Some consider it to be an extreme form of tetralogy with an atretic main pulmonary artery. If there is a remnant of the pulmonary artery leaving the right ventricle and pulmonary blood flow is supplied by the aorta via a ductus, it is pulmonary atresia.

The saturation of blood in both the pulmonary artery and aorta is the same; the degree of systemic arterial oxygen saturation depends on the ratio of the pulmonary to systemic blood flow. Both ventricles eject their blood at systemic pressure into the truncus, with the result the pulmonary vascular tree is subjected to systemic pressure. In the presence of normal pulmonary vascular resistance, the blood flow to the lungs is much increased, and much greater than the systemic flow, and the saturation is higher, the arteriovenous oxygen difference is small, and cyanosis is absent or minimal. When pulmonary vascular resistance is high due to pulmonary vascular obstruction or very small pulmonary arteries pulmonary blood flow is reduced, oxygen saturation is low, the pulmonary flow is inadequate, and cyanosis is intense. If pulmonary arteries areabsent, pulmonary flow via the collaterals is inadequate, and cyanosis occurs early. The systolic pressures in both ventricles are identical to that in the aorta.

CLINICAL FEATURES

The clinical picture is variable due to variable hemodynamics. In the majority of pts, the pulmonary flow is torrential; therefore, these patients do well and function similarly to a patient with large VSD and pulmonary hypertension. The clinical picture is dominated by dyspnea, fatigue, heart failure, recurrent respiratory infections, and poor physical development. Cyanosis is usually absent, the nailbeds are commonly dusky.

The heart is enlarged precordium hyperdynamic, and the hyperactive impulse felt hot at the apex, and over the xiphoid process Systolic thrill is present at the low left sternal border; there is a pansystolic murmur best heard over the left low sternal border. The murmur is preceded by a loud early systolic ejection click. The first heart sound is normal, and 2nd sound is single and loud. A mid-diastolic apical flow (rumbling) murmur is audible, mitral flow murmur. In older children with decreased pulmonary blood flow, there is progressive cyanosis that becomes marked,polycythemia, clubbing, retardation of growth and development, easy fatiguability, dyspnea, on exertion, and CC'F development. These patients do very poorly.

The heart is not unduly hyperactive, both the sounds are loud, and a systolic murmur is heard, but there is no diastolic murmur. When there is hypoplasia or absence of pulmonary arteries, cyanosis anddyspnea are present from infancy, cardiomegaly is moderate, and a continuous murmur of bronchial collateral vessels may be heard. A very loud systolic ejection click is commonly heard. There may be a diastolic aortic murmur along the upper right sternal border due to aortic runoff. The runoff of the blood from the truncus to the pulmonary artery may result in wide pulse pressure.

Truncus arteriosus is one of the causes of mildly cyanotic heart disease and' COF at an early age. ECG usually has a normal axis, but rarely left axis deviation may occur, and there is evidence of RVH or combined ventricular hypertrophy commonly, only rarely LVJ. X-ray appearance is variable. Cardiac enlargement is due to the prominence of both ventricles. The truncus may produce a prominent shadow that follows the normal course of the ascending aorta and aortic knob, and in el/2 pts, it arches to the right. The shadow of the main pulmonary artery is not clearly discerned. Sometimes a high bulge seen to the left of the aortic knob is produced by the main left pulmonary arteries. The pulmonary vasculature is prominent in most cases; it is increased in the presence of normal pulmonary vascular resistance and increased flow, but it decreases as the resistance increases. The most common picture is a boot-shaped heart, the absence of the main pulmonary artery segment, and a large aorta that frequently arches to the right. A diffuse reticular pattern in the lung fields with retro esophageal vessels demonstrated by the barium esophagogram may be seen in PTA with bronchial collateral blood flow to the lungs. Sometimes there is a difference in the vascular markings of the 2 lungs.

Angiocardiography reveals; the presence of a VSD and a single vessel arising from the heart. The origin of the pulmonary arteries is also revealed sometimes; the condition may not be differentiated from pseudotruncus (pulmonary atresia and VSD). The catheterization shows the shunting and that the pressure in both ventricles and truncus is similar.

TREATMENT

Treatment consists of anti-congestive measures and pulmonary artery banding- in cases with torrential blood flow and CCF. Corrective surgery is done by closing the VSD and insertion a conduit to act as. a pulmonary valve and main pulmonary artery. Severe pulmonary vascular obstruction or hypoplastic pulmonary arteries preclude surgical treatment. Aortic homografts for total correction of the truncus have been attempted.

The prognosis depends mainly on the status of the pulmonary circulation Patients with low pulmonary blood flow do poorly and usually die within a year. If suitable pulmonary blood flow occurs; via collaterals, patient may survive well into adult life with little incapacity (some have survived into 3rd decade). The majority of p succumb during the first 2 years from CCF, hypoxia, SABE, or brain abscess.

ANOMALOUS PULMONARY VEKOUS DRAINAGE (TOTAL)

This is due to abnormal development of the pulmonary veins, and all the blood returning to the heart via the pulmonary veins is drained into the right atrium either directly or via a systemic venous connection, and there is no venous drainage into the left atrium. Usually, the pulmonary veins form a single trunk before entering the systemic venous circuit; in the majority of cases enters the left SVC (persistent anterior cardinal vein) or right SVC, or into the corona sinus, right atrium, and if there is an entry below the diaphragm, it is the portal vein, ductus venosus, or IVC. Rarely there may be multiple entries there before in order of frequency, and the entry is into the left SVC coronary sinus, right atrium, right SVC, portal vein, or ductus venosus. A right-to-left shunt is always present at the atrial level CASD or PFO). Complete mixing of systemic and pulmonary venous return occurs in the right atrium Eid, therefore, left atrial, and hence the systemic arterial saturation levels are approximately equal to that of the right atrium saturation. The degree of saturation of the blood, and thus the degree of cyanosis, is determined by the ratio of the quantity of the pulmonary blood flow to that of the systemic blood flow. If pulmonary vascular resistance is normal, the flow of blood into the pulmonary artery is much greater than the flow into the left of the heart; in this case, there is a much greater return from the pulmonary circulation. Therefore, the saturation within the right atrium is very high. Such patients will function very well, with relatively normal pulmonary artery pressures, and at least physiologically are very similar to patients with very large ASD and normal pulmonary return if pulmonary vascular resistance is elevated, the ratio of pulmonary to systemic blood flow is much, lower, When the pulmonary vascular resistance equals that of systemic vascular resistance, equal amounts of flow are got in the two directions marked desaturations of the mixed blood develops, and the patient is markedly cyanotic. Such patients does not do well and eventually develop severe right heart failure.

The complete form of anomaly is frequently associated with asplenia and polysplenia syndrome. Blood flow into the systemic circulation is maintained by an ASD or PDA.

CLINICAL FEATURES.

Symptoms usually occur early, and most of the patients present in the first 2 years oflife. Symptoms depend on the underlying hemodynamics and associated lesions.

a) In patients with normal pulmonary vascular resistance (where there is no evidence of pulmonary venous obstruction), symptoms appear during the latter part of the neonatal period, with tachypnea andspeeding difficulties appearing. This progresses to frank cardiac failure associated with respiratory infections and failure to thrive. These patients are usually thin and small, resembling patients with a large VSD. They do relatively well after early infancy is passed except for frequent Respiratory infections

Cyanosis in them is mild, and duskiness of the nail beds and mucous membranes is present, but definite cyanosis and clubbing are not present. They may h/o cyanosis during the neonatal period. JVP shows a definite- V wave. Mild cyanosis becomes apparent after crying. The patient is a-scrawny irritable infant with dyspnea and tachypnea. The left side of the chest is prominent, the precordium is hyperactive, and a right ventricular have present. The first sound is-normal to slightly louder, 2nd the sound is widely split and fixed. Gallop rhythm is usual, and frequently there is a 3rd and 4 the sound, which produces a quadruple or quintuple rhythm. The pulmonary part of the 2nd sound is normal.

In most cases, a systolic ejection murmur heard maximally along the left sternal border is heard, best heard over the pulmonary area but radiates diffused over the lung fields anteriorly and posteriorly. A diastolic murmur (early to mild diastolic) may be heard at the lower sternal border inthe 3rd and 4th space (a tricuspid flow murmur). A continuous murmur with the quality of venous may be audible over the pulmonary area and under the right clavicle. Clinical signs of pulmonaryedema may be present. There is cardiomegaly. X-ray of the chest shows cardiomegaly primarily involving the right atrium, right ventricle, and pulmonary artery. X-ray is pathognomonic if pulmonary veins enter the innominate vein and persistent left SVC (55% cases). This produces a marked enlargement of the super mediastinum (large superior cardiac shadow). The supracardiac shadow is produced by the dilated left SVC, left innominate artery vein, and right SVC; this produces a figure-of-eight or snowman appearance. There is a marked increase in the pulmonary vascular markings if the pulmonary vein drains elsewhere, the heart is enlarged, the pulmonaryartery and right ventricle are prominent, at the pulmonary vascularity increases.

EEG

ECG shows right axis deviation and varying degrees of right atrial and right ventricular hypertrophy. There is usually a QR pattern over the precordial leads (V4R and VI).

1. In cardiac catheterization, the oxygen saturation in both atria, both ventricles, and the aorta is almost similar and higher than that in the peripheral systemic level. In infancy, pulmonary hypertension is usual, but in older pts, the pulmonary pressure is moderately elevated. Angiocardiography in the pulmonary artery is usually diagnostic, with the pulmonary venous return being delineated during the levophase study. Echocardiographic demonstration of a chamber posterior to the left atrium is diagnostic of the anomaly.

2. Infradiaphragmatic total venous return; The clinical picture of infra diaphragmatic drainage (differs somewhat from the usual picture. Symptoms are present within the first few months of life and are dominated by greyish cyanosis and symptom of increased pulmonary venous pressure (pulmonary edema). X-ray shows a normal size heart with stippled pulmonary vasculature because of the prominent pulmonary veins and pulmonary edema. The chest filmsmay superficially resemble those of newborns with hyaline membrane disease.

3. Patients in which the pulmonary veins drain into a systemic vein below the diaphragm and those in whom the venous drainage is into the systemic vein above the diaphragm (supracardiac, cardiac, and intracardiac drainage) associated with increased pulmonary vascular resistance present differently from those in whom there is pulmonary vascular

obstruction. These infantsare quite sick cyanosis common at birth and are quite evident by the first week. Another common early symptom is severe tachypnea. COF develops later. Examination reveals a cyanotic, very tachypneic baby, a striking right ventricular impulse, a shock of the 2nd sound, the loud first sound, a very loud 2nd sound, which is single, a systolic ejection murmur heard over the pulmonary area, radiating well over the lung fields. In many cases, there is no murmur.

In the obstructive type, the heart is small or normal with severe pulmonary congestion in the pulmonary fields. ECG again shows right axis deviation, right atrial hypertrophy, and right ventricular hypertrophy. Prognosis is usually poor in the total anomalous venous return, and survival beyond infancy is unusual. Death is due to CCF. Patients who survives beyond 2 years of age may have surprisingly few symptoms. Patients with normal pulmonary vascular resistance may do quite well through 2nd decade, but eventually, progressive increase in pulmonary vascular resistance and pulmonary hypertension occurs. Patients with increased vascular-resistance and pulmonaryhypertension do very poorly; 1/2 die within the first 6 months, and untreated, most die before their first year; in the intracardiac drainage (where the 4 veins join behind the heart and drain through the diaphragm, usually connecting with the portal vein; this type is usually associated with pulmonary venous obstruction is extremely poor.

Treatment: Surgical treatment is possible; until recently, surgical mortality was more than 90%, but now surgery is done under cardio-pulmonary bypass or deep hypothermia (cooling to 20C), and still the risk is 30-60%, but must be undertaken very early after COF is treated. If the surgery is not done immediately, atrial septostomy is done at the catheterization. The treatment consists of anastomosis of the common pulmonary vein to the left atrium while the ASD is closed. The high operative risk in symptomatic infants is due to hypoplastic ventricle which cannot sustain cardiac output after correction, and poor lung compliance due to pulmonary hypertension and edema Patients surviving past the first year may be electively operated on later at lower mortality.

PARTIAL ANOMALOUS PULMONARY RETURN

One or more of the pulmonary veins enter the systemic venous circulation or the right atrium, resulting in L-R shunting of oxygenated blood, which is frequently increased by the association of a VSD. One or all the veins of only one lung (mostly the right one); again, the site of drainage can be any of the previously mentioned sites, but most commonly, it is the SVC. The history, physical signs, ECG, and X-ray are indistinguishable from the findings of ASD (Secundum). Symptoms rarely develop in children if there is no associated defect. The examination is identical to ASD, but the fixed splitting of the 2nd heart sound is not present. ECG shows an incomplete right bundle branch block, or maybe normal peaked P waves may suggest right atrial hypertrophy. X-ray shows a normal-sized ‘heart; the right atrium and pulmonary artery may be prominent. If the anomalous is draining into the inferior vena cava, it may be seen as a crescentic vessel shadow close to the right atrial border, coursing toward the diaphragm (Scimitar syndrome). Cardiac catheterization may show entry of the catheter into the anomalous vein from the superior vena cava or the right atrium; ASD is demonstrated; Indicator dilution curves also are very helpful. Selective pulmonary arteriography is also very helpful. (demonstration of the pulmonary veins and their drainage shown by right and left pulmonary arteriography). The prognosis is also like the ASD (Secundum); if there are no other abnormalities and a small L~R shunt, the prognosis is excellent when several pulmonary veins are involved, and shunting is large, the natural history is of an ASD. Treatment is surgery under cardiopulmonary bypass, and ASD is also closed.

COARCTATION OF THE AORTA

Constrictions of varying lengths may occur at any point between the arch and the bifurcation of the aorta, but 96% of these constrictions occur as a localized structure just below the origin of the left subclavian artery. Males are affected times more often. In most cases, coarctation occurs in the thoracic portion of the descending aorta (rarely abdominal aorta is involved). In coarctation of the aorta, constriction occurs distal to the origin of the brachiocephalic vessels. The right end left subclavian artery may arise anomalously either at or below the coarctation. This anomaly is divided into lesions occurring at or below the ductus (postductal type or adult type) or those found above the ductus (preductal or infantile type). Many lesions are juxtaductal. Most of the symptomatic infants will have associated PDA, tubular hyperplasia of the aortic isthmus (due to paucity of blood flow in the fetus, which often spontaneously enlarges with postnatal growth), VSD, and bicuspid aortic valve. The section of the aorta immediately distal to the coarctation is often dilated (post-stenotic dilatation).

POSTDUCTAL TYPE

Postductal coarctation is usually diagnosed after 1 yr of age. it exhibits no symptoms generally during infancy and the first decade, but the symptoms can occur at an age and are the result of a hypertensive state, decreased myocardial performance, or a deficient circulation in the legs. Thus, hypertension may cause epistaxis, throbbing headaches, or symptoms of left ventricular or frank COF may occur secondarily to the hypertensive state, and there may be exercise intolerance and fatigue, and painful calves on running, intermittent claudication and cold feet are due to deficiencycirculation to the legs. Hypertensive cardiovascular disease hypertensive encephalopathy cerebrovascular accidents and aortic rupture are the rare complications that can occur in the adults.

SIGNS OF POSTDUCTAL COARCTATION:

CHILDREN WELL DEVELOPED PULSES

Radial arteries are easily palpable and strong, while as the femoral, popliteal posterior tibial, and dorsalis pedis pulsations are either absent or every weak and delayed (in contrast to the boundingpulsations in the upper limbs and carotid vessels). Many infants will have initially equal upper andlower limb pulses until the coexistent ductus arteriosus closes.

Normally blood in pressure in upper limbs is slightly higher than in the lower- limbs during the firstfew months of life only, latering normal persons, the systolic pressure in the lunge legs is 20-40 mmHg (cuff method) than that in the arms. After 1 yr of age, BP higher in arms than legs are suggestive of coarctation. In coarctation, the pressure in the legs is much more than that in the arms and frequently cannot even be recorded. The actual level of pressure in the arms may be moderate to severely increased. There is also a rise in BP following exercise.
The left subclavian artery is occasionally involved in the coarctation, in which cases the left brachial pulse is weak, and there is a difference of more than 30 mm in two arms; therefore, it isessential to take Bp in both the arms. In the presence of CCF, the differences in pulses may not become apparent, but once compensated, the difference becomes obvious(when the pulses in the legs remain feebly palpable or absent, and the pulse in the arms becomes stronger than normal – Collareals; Owing to the obstruction of the aorta, extensive collateral circulation usually develops, chiefly from the branches of the subclavian artery, the superior intercostal artery, and theinternal mammary artery with its intercostal,

superior epigastric, and musculophrenic branches. The thoracic and subscapular branches of the axillary artery may also enlarge as the collaterals. These vessels unite with the intercostal branches of the descending aorta and inferior epigastric branches of the femoral artery to create a channel for arterial blood to bypass the area of coarctation. The vessels contributing to the collateral circulation become enormously enlarged and tortious by early adulthood. The BP is elevated in the vessels arising proximal to the coarctation below it the amplitude of pulsation is diminished, and the pressure below the constriction is lower than that above it.

Hypertension is not only due to mechanical obstruction, and renal ischemia also does not play a large role. Cardiac signs are more striking after the first decade; heart sounds are normal. The aortic component of the 2nd sound is often louder. A soft systolic ejection murmur may he audible at the aortic area or the midsternal left border and is well transmitted to the back along the course ofthe aorta. A systolic murmur may also be heard in the **2**nd or 3rd at right space with transmission to the neck, due to the bicuspid aortic valve, which is present in the majority.

The collateral arterial circulation may give rise to visible pulsations and to systolic murmurs bestheard in the back between the scapulae (in the interscapular area) and at their angles (i.e., over the area of the coarctation). Cardiac enlargement with a left ventricular tap is also present in the olderchild. Murmurs are variable in location intensity and quality, but the common murmur is systolic in time, ejection in nature, maximal over the base of the heart, and radiates down the sternum to the apex and to the interscapular area and frequently is loudest at the back. (The murmur may be produced by the coarctation, by tortuous collateral vessels, by abnormalities of the aortic valveor by the asociated structural anomalies of the heart, as septal defects. Occasionally there is a diastolic element which may be due to aortic insuffiency (congenital or rheumatic); it is best heard over the base of the heart and down the left sternal border. A continuous murmur over thepulmonary area radiating to the left clavicle suggests an associated PDA. Rarely a diastolic murmur is heard in the back; a rumbling diastolic (apical) diastolic murmur of uncertain origin may also be present.

X-RAY:

X-ray may be normal or there may be slight to moderate left ventricular enlargement usually left atrial and left ventricular enlargement is present. The ascending aorta is usually normal in size, but the descending aortic arch has the appearance of a double-aortic-knob resulting in figure-3 sign. On barium swallow, the esophagus has a characteristic E-shape; the first arc of this E is due to dilatation of the aorta just proximal to the coarctation, the **2**nd arc is due to post stenotic dilatation of the aorta, the middle bar of the E is due to the coarctation of aorta itself. The enlarged left SC artery is seen as a prominent shadow in the left superior mediastinum.Notching of true inferior border of the ribs due to pressure erosion by the enlarged collaterals is seen by late childhood, only the first and last 2-3 ribs are spared (Usually 3rd to 9th ribs). Rarely erosion is due to unilateral and is due to one of the SC arteries arising below the area of the coactation. The indentations produced on the barium filled esophagus in addition to the upper onedue to aortic knob and left SC artery and the lower from the post stenotic dilatation; there mayin addition be prominent serrations on the posterior aspect of the barium-filled esophagus suggesting the 'presence of large intercostal arteries entering the aorta below the coaction. Occasionally scalloping in the soft tissue is seen retrosternally.

ECG:

ECG is normally usually, showing right ventricular preponderance in infancy, later theremay he evidence of left ventricular hypertrophy and occasionally of left bundle

branch block. Cardiac catheterization reveals an elevated ascending aortic pressure with a pressure gradient localizing the site of the obstruction when the catheter is withdrawn below the coarctation.
Angiocardiography in the ascending aorta defines the area severity and extent of coarctation. Most often the diagnosis is made by physical examination alone routine examination of all hypertensive subjects, and of all infants, in whom CV defects are suspected should include palpation of all the major accessible peripheral arteries. Aortography or angiocardiography areseldom indicated especially when the site of Obstruction is unusual as abdominal aorta.
Associated defects may produce gross signs-aortic valve abnormalities occur in 75% of cases, mostly bicuspid aortic valves, but usually do not produce signs unless aortic incompetence or stenosis develops. Rheumatic mitral stenosis or aortic incompetence are rare complications, and VASD, ASD and PDA may be associated severe neurologic damage or even death may occur from the associated cerebral vascular disease. Subarachnoid or intracerebral hemorrhage may occur from the rupture of congenital aneurysms in the circle of Willis, of other vessels with defective elastic and medical tissue of vessels, or even the normal tissue. These accidents are secondary to the hypertensive state.
Abnormalities of the SC arteries may also occurand include involvement of the SC artery around the coarctation, stenosis of the orifices of the left SC artery, and anomalies in the origin of the right subclavian artery.

PROGNOSIS -

The isolated coarctation, the child develops normally and usually does not develop any symptoms during childhood. Thus, children who survive the neontal period without developing COF do quite well throughout childhood and adolescence. Starting in the 3rd decade, the patient may develop easy fatiguability, dyspnea on exertion, cardiac enlargement, and left ventricular failure. Symptoms may appear in infancy, but usually develop later, and by 25 years, all have symptoms. Most of the untreated cases will die between the ages of 20-40, and only ¼ of the patients live through the 4th decade. Hypertensive cardiovascular disrase and SABE lead to death. The common seruous complications are related to the hypertensive state, which may result in COF orintracranial hemorrhage. Heart failure is frequently related to the complicating anomalies bicuspid aortic valve with aortic stenosis or insufficiency. Subacute bacterial endocarditis, or endarteritis is a frequent complication and most commonly involves the abnormal aortic valves. Rupture of the aorta, if it occurs, is due to defective elastic and medical tissue. Aneurysms of the descending aorta or of the enlarged collateral vessels is not usually unusual. The natural course inany individual case is unpredictable. Almost all the complications are rarely encountered before adolescence, including SABE.

TREATMENT.

Most patients should be treated surgically, the optimum age for correction being between te8-15 years, because at this time, the aorta has good elasticity and no degenerative changes, and the lumen after the anastomosis is adequate to carry the patient through adult life, and the mortality rate is less than 2%. After the 2nd decade, the operation is more hazardous due to decreased cardiac reserve and degenerative changes or even aneurysms around the area of the coarctation; the mortality rate is 5% after the 2nd decade. Treatment is gross excision of the area of the coarctation and end-to-end anastomosis, which or without grafting. If the length of the constriction does not allow primary anastomosis Dacron grafts aeused. (Crafford-Gross). After the Operation, there is a striking improvement in the amplitude of pulsations in the femoral pulsations in the femoral arteries Patients also note a definite increase in temperature in their legs. Headaches and epistaxis disappear, and symptoms of cardiac failure are improved. The relief of hypertension may be delayed for 3-4 weeks. Murmurs may not disappear after operation; they are probably due to persistent enlargement of the collateral vessels or aortic valvular disease.

POSTCOARCTECTOMY SYNDROME

Postoperative mesenteric arteritis may cause hypertension with abdominal pain in the immediatepostoperative period. There is pain with anorexia, nausea, vomting, leukocytosis, and even signs ofsmall bowel obstruction. These patients respond to antihypertensive drugs, intestinal decompression, and cortico steroids. Though most of the patients are asymptomatic after the operation, they should hobe observed for years to come because of the frequency of the associated aorticvalve abnormalities. Also, hypertension may persist or recur after many years, and the blood pressure Response to exercise is abnormal (systolic hypertension with wide pulse pressure).

PREDUCTAL (INFANTILE) CORACTATION SYNDROME

Symptoms occur in infancy, usually before 6 weeks of age, may be due to a high incidence of associated defects such as VSD; associated defects are frequently found as PDA VSD, ASD, aortic valvular disease, and transpos of great vessels. In infants, coarctation is a common cause of heartfailure Endocardial sclerosis may complicate this anomaly in older infants with coarctation. The clinical picture varies and depends on the associated defects and pulmonary vascular resistance. Infants fail to thrive, have feeding problems, are dyspneic, and show other symptoms ofcardiac failure. In the isolated coarctation, the classical signs are present. The infant is dyspneic, tachypneic,tachycardiac, and anxious; signs of cardiac failure as hepatomegaly and congested lungs, are present. Cicumoral cyanosis may be present peripheral pulses are weak, and femoral pulses may be absent. Blood pressure in the arms is higher than in the legs. The heart may be hyperactive, and agallop rhythm may be appreciated. A systolic ejection murmur may be heard along the left sternal border. In the presence of a large VSD, pulmonary flow is increased, and pulmonary hypertension isusual. These infants are seriously ill, with signs of heart failure and pulmonary edema superimposed on those produced by both the coarctation and VSD, but the reaction of pulmonary bed is variable hypoxia resulting in pulmonary vasoconstriction. Therefore, the clinical picture is variable. Ciritical left ventricular outflow obstruction produced by complicating stenosis of the aortic valve may be associated with endocardial sclerosis and a thick-walled left ventricle with a smallcavity. These patients are critically ill with severe COF and pulmonary edema.

Coarctation of the aorta and transposition may result in differential cyanosis (the lower body being less cyanotic than the upper in patients with an associated PDA. In some pts, differential cyanosis is seen with lower limbs more cyanotic than the upper. The direction of flow across theductus depends primarily on the pulmonary vascular resistance, and the shunt is from the aorta to the pulmonary artery if the pulmonary resistance is lower than the systemic. (This occurs irrespectiveof the site of the aortic opening of the ductus. inserting in relation to the coarctation). In babies with a large ductus inserting distal to the aortàc coarctation and with greatly elevated pulmonary vascular resistance, right ventricular blood is ejected through the ductus to the descending aorta. Thus, the clinical picture in them is confusing; since femoral pulses are readily palpable because the right ventricle is acting as a systemic ventricle, therefore, one of the cardinal signs of coarctation is absent.

Symptoms occur early, and include cyanosis, dyspnca, superimposed pulmonary infections, feeding difficulties;

COF occurs early. Because the descending aorta is supplied with venous blood, differential cyanosis may be expected below the pelvic brim and normal color of the upper half of the body. The heart is enlarged; the murmur is systolic, is heard over the whole precordium, and is usually followed by a loud 2nd sound. ECG shows right ventricular hypertrophy (with or without left ventricular hypertrophy); with associated lesions, ECG may get altered. X-ray There is a markedly enlarged heart, witii increased pulmonary vascularity. Cardiac cathetrization shows right ventricular and pulmonary arterial hypertension. The pulmonary wedge pressure is markedly elevated. Right to left shunting may be noticed through the PDA into the descending aorta. Angiocardiography performed in the ascending aorta defines the area of coarctation and the extent of the lesion. Prognosis is poor untreated patients who develop COF within early infancy die within the first few months of the life. If they survive this period, they do very well later, and can be repaired later.

Treatment consists of vigorous anticongestive measures. Dilatation of the associated PDA with a constant infusion of prostaglandin may stabilize the critically ill infant until an operation can be done. Hypoglycemia is frequent and is due to compromise of the hepatic arterial perfusion because of intermittent or permanent closure of the ductus. If there is no Response to therapy, or if there is the recurrence of symptoms with the progression of heart failure, surgery is done though the riskis greater resection of the coarctation, division of the ductus, and pulmonary artery banding if severe hyperkinetic pulmonary hypertension is due to a large VSD) COF due to isolated coarctation may respond to medical therapy alone so that surgery can be postponed to childhood (after 5 years significant hypertension during infancy may require treatment usually within diuretics. Many with isolated coarctation and no associated lesions do well and need no surgery during infancy. In infants with striking

COF and without associated lesions, severe hypertension isa contributing factor. Reduction of afterload with IV nitroprusside or propranolol followed by chronic propranolol may be lifesaving Infants with associated defects need immediate surgery but may need revision of the recoractation later in life (some use a subclavian flap anastomosis reducing the likelihood of this late complication.

PRIMARY PULMONARY HYPERTENSION

A disease of unknown origin characterized by hypertension of the lesser circulation and right sided heart failure, which may occur at any age. There is precapillary obstruction of the pulmonary vascular bed due to hyperplasia of the muscular and elastic tissues and the thickenedintima of the small pulmonary arterioles and arteries. Atherosclerotic changes may be found in the larger pulmonary arteries. Other cause of pulmonary heart (Chronic or Pulmonarynale) is absent, and there is no evidence of emphysema, pancreatic fibrosis, or kyphoscoliosis. Recurrent pulmonary emboli may produce the same clinical picture but is rare in children. Severe pulmonary hypertension may result from myriads of minute micro emboli from the Cardiac end of a ventriculojugular shunt tube inserted for hydrocephalus. Significant pulmonary hypertension may also result from persistent obstruction of the upper airway (gross enlargement of the tonsils or adenoids or may accompany gross obssil as in Prader-Willi syndrome. Pulmonary hypertension places a mechanical burden on the right ventricle and that pulmonary artery with resultant right ventricular hypertension and dilatation of the pulmonary artery. Frequently cardiac output is reduced. Later right sided heal failure develops, sometimes with tricuspid insufficiency.

The predominant symptoms are effort intolerance and fatigability, occasional patients c/o precordial pain, dizziness, or syncope. Peripheral cyanosis may be present, and is associated with cold extremities, with a near normal oxygen saturation. It rt-sided heart failure develops, JVP is raised, and there is edema and hepatomegaly. In the jugular vein A-wave is seen, and if tricuspidincompetence is associated a c-wave is also added with systolic hepatic pulsations. Heart is enlarged, with right ventricular tap. The first heart sound is followed by a pulmonary ejection click. The systolic murmur is soft and short and sometimes followed by a blowing diastolic murmur due to pulmonary incompetence. The 2nd heart sound is closely split, loud (sometimes, booming), and frequently palpable. A presystolic gallop rhythm may be heard down the left sternal border. X-ray shows a prominent pulmonary artery and right ventricle. The pulmonary vascularity in the hilar areas is prominent whileas the peripheral lung fields are clear. ECG shows RVH with peaked spiked P waves. Cardiac catheterization is diagnostic, by showing right ventricular and pulmonary hypertension with a normal pulmonary arterial wedge pressure. The cardiac output is low and the arterial oxygen saturation near normal.

Cardiac catheterization demonstrates the size, direction, and magnitude of the shunt, which has resulted in pulmonary hypertension; in these conditions, the pulmonary arterial pressure- wedgepressure is elevated significantly in Eisenmenger's syndrome. If primary hypertension is associated with a reversed intra-atrial shunt through a foramen ovale, the clinical picture simulates Eisenmngers syndrome. Pulmonary hypertension is progressive, and treatment provesdisappointing; some cases benefit from, the treatment of CCF.

DEXTROCARDIA AND LEVOCARDIA

Dextrocardia is a right-sided heart with or without reversal of the position of (both organs (situs inversus). Isolated dextrocardia usually has other severe cardiac defects associated when there is dextrocardia with situs inversus, and the heart is usually normal. Dextrocardia is frequently complicated by severe malformations as a combination of a single ventricle, arterial transposition, pulmonary stenosis, VSD and ASD, complete atrioventricular canal, anomalous pulmonary venous return, tricuspid atresia, pulmonary arterial hypoplasia, and atresia. The patient with cyanosis and signs of pulmonary stenosis generally has arterial transposition, pulmonary stenos, and VSD in addition to dextrocardia. Dextrocardia with situs inversus and VSD with normally related great arteries (Mirror-image dextrocardia) is associated with a functionally normal heart. Some of the patients have Kartageners syndrome (complete situs inversus, paranasal sinusitis, and bronchiectasis).

Atrial localization is facilitated by radiologic demonstration of the position of the abdominal organs and tracheal bifurcation for recognition of the situs of the right and left bronchi. Usually, the atrial situs is at the same level as the visceral situs; if the viscera are in a normal position, the atria have a normal position. Abdominal situs inversus is associated with the left atrium to the right and the right atrium to the left. If the abdominal situs cannot be determined, as with the centrally located liver, atrial localization is difficult, and asplenia or rudimentary spleen is common.

Localization of the ventricles and great arteries depends on the direction of development of the embryonic cardiac loop. Initial protrusion of the loop to the right (d-loop) carries the future right ventricle to the right, and the left ventricle remains on the left (l-loop) and carries the future right ventricle to the left, and the left ventricle is on the right. In both types of the loop, the relations of the great arteries may be normal or transposed. Angiographic demonstration of the relations of the aorta and pulmonary artery indicates the type of the cardiac loop and the relative location of the ventricle. The clinical picture of the abnormal cardiac position is dominated by the associated cardiovascular anomalies. Apical impulses and sounds are heard on the right side of the chest. X-ray shows a cardiac silhouette on the right side. On ECG, inverted P waves in the lead I show atrial inversion. Deep Q waves or QS in V1, V2, and all are seen in patients with dextrocardia and normally related arteries. QRS is predominantly down in the lead I; lead II resembles normal lead III and vice versa.

LEVOCARDIA WITH VARYING DEGREES OF VISCERAL HETEROTAXY

(Partial or complete situs inversus) This is usually associated with severe cardiovascular defects, frequently of the cyanotic type; these include combinations of abnormal systemic venous return (bilateral superior vena cava), absence of the inferior vena cava with venous drainage of the lower part of the body into the azygous system), anomalous pulmonary venous return, arterial transposition, pulmonary stenosis or atresia, ASD and VSD, common atrioventricular canal, single ventricle, and PDA. These patients have a high incidence of asplenia or rudimentary spleen, which may be suspected when Howell Jolly bodies (nuclear remnants) or Heinz bodies (precipitated hemoglobin) are seen in the red cells. Treatment is determined by the underlying defects. Cyanotic infants with pulmonary stenosis and VSD as a part of the malformation improve after anastomosis of the systemic and pulmonary blood supplies ASD, VSD, and tetralogy is repaired successfully.

PRIMARY PRESENTATION OF CARDIAC DISEASE IN INFANCY

Which primarily present at birth

-Acyanotic: Primary myocardial disease (endocardial fibroelastosis, viral myocarditis)
, conduction disturbances (complete heart block, supraventricular tachyarrhty thmias),abnormalfetal pathway (premature closure of PFO, and premature closure PDA) – Cyanotic: Pulmonary atresia, tricuspid atresia, pulmonary stenosis, and transposition of great vessels, which primarily present during the first week.:
-Acyanotic: Hypoplastic left heart syndrome, Coarctation, AS, PS, endomyocardial disease, rhythm disturbances, conduction disturbances, AS, total anomalous pulmonary venousreturn.
Cyanotic: TGA, total anomalous pulmonary venous return, Pulmonary artesia, PS, tetralogy ofFallot, tricuspid atresia. Which primarily present from the 2nd-6th week:
-Acyanotic: VSD, PDA, persistent truncus, TGA, complete atrioventricular canal, singleventricle, aortic stenosis, pulmonary stenosis, total anomalous pulmonary venous return.

Cyanotic: Pulmonary atresia, pulmonary stenosis, tetralogy

of Fallot, and tricuspid atresa.

PRESENTING SIGNS AND SYMPTOMS IN CONGENITAL HEART DISEASE.

Diagnosis	Age	Pres Signs	Auscul	X-RAY	ECG
TGA with intact septum	First hr or days	Cyanos is	Unremarkable	Cardiomeg aly, Pulmonary Vas+	RVH
VSD	First weeks	CCF	Pansystollic and stenotic mirmur	Cardiomeg aly, Pulmonary Vas++	ComVH

Selective Diagnosis and Causes of Death

VSD and PS	First days or first week	Cyanos is	Pansystolic and stenotic murmur	Cardiomeg aly, Pulmonary Vasc-	ComVH
2 Fallots tetralogy	First days or first week	Cyanos is	Early Stenotic murmur single S2 at	Cardiomeg aly not seen Pulmonary Vasc-	RVH
3PS Pure	First weeks or months	Cyanos is	Late stenotics widely split S2 faint P2	Cardiomeg aly+, Pulmonary Vasc-	Marked RVH
4 Hypoplastic heft	First Days	Cyanos isand COF with femora l pulses	Late systolic murmur single S2	Cardiomeg aly++, Pulmonary Vasc++	Marked RVH
5VSD	First weeks	CCF	Pansystolic murmur narrowly split S2 loud P2	Cardiomeg aly+, Pulmonary Vasc+	ComVH
6Coarctation	First weeks	COF with hyper	Stenotic Murmur	Cardiomeg aly+, Pulmonary Vasc+-	RVH
		tension	across back		
7 PDA with pulmonary	First weeks	CCF boundi ng pulses	Cresentric systolic murmur early diastolic murmur SplitS2 Loud P2	Cardiomeg aly+, Pulmonary Vasc+	ComVH

PAROXYSMAL SUPRAVENTRICULAR TACHYCARDIA

Parosxysmal tachycardia is caused by ectopic beats arising from the same focus in rapid succession. The ectopic focus may be anywhere in the atrial, junctional, or ventricular tissue, Paroxysmal tachycardia may occur at any age, and has occurred in the last month of fetal life also. In most cases, the ectopic focus is situated in an atrium (paroxysmalatrial tachycardia or flutter). Paroxysmal ventricular tachycardia is rare in infants and children.

In the supraventricular tachycardia, a hyperirritable focus is located below the sinoatrial mode (in the atria or AV node), discharges at a very rapid rate, and takes over the function of cardiac pacemaker for a period ranging from several seconds to several days.

CLINICAL FEATURES:

Characteristically, paroxysmal supraventricular tachycardia comes suddenlyand goes suddenly (both onset and the ending are abrupt); the cardiac rate is usually more than 100 and maybe more than 300/min, but generally, the ventricular rate is 140-240 /min. The arrhythmias may be paroxysmal, repetitive, or occasionally sustained and may occur in uetro. Ifthe attack is not witnessed, its occurrence can be elicited by an accurate history.

It may occur in association with many conditions such as rheumatic fever, digitalis toxicity, cardiac failure, hyperthyroidism, or CHD as Ebstein's anomaly, or during cardiac catheterization, may be precipitated by an acute infection. Frequently it is associated with Wolff-Parkinson syndrome. An older child may have no symptoms at all, except that he is aware of the rapid heart rate. During early phase, older child complains of a fluttering within the chest and is quite irritable and fearful, with exceptionally rapid rates in the early phase or when the attack is prolonged, precordial discomfort and COF may supervene.

3 factors influence the development of CCF

- The rate of tachycardia; COF did not occur in patients whose rates were less than 180/min. The more the heart rate, the more likely the development of COF –
- The duration of tachycardia; the longer the tachycardia persisted, the more likely COF was to develop. COF was not found in patients whose tachycardia did not persist for more than 24 hours. Morethan half got COF after 48 hours.
- The age of the patient the younger the pt, the higher the incidence of CCF.

When the rates exceed 200, patients frequently look ill, with pallor, anxiety, mild cyanosis, dyspnea, chest pain and syncope, and CCF. The attack usually lasts for a few hours, seldom exceedsdays, but may last from a few seconds to several weeks.

In infants, the normal cardiac rate is rapid and increases much with crying, but persistent tachycardia during quiet periods or sleep suggests the diagnosis. Infants frequently have rates in the range of 300 and go into COF within a few hours, and once the COF develops, the infant is quite ill, has an ashen and cyanotic color (slight to marked cyanosis), is restless and irritable, and has as signs of COF tachypnea and hepatomegaly. Pulses are difficult to count because these are very rapid and thready; the extremities are cold and clammy; the heart rate is extremely rapid, and heart tones poor. Pales are present in the lung. There may be fever and leukocytosis. The older child is not so ill when first seen because arrythmia is recognised early in the course. X-RAY of the chest is normal in the early phase, but when COF supervenes, there is significantcardiomegaly and pulmonary venous congestion.

ECG:

This is the most important diagnostic tool and shows the nature and site of origin of the ectopicbeats. There is a very rapid heart rate which can be anywhere between 140-

320/min.
The rhythm is extremely regular; there is no variation in the R-R interval throoughout the entire tracing P waves may be absent or indiscernible. If P waves are present, there is no variation in theappearance of the P wave or in the PR interval. P waves may be difficult to find because they are superimposed upon the preceding T wave. If the focus is located within the AV node, the P waveswill not be seen. QRS complex is usually the same as in normal sinus- rhythm, but may be widened due to aberrant conduction, in such a case, it is confused with ventricular tachycardia (supraventriculartachycardia with aberrant ventricular conduction). There may be secondary ST and T wave depression. Termination of the tachycardia is characterised by a normal sinus rhythm, and varying degrees of AV block donot help as in the atrial flutter.
Treatment: The attack may terminate spontaneously suddenly through simple procedures of vagalstimulation, such as pressure over the eyeballs or over the carotid sinus (unilateral carotid massage), or other procedures applied by the older children, such as self-induced vomiting, breath-holding, Valsalva's maneuver, breath-holding, drinking ice water, or the adaption of a particular posture can abort the paroxysm and affect a conversion to the normal sinus rhythm. In some children these measures fail, and these cannot be applied in the infants or fail.

When these measures fail digitalis in full doses is used and this drug always achieves conversionof arrhythmias. Digoxin is the choice for its rapid effects This drug suceeds in more than 95% cases. Again, ½ of the calculated dose is given initially, then the rest is given in two divided dosesover the next 8 hours. In infant's digitalis, should he given even if paroxysm was abolished by vagalstimulation since recurrence rate is high and the therapy should be maintained for 1 yr after the paroxysm.

If, in rare instances, digoxin fails and COF progresses, other measures are used xBeta-adrenergicantagonists such as propranolol 1 mg/kg.
Infusions of phenylephrine, one 10-mg ampule in 1 dl=100 microgram/ml IV.Diphenylhydantoin, procanamide, oral quinidine sulfate, prostigmine, lidocaine, tensilon, verapamil may be used.
If drug therapy fails, DC cardioversion is used.

It is important to relieve the apprehension associated with the paroxysm by sedation, preferablywith morphine.

PROGNOSIS:
If supraventricular tachycardia persists without treatment, CCF, cardiovascular collapse, and death are the result, but if the tachycardia is successful, the great majority of cases do quite well, and signs and symptoms of heart failure clear up rapidly. Cardiakegaly may persistfor days on X-ray; ECG changes, including the abnormalities of the P wave, ST, and T wave changes, may also persist for up to 1 week.

Recurrences are common, especially within the first year of the attack (first attack); this is especially true with cases of WPW syndrome (pre-excitation syndrome); therefore, it is recommended all patients should- remain on digitalis therapy for 1 -2y. In most cases of paroxysmal tachycardia, there is no underlying structural anoma lies or cardiac disease. If cardiac failure supervenes, cardiac function rapidly returns to normal after cessation of the attack. Between attacks, some children may exhibit ECG signs of WPW syndrome, which is due to an anomalous connection between the right atrium and ventricles. By special conducting fibers. ECG shows a widened QRS complex at the expense of a shortened PR interval as measured from the beginningof the P to the end of the S is normal. In most cases, there is no underlying cardiac disease. Paroxysmal atrial tachycardia occurs in 50% of cases; of WPW syndrome and 5% pts, withparoxysmal atrial tachycardia exhibiting this syndrome between attacks of tachycardia. Ditethe conversion to a normal rhythm, infants who have been in severe COF for prolongedperiods, with evidence of cardiovascular collapse, may still occur; therefore, treatment must beinstituted early especially in infants.

VENTRICULAR TACHYCARDIA

Spontaneous ventricular tachycardia is rare in children and is usually associated with serious; heart disease and may be seen after the immediate period after cardiac surgery or occasionally during severe myocarditis. It cannot be tolerated for long without the development of signs of inadequate cardiac output Patients are critically ill with restlessness, pallor, and hypotension. The diagnosis is confirmed by ECG- which reveals wide QRS complexes without preceding P waves. Treatment should be given immediately, most ideally, and electrical cardioversion should be done. Drugs may be used, such as lidocaine (as an intravenous bolus of 1-2mg/kg, followed by continuous infusion of 15 microgram/kg. others used are procainamide and quinidine sulfate.

ATRIAL FLUTTER

This is due to abnormal rapid but regular atrial contractions, which is rare in childhood and can occur at any time but is more common during infancy, it may occur in normal hearts but is most common in patients with organic heart disease. The abnormal contractions are supposed to be due to a circus movement in the atria or due to an irritable focus in the atrial muscle like that of paroxysmal atrial tachycardia and atrial extrasystoles. There is an extremely rapid heart rate ranging from 250- 400/min. Since the AV node can transmit such rapid impulses, the ventricles respondto every 2nd, 3rd, or 4th atrial beat. Thus, in contrast to supraventricular tachycardia, varying degrees of heart block exists.

Many cases complicate myocarditis of any cause or occasionally acute infectious diseases and has followed palliative or corrective intraatrial surgery as for TGA, ostium scandium or total anomalous pulmonary venous return. It should become suspected if regular tachycardia is not influenced by emotion, effort, or posture.
Symptoms and signs depend on the ventricular Response ; if there is a rapid ventricular Response with a heart rate greater than 200/min, COF ensures its sign; and symptoms. If the patients ventricular Response is slow (one ventricular beat for 3-4 atrial beats), the patients status remains unchanged, and there is no symptom. Carotid sinus pressure produces a slowing of the heart rate. ECG shows rapid and regular atrial flutter (f-waves). If the ventricular rate is rapid, digitalization is done. which first converts flutter into fibrillation and then into the normal sinus rhythm, butsometimes it merely increases the AV block, in patients with organic disease, if normal sinus rhythm is not achieved ventricular rate.

CYSTIC FIBROSIS

Cystic fibrosis is characterized by a triad of chronic pulmonary disease, pancreatic achylia, and abnormally high sweat electrolytes (chloride more than 60mEq/l). It is a genetically transmitted autosomal recessive disease with a gene frequency of 1:20 (5% Caucasians are carriers), whileas anincidence of 1:1600(affected infants). Siblings are frequently affected (this disease is rare in negroes and unknown in the Asian population. The sex distribution is equal. There is Widespread involvement of exocrine glands, and multiple organ systems are involved, lungs, GIT, sweat glands, and testes.

ETIOLOGY:

Host exocrine secretions are affected. Therefore, it is called dysextcrinopathia. Recently finding of accumulation of a metachromatic substance in the fibroblasts of tissue cultures from skin biopsies shows it is a more generalised disease. The primary defect is still unknown. Disturbed transepithelial transport of water and electrolytes is responsible for all clinical findings. All mucus glands produce glycoprotein-rich secretions due to sparse water excretion; due to high viscosity, the flow of mucus is disturbed, causing the obstruction. Reduced reabsorption of electrolytes causes a high NaCl content of secretions from several non-mucus glands, including sweat, salivary and tear glands. In the lungs, there is the production of abnormally viscous mucus, and the Respiratory cilia are unable to effectively clear this tenacious mucus.

Therefore, is progressive obstruction of the airways, beginning with the small bronchio-les, leading to air trapping and atelectasis. Secondarily acquired lung infection occurs and predisposes to destruction of the reap epithelium and airways resulting in bronchiectasis. The bacteria most cultured from the decctorated sputum are pseudomonas aeruginosa, staph areus, hemophilus influenzae. They are also prone to get viral lower Respiratory infections.

EVALUATION AND DIAGNOSIS:

The findings vary according to the age of the patient at the time of diagnosis. In neonates, it presents as meconium ileus, rectal prolapse, and prolonged jaundice can be seen. In infants, the course is severe with tachypnea retractions, and a prominent tympanitic abdomen is typical; often, he presents as bronchiolitis picture. Some may remain asymptomatic till childhood or adolescence. In them isolated lung disease may be the only manifestation. Diffuse rhonchi and rales and clubbing of the fingers may be found. Nasal polyps and recurrent sinusitis are associated findings. Any patient with repeated pulmonary infections should be suspected of having cystic fibrosis, as should be a case of malabsorption.

In severe disease, patients has a foul-smelling bulky frequent fatty stool (chronic diarrhea), failure to thrive, and frequent pulmonary infections, with marked exercise limitation and chronic cough productive of purulent sputum. Pancreatic insufficiency occurs in 85% pts, and if not present at birth, it develops during infancy or soon after. The pancreatic ducts becomeobstructed by inspissated secretions masses. The ensuing pressure and dilatation of tracing causes degeneration of the secretory cells and replacement by fibrous tissue. Although the destruction of the pancreas is progressive, insulin production is usually sufficient.

Heconiumileus presents with intestinal obstruction with sticky tough meconium often associated with ileal atresia in the immediate neonatal period in 10-15% of neonates. Sometimes there is volvulus as well. Perforation resulting in meconium peritonitis may occur and has a highmortality. The treatment of meconium ileus is usually surgical, but enemas containing proteolyticenzymes or mucolytic agents (N-acetylcysteine) may be used. The sweat test is not diagnostic in the first week of life; thus, the diagnosis may not be definitive until later.

Meconium ileus equivalent is the intestinal obstruction in the older child presenting withabdominal pain and way be associated with intussusception. Infants with mild disease may present with asthma at a later stage. Occasional patients has no symptoms till adulthood.

Physical examination may be normal or may reveal signs of pulmonary involvement and malnutrition. Manifestations of the associated lung disease include hyper expansion of the thoracic cage with the use of the auxiliary muscles of respiratory, rales, rhonchi, wheezes, unevenly decreased breath sounds in different parts of the chest, cyanosis, digital clubbing, patients with moderate to severe lung disease may have significant accentuation of the pulmonary component of the 2nd heart sound, physical signs of the malabsorption include poor growth (weight gain is more impaired than linear growth), decreased SC tissue and muscles mass.

Pulmonary involvement is seen in all patients (although it may take some time to become evident), the typical finding is a pertussis-like cough with abundant production of mucus, here isa tendency to overinflation of the lungs, and there may be a picture of asthmatic bronchitis. Parts of the lung become emphysematous; others become atelectatic. Complications of chronic bronchitis (cardiopulmonary complications) are pneumothorax, pulmonary abscess, pulmonary aspergillosis, hemoptysis, empyema, nasal polyps, sinusitis, pulmonary hypertension corPulmonarynale, respiratory failure , and pulmonary osteoarthropathy. Bronchiectasis and recurrent pneumonia are common, the bacteria mostly being staph and pseudomonas. The ultimate result is pulmonary fibrosis causing together with chronic infection, severely decreased lung function, chronic hypoxia, and hypercapnia. Treatment slows down or arrests this development.

The liver edge may be palpable well below the right costal margin, being due to a flatteneddiaphragm lowering the liver, although it can occasionally be caused by corPulmonarynale, in which case it would be associated with gallop rhythm. Cirrhosis of the liver develops in 15-20% of cases (Cystic fibrosis is one of the main causes of hepatic cirrhosis in children in the West). Elevated alkaline phosphatase may be the first sign of hepatic involvement. Subsequent development of portal hypertension is common. Rectal prolapse is a common presenting feature(vert diabetes mellitus occurs in 1% of cases. Ketoacidosis is rare. Gallstones occur in nearly 1/3 of all cases, but acute cholecystitis develops in only a few. Thus, intestinal complications include intussusception, ımpaction, rectal prolapse, recurrent abdominal pain, portal hypertension, oesophagal varices, hematemesis, failure to thrive. Nearly all males are sterile. In hot weather,the massive salt loss through sweat may lead to serious hyponatremia.

LABORATORY DATA

The earliest lab signs of the associated pulmonary disease are a decrease in arterial oxygen tension and abnormalities of pulmonary function tests of the small airway patency, such as the forced expiratory flow rate from 75% to 25% of vital capacity (FEF 25-75) the flow volume loop, and the single breath oxygen test. With the progression of pulmonary disease, pulmonary function testing demonstrates increasing obstructive lung disease with further decreased maximal flow rates and vital capacity and increased absolute lung volume (first residual volume, then functional residual capacity, then total lung capacity, are increased) and airway resistance. With very severe diseases, there may be a decrease in total lung capacity.

The sweat test is performed using the pilocarpine iontophoresis technic. Demonstration of an abnormal content of electrolytes in sweat in patients with chronic pulmonary disease or malabsorption is important. A sweat chloride concentration of more than 60mEq/l is diagnostic in children, and 50-60 mEq is suggestive, whereas less than 50 is normal (if at least 50mg of sweat has been collected). In neonates, conc of 40 mEq/1 is highly suggestive. The levels of sweat sodium are generally about 10mEq/l higher than those of Cl. Less consistent is a demonstration of a lack of pancreatic enzymes (usually trypsin) in duodenal aspirates. Demonstration of low chymotrypsin activity in feces is a good sweating- screening test. Fat balance studies usually reveal massive steatorrhea v/ith a fat absorption varying from 20- 60% of the ingested fat. There is increased fat excretion in feces. Fecal nitrogen is also increased and may account for more than 50% of the ingested nitrogen. Starch hydrolysis is grossly impaired. With more severe disease ECG and echocardiogram may demonstrate abnormalities of the right ventricle due to pulmonary hypertension. Although liver involvement is histologically demonstrated at an early stage in the disease, lab evidence of liver involvement (increased liver enzymes and decreased liver-dependent clotting factors) does not appear till late.

The earliest changes on the chest X-ray are mild hyperinflation, best seen as the loss of diaphragmatic doming on the lateral chest x-ray-, and increased bronchovasular mornings, especially in the upper lobes. Later there are diffuse infiltrates, marked hyperinflation, and areas of atelectasis interspersed with areas of emphysema, giving a picture of cystic lung changes., Extreme fibrosis and hilar adenopathy maybe soon. Occasionally, the changes tend to be confined to one or 2 areas of the lung. Sinus X-rays show a high incidence of sinusitis, and X-rays of the long bones may demonstrate pulmonary osteoarthropathy in patients with severe pulmonary disease-Sputum a typically thick and viscous; frequently, pseudomonas aeruginous and staphylococcus areas are isolated from sputum cultures.

TREATMENT:

Treatment of pancreatic insufficiency:

Pancreatic preparations are required by 85% of cases (all these who have steatorrhea). Severalpancreatic extract preparations are available, in capsule, tablet, or powder form, to be taken at mealtime'. The dosage should be individualized to produce 1-2 formed stools daily. One or 2 capsules are given with every meal in high doses. Fat absorption improves but does not return to normal, even with massive doses. Excessive dosage may lead to meconium ileus equivalent (recurrent abdominal pain, palpable feces masses and obstruction). Overdosage causes anorexic obliteration. Dosage is only established by trial. The enzymes may be mixed with someform of fruit (applesauce). The requirement decreases or increases with age. Persistence of marked diarrhea in the face of adequate replacement therapy should make one suspect other cause. Disaccharidase deficiencies and celiac disease have been reported in rare patients with cystic fibrosis. Pancreas contains pH-sensitive microspheres and seems to be most effective in many pts.

Diet should be high in protein and carbohydrates, but low in fats (about 30-40 g fat/day in older children) is indicated. Medium chain triglycerides (MCÏ) are more readily absorbed than long-chain fats and are an important source of calories. MCT supplementation should be given in patients with poor weight gain and is especially useful in small infants. Glucose polymers and high protein snacks are useful in caloric supplementation. Infant formulas supplemented with MCT are usedfor infants. Some infants especially those receiving soy-based formulas, may present a with hypoproteinemia edema due to difficulty in absorbing the protein. Multivitamins are given daily. Vitamin E (50 iu/d till 3 years, and 100 ip after 3rd yr) should be given to all pts) Vitamin K(2.5 mg till age lyr biweekly) After 1yr of age, indicated only if liverdisease is present or when PATIENT is prolonged.
-Salt supplementation: In hot weather and fever, when sweat loss is great, and patients with hyponatremia, should be given additional salt; 1g daily till 2 yr of age, and 2g/d over 2 years.

TREATMENT OF PULMONARY INSUFFICIENCY:
-All patients have impaired lung clearance mechanisms and accumulate viscous mucus in the airways, postural drainage, and chest percussion in 9 different positions at least once daily. Chest physiotherapy is carried out by the pt, a therapist, or by an electric vibrator. Chest physical therapy (postural drainage) is indicated in any clinical situation when excess fluid is not removedby the normal cough or ciliary action of the airways is usually possible to nave it performed at least once or preferably twice daily without any great

change in the family routine. The frequency depends on the severity of the illness. The best method of learning the technique is forthe parents and patient by a qualified physical therapist. Physical activity should be encouraged as increased respiratory helps to bring up the bronchial secretions, many are helped by bronchodilators prior to postural drainage.
-Adequate hydration is of prime importance; mobilization and loosening of secretions areessential.
-Mist tends are no longer used, because of the lack of particle deposition in the small airways andworsening function tests. If used the patient is placed in the mist tent during the night, the mist consisting of mist dilute saline.
-Oxygen therapy is often indicated to maintain adequate arterial oxygen tension during acute exacerbations. In addition, severely affected patients may benefit from chronic oxygen administrationat home at night. Recurrent morning headaches will often disappear when night-time Oxygen therapy is initiated.

Aerosol drugs: Any generator properly suited to deliver medication can be used. Most of the preparations induce normal saline as the base solution. Saline given directly as an ultrasonic aerosol may liquefy secretions, but occasionally may cause bronchospasm. Particle size is critical(2-5microns). Particles 5 microns are best, since they are most likely to enter the smallairways when inhaled through the mouth. Aerosol therapy should be given just prior to chest therapy, especially in patients who have difficulty raising sputum.
Acetylcysteine, the most effective mucolytic agent, acts by breaking disulfide bonds in the mucoid secretions, but it may cause bronchospasm (especially in patients with asthma). It loses activity rapidly if in a solution of less than 10% concentration or if in contact with rubber or metal. It inactivates many antibiotics given by aerosol, it is given as a few ml of 10% N-acetylcysteine or 10% propylene glycol through a nebulizer 2-3 times a day. Properly administered- it

often resultsin a great outpouring of secretions, which requires mechanical softening, if the patient has an inadequate cough, or inadequate ciliary action or both. Children object to its taste and odor. It works best if given with a bronchodilator.

***BRONCHODILATOR*:**

Isoproterenol has a mechanism of action and side effects like that of epinephrine. It causes a fall of 5-1Omm in p02. Therefore, it may be dangerous to have a patient use handheld recharged nebulizers during a severe attack, especially if oxygen is not being administered. Also, in an occasional aerosol pt, bronchospasm increases following the administration of isoproterenol by aerosol. This rare complication may be detected using pulmonary function tests before and after administration. Increases cyclic AMP, leading to a relaxation of bronchial smooth muscle and a decrease in. bronchial hypersecretion; side effects are cardiac arrhythmias, dryness of secretions, anxiety, restlessness, and headaches in a hypoxemic pt.

Xanthines are phosphodiesterase inhibitors, which result in an increase in cyclic AMP, stimulate CNSand cardiac muscle and relax smooth muscles. Oxygen therapy is often indicated to maintain adequate arterial oxygen tension during acute excernations. In addition, severely affected patients may benefit from chronic administration at home, at night. Recurrent morning headaches will often disappear when nighttime oxygentherapy is initiated.

Expectorants: Iodides are not used; glyceryl guaiacolate is of questionable value (Dose is 5ml 4-6 hourly). Antibiotics play an important role but are not given just because of a positive culture, but only when there are signs of active infection such as fever, X-ray changes, or elevated ESR. Antibiotics are selected on sputum cultures and organism sensitivities, although any child with cystic fibrosis (advanced) will harbor

H influenzae, S aureus, and F aeruginosa. The most effective oral antibiotics are cotrimoxazole(8-20mg/kg/d of trimethoprim in 2-3 doses), dicloxacillin (25- 50mg/kg/d), chloramphenicol(50mg/kg/d), and for older children, tetracycline (24-40mg/kg/d) Appropriate antibiotics for IV administration are gentamicin (7mg/kg/d in 3 divided doses;), and carbenicillin (500mg/kg/d) methicillin and ticarcillin (200mg/kg/d), and tobramycin (G- 5mg/kg/d). Since unless nave increases clearance and raxes of these drugs (aminoglycosides), larger doses may be needed. Patients should be hospitalized when on iV therapy. Long-term use will disturb Bacterial Balance and cause an overgrowth of resistant pseudomonas, proteus, staph, and fungi.

Severely affected patients may some degree, oo univentricular cardiac failure and may benefit fromdiuretics or digitalis. Oral ueoncniodilator therapy (tneopny limej4-6mg/kg/d) is helpful in some cases. electrolyte abnormalities(hypocnloremic alkalosis)are seen more frequently in patients with receiving large quantities of car Denecillin, and nypocalcemia and Hypomagnesemia are occasionally seen in associated with gentamicin therapy. There is an increased risk of atopy in these children with cystic fibrosis, and some benefit from intermittent antihistamine therapy. antihistamines on the contrary increase viscosity of respiratory secretions.
p) Intestinal obstruction due to uncomplicated meconium ileus in neonates can be relieved bydiatrisoate sodium or acetylcysteine enemas, when surgery is necessary, intestinal atresia or volvulus requiring resection may be seen in proximal region or meconium ileus.
recal impaction (meconium ileus equivalent) and intussusception in older cnilc which cause intestinal obstruction and abdominal pain in older child can be relieved without surgery, -The inspissated feces can be softened by oral acoty Icysteine, liquids or mineral oil. Intussusception can be reduced by enemas, surgery being required

occasionally.

PROGNOSIS:

Prognosis depends mainly on the bronchopulmonary involvement; treatment of the lung changes is most important. Average life expectancy in them is 18-20 years., and an optimisticoutlook must be maintained. Pulmonary involvement usually determines the fate of the pt. At present, only 505' patients can live to 20 years.

BRONCHIAL ASTHMA

Bronchial asthma is manifested by paroxysmal or chronically exacerbating dyspnea characterized by bilateral wheezing, prolongation of expiration, hyperinflation of the lungs and cough; restoration of abnormal pulmonary function towards normal by injection or epinephrine ,inhalation or adrenergic aerosols, or other therapeutic measures; eosinophillia or sputum andblood positive immediate skin test to provoking allergens and recurrent, attacks or dyspnea, coughing, wheezing caused by specific irritants and exercise. Bronchial asthma is a largely reversible obstructive process of the tracneobronchial tree causedby mucosal edema, increased and viscid secretions, and smooth muscle constriction.

Prior to puberty males are twice as prone as girls, but by adolescence and later, Incidence is similar in both sexes. Asthma is a reversible airway obstructive disease, emphysema is irreversible diffuseobstructive disease, but is rare in children. Both small (less than 2mm in diameter) and more larger airways are involved, in most cases of childhood asthma, the onset is by the 7th yr., but it assumes importance in second 6 months.

PATHOGENESIS:

The elements causing airway obstruction are edema of the mucus membranes, increased mucus secretions, and spasm of the smooth muscles. With sudden onset, and in early phase, spasm of the smooth muscle plays a major part. Later mucous edema and increased mucosal secretions dominate the obstruction. Those who die in the status, asphyxiate from complete occlusion by theairways by mucus plugs. All the asthmatics have a hyperreactivity or the airways to many environmental factors including irritants of various kinds (SO2, tobacco smoke, other pollutants), strong odors as wet paints, cold air, and rapidly changing temperature and humidity conditions. There are some whose inhalant allergens cannot be defined identified by history or skin testing, and Ig-E mediated allergy is not related to the – pathogenesis.

The commonest allergens in children are House dust, indoor molds, insects, epidermal (feathers,saliva and dander of cats, dogs, horses, cattle), airborne pollens (tress, grasses, weeds) and out-of-door seasonal molds, molds may provoke as trim an especially in infants (less common in childhood). Many children with initial hay fever develop asthma.

Main feature of asthma is an extraordinary hyperreactivity of the tracheobronchial tree to variouschemical mediators (acetylcholine, histamine, prostuagland inà), and agents that cause liberation oractivation of these substances, upper and lower Respiratory tract infections of viral orogms trigger or aggravate asthma. Other triggering factors are rapid changes in temperature or barometric pressure, the common air pollutants in cities, cooking odors, smoke, paint fumes, and exercise.

Psychologic factors are important. Aspirin idiosyncrasy may lead to Asthma.

Several factors play their part.

- Biochemical factors: Epinephrine administration causes hyperglycemia and lactacidemia because of activation of beta-2 receptors in muscle and liver in normal persons. In asthmatics, due to abnormality in Structure or function of beta-ädrenergic receptor-adenyl cyclase complex thereis blunted hyper glycemie Response and absent lactacidemia (plasma lactic acid does not increase'Their leukocytes are also deficient in caMP synthesis.

- -n extrinsic(allergic)asthma, attacks follow exposure to dust, pollen, dander and foods, with increase in Ig-E increase(both total and specific),in intrinsic or nonimmune asthma (mostly seenin first years, and in women about the time of menopause)there is no such involvement of IgE. These are clinically similar.
- Respiratory infections provoke attacks especially in intrinsic variety. Viral infections as RSV and parainfluenza virus lead to exacerbation of attacks especially in young children, (adenovirus, and A2influenza virus didnot do it showing specificity 0f infective precipitators).
- Asthma may got exacerbated with menses especially premenstrual) or menopause in some it improvesat puberty, similarly, there is an increased risk of Addisons disease in them, and those with thyrotoxicosis does not improve unless their endocrine problem is dealt with (these show some endocrinal influence).
- Emotional factors play an important role: in children.

CLINICAL FEATURES:

Onset may be as early as the first few weeks of life. In infancy, the first attack is associated with anURI or bronchiolitis, as the age increases, the episodes are more related to inhalant allergens and irritants. A h/o atopi dermatitis, or allergic rhinitis may be got. A family h/o atomic diseases, as allergic rhinitis and bronchial asthma are got.

Asthma can occur in the absence of overt wheezing, and there may be h/o chest congestion torecurrent cough.

- -The onset of asthma may be insidious or abrupt. Sudden onset is often usher in by a spell of coughing, which may be associated with itching of the chin, anterior part of the neck or chest. The onset is gradual, and resolution slower when the asthmatic attack complicates a Respiratory infection; wheezing may apnea a day or more after rhinorrhea and may resolve over a period of hours or day. The asthmatic paroxysm is characterized by increasing dyspnea, with prolongationof the expiratory phase of respiratory, by wheezing and. coarse and fine rhonchi (these diminish intensity as the obstruction becomes more severe). A severe paroxysm greatly limits the pulmonary ventilation; the resulting hunger leads to flaring of the alae nasi, use of accessory muscles of respiratory, cyanosis, and at times hypercapnia. There is tachypnea and tachycardia, restlessness, apprehension, fatigue, drowsiness, even coma; profuse sweating, flushed moist skin, pallid cyanosis, dry mucus membranes, With distressing cough there is abdominal pain also, and child vomits with a temporary relief from dyspnea. Sputum is tenacious and scanty unless treatment is given when it becomes abundant and loose, and spirals of mucus containing eosinophils are coughed up. Initially there may be hypertension but later hypotension, sings cardiac failure, and pulsus paradoxicus may result.

- -The chest is hyperresonant, hyperinflated, with wheezing and ronchi in mainly expiratory phase. -Physical examination with chest auscultation in a forced expiratory maneuver rather than on simple tidal volume, or pulmonary function tests can be highly revealing even in atypical cases. Breath sounds may be suppressed, and sometimes restriction of the tidal air is so great that breathsounds are barely audible. (an ominous sign). Physical findings are those of generalized obstructive emphysema. If atelectasis, pneuraothorax,'or pnepmomec astinum occur, chest findings are altered, with a shift of mediastinum. When emphysema occurs, and is severe, liver and spleen may be felt below the cost margins, many attacks of asthma over a long period may lead to chronic emphysema, which may be reversible with therapy during childhood. Children with chronic asthma have fine lanugo hair over the shoulders and arms. Pulmonary osteo arthropathy is rare, but allergic rhinitis and sinusitis are common. -Episodes of asthma in association with infections are frequently insidious in onset and prolonged; those due to specific identifiable allergens tend to be acute and brief if the causative agent is removed.

-

ASTHMA IN EARLY LIFE:

Bronchial asthma in infants (under 2 years.) has some peculiarities. The first attack usually follows by a few days the onset of a respiratory infection; some degree of cough or wheezing may persist for prolonged periods and becomes worse with subsequent colds. In infants, the predominant symptoms may be dyspnea, excessive secretions, noisy and rattly breathing, cough and some intercostal and suprasternal retractions(rather than the typical pronounced expiratory wheezes that occur in older children. Initial and repeated diagnoses of these episodes are made as bronchiolitis, croup, pneumonia. Recurrent episodes of coughing and wheezing are highly a suggestive of asthma regardless of age. There are many other causes ofpartial airway obstruction resulting in wheeze in early life.

Congenital anatomic malformations may lead to intrinsic or extrinsic obstructions; these includegastrointestinal, respiratory(lobar emphysema) and CVS (aberrant vessels). aspiration of FB can usually be suspected based on a careful history of onset of first attack, and in addition a FB almost always produces pneumonitis on an X-ray. Nonopaque materials(plastics)are not visualized, but fluoroscopy may be useful in diagnosing a unilateral obstructive process due to a FB. -Respiratory infections (bacterial and viral) during early life, commonly cause symptoms of airway obstruction. Contain viruses (RSV, parainfluenza) are pronecause airway obstruction in infants and young children. Bacterial infection: of lower Respiratory tract are rare- A child with recurrent episodes of cough with bacterial infections and wheezing associated with, bacterial infections., should be investigated for cystic fibrosis of the pancreas or immunologic deficiency syndrome.

Inhalants and foods may be cause of wheeze in early age as

milk, wheat, eggs, and chocolates. Diagnostic clues in recurrent wheezing are concurrent illness in the community, past h/o atopicdisease, family h/o atopic eosinophilia of blood or nasal and bronchial secretions, skin testing to relevant allergens, Response to epinephrine, and Response to corticosteroids. Each of these areas should be examined in assessment.

A system of bronchial cough, tracheal in origin (irritable trachea) occurs and since bronchodilator may help, it is difficult to distinguish from Asthma Wheezing is absent generally, and there are no signs of lower Respiratory tract obstruction. This allergic cough is usually precipitated by a viral Respiratory infection but may presage asthma in later life.

-Bronchial asthma may be confused with middle and lower Respiratory tract infections (laryngotracheobronchitis, acute bronchiolitis, bronchopneumonia, and pertussis) especially in the very young. Nasal wheezes may be transmitted to the chest especially in infants, from upper airway edema, increased secretions, or other obstructing factors as allergic rhinitis, upper RTI, adenoidal hypertrophy, FB, choanal stenosis, and nasal polyps(incidence high in cystic fibrosis). Congenitallaryngeal stridor is usually associated with other anomalies. In tracheal or bronchial FB, dyspnea, or wheezing is usually of sudden onset, but not always unliteral. Characteristic X-ray findings are not always present.

Cystic fibrosis and bronchial asthma are differentiated based on high sweat sodium andchloride, a h/o serious pulmonary infection since birth (often in cystic fibrosis), a personal or family h/o associated intestinal disturbances with profuse bulky stools and pancreatic enzymedeficiency both the conditions can coexist.

Tracheal or bronchial compression by extramural forces may resemble asthma and may be due toa FB in the esophagus, aortic ring, anomalous, vessels, or inflammatory or neoplastic lymphadenopathy.

Chronic recurrent bronchial asthma may lead to organic and psychological invalidism, barrel chest, and distensive emphysema; atelectasis and massive pulmonary collapse, mediastinal emphysema, and pneumothorax; and death due to Respiratory failure or misused drugs (oversedation, misuse of adrenergic aerosols, theophylline, tranquilizers, narcotics.) . Severe asthma may have acomponent of irreversibility.
-Lab findings: Eosinophill accumulation clumps of eosinophils on sputum smear) and peripheralblood eosinophilia are commonly found but are absent with infection or if corticosteroids are being given. Hematocrit can be elevated with dehydration (as in prolonged attacks) or in severe chronic disease. In severe asthma the first sign is hypoxemia without C02 retention. Respiratory acidosis and increased C02 tension may ensue. Moderately severe hypoxemia may occur with low C02 tension due to a combination of hyperventilation and ventilation perfusion disturbances.

X-RAY

X-ray shows bilateral hyperinflation, bronchial thickening and peribranchial infiltration, and areas ofdense, patchy atelectasis and associated bronchopneumonia. Patchy atelectasis is common and misread as pneumonitis. Pulmonary arteries may appear prominent.

The physiological abnormalities seen in pulmonary function testing in asthmatics reflect obstructive process in the small airways. Tests that measure expiratory flow rates EFR, forced expiratory volume in 1 second FEV1, maximal mid-expiratory flow MMEF, and peal expiratory flow PEFR show evidence of obstructs airways. Testing- the child before and after administration of a bronchiodilatic is useful in establishing reversibility of the process. More sophisticated testing shows increased total lung capacity and increased airway resistance, and uneven distribution of gases and air-trapping (body plethysmography and helium or nitrogen washouts respectively). Measurement of closing volume and MMEF determines involvement of small airways (less than 2mm in diameter). Series measurements of pulmonary functioning are much more valuable than isolated tests since findings vary because reversibility is the main feature of childhood asthma. Thus increased airway resistance with a decrease in flow rates, decreased vital capacity, and increased functional residual capacity and residual volume.. VC, FRC, and flow rates may be normal in asymptomatic intervals, but frequently there is residual hyperinflation chronically. Blood gases and pH during an asymptomatic period are characteristically normal. During a symptomatic period, especially with severe symptoms, hypoxemia ofsome degree is always present. Measurement of blood gases and pH are most important in following the progress of the child hospitalized for status asthmatieus. Positive skin reaction (immediate wheal and flare reactions.) to injected alleiens are frequently present. Provocative tests are positive. Positive clinical reactions usually occur within hours afteringestion. A positive reaction usually occurs immediately after inhalation but may not occur untila few hours after challenge. Asthma may occasionally be provoked by skin testing with appropriate allergens.

TREATMENT:

As far as possible contact with proved or suspected irritants and allergens should be avoided. Exposure to nonspecific irritants should be minimized as with tobacco smoke, strong odors suchas wet paints and disinfectants, and by the avoidance of ice cold drinks and rapid changes in environment and humidity, proper maintenance of humidified air is especially important in dry cold climates in the winter. If clinical history suggests IgE mediated sensitivity to inhalant factors which cannot be avoided, hypersensitization therapy should be instituted (with pollens, seasonal molds, and house dust).

-Parents and patients should understand the asthmatic process and prevention. -Adequatehydration should be maintained by encouraging, adequate fluid intake or give IV fluids if necessary- Postural drainage preceded by an adrenergic aerosol up to every 4 hours may be useful. Role of expectorants is dubious.

- -If present, metabolic acidosis should be corrected- by giving an energy source (to reduce ketosisby using 5% dextrose iV), food if tolerated, and bicarbonate.
- -Use of bronchodilators is the main stay of treatment. Theophylline and bronchodilators are usedalone or in combination. Aerosols are extremely useful if not abused.

*An acute episode of asthma of sufficient severity to cause obvious distress is effectively treated by SC epinephrine :0.01 ml/kg SC or IK up to a maximum c of 0.25ml(in infants and small children,0.05ml suffice, in older child 0.1-0.2 ml of a 1:1000 solution); may be repeated at 20 minintervals up to 3 doses.to get optimal relief. If no more than 9.2 ml are given/dose, pallor, tremor, etc. can be frequently minimized- Long-acting epinephrine repository ,as epinephrine suspension gives a more sustained relief; as Sus-phrine,1:200 thioglycol ate suspension of epinephrine, given 0.1-0.0-2 ml SC 8-12 hourly- Inhalers as isoproterenol sulfate inhaler, inhalations from pressurized aerosol, can be repeated 3-4 hourly gives rapid relief of symptoms. Isoproterenol hydrochloride, 1:200 solution may be used by a nebulizer so that rihemethanesulfonate, metaproterenol, and salbutamol inhalers can be used again 3-4 hourly, without avoiding excessive use.

If the Response to epinephrine and isoproterenol is not satisfactory, one of the theophyllines shouldbe used. Aminophylline (85% theophylline and 15% ethylenediamine) is given IV 4-6mg over 5- 15 minutes at a rate of not more than 25mg/min; can be repeated every 4-6 hours repeatedly.

The drug is quite safe in patients who had no theophylline in past 8 hours., and generally relieves symptoms. Aminophylline tablets are well absorbed from the GIT, and a safe and effective dose is 5mg/kg/6hourly. Since it has a short half-life, the dose should be given not more than 8 hourly, since such administration load to fluctuations of plasms level, and thus inadequate therapeutic response. Since theophylline is eliminated from the body by biotransformation in the liver; liver disease anddrugs affecting its metabolism will alter the plasma half-life in patients also vary in there rate of metabolism., therefore children receiving theophylline should be watched for theophylline toxicity(early signs being vomiting, especially of blood hemorrhagic gastritis, along with such CNS signs and symptoms as restlessness irritability, agitation, and later seizures.

- -Other drugs that are used in day-to-day management of asthma include-oral theophylline, pseudoe-i-hedrine and ephedrine 'terbutaline, metaproterenol (orciprc naline) and antihistaruinics. In the majority of children who have only intermittent episodes of asthma, oral theophylline(5mg/kg/6hrly) during symptomatic periods suffices. Ephedrine (0.5-1 mg/kg/d) in 4hourly doses is added for additional bronchodiator activity. Children with acute exacerbations of coughing and wheezing who have continuing symptoms of airway obstruction as night cough or coughing and wheezing on exercise will benefit from regular round the clock bronchodilator therapy. Theophylline 6 hourly with or without ephedrine is sufficient lessens cough, improves exercise tolerance, and wellbeing and lessens the number of acute exacerbations. In severe chronic asthma unresponsive to other measures, corticosteroids may be given. Adequate doses as 2mg/kg/d of prednisolone should be given. When chronic use is necessary for control of asthma, alternate day prednisolone or other short acting equivalents given before 8 AM on alternate days should be attempted. Bedomethasone dipropionate by topical aerosol can be given in dose of up to 600micg/d. After use in acute attack, they should be promptly discontinued for return of normal hypothalamus pituitary adrenal function quickly .When continuing use of bronchodilators in maximal doses limiting the normal life of child ,alternate day costicosteroids are very helpful. The patient is given an intensive daily therapy for a few days and then switched on to an alternateday regimen with prednisolone or methylprednisolone. Administering early in the morning mimics the circadian rhythm of endogenous cortisol secretion. When the patient responds well, prednisolone is reduced by 5mg/dose every 10 days until the lowest dose compatible withcontrol of symptoms.

Bronchodilator therapy should be maintained at the same time, since it results in less need for steroids, and thus a reduced dose. Low dose alternate day therapy is successful without adverse effects. The new group of corticosteroids for topical use have minimal risk of systemic absorption., since they have a minimal solubility. Before starting corticosteroids, cromoglycatesodium,20 mg by inhalation 4 times a day, should be given a trial for 1 month at least.
It is a white powder that is. aerosolized by a special device, mainly useful for extrinsic variety, some with intrinsic type also benefit. Disodium cromoglycatG (cromolyn sodium) is used prophylactically in asthma.
If there is evidence of bacterial infection, antibiotics should be given. Leukocytosis of up to 15000/ml is common in severe asthma without any evidence of bacterial infection. Even highercounts are seen after epinephrine administration. Patchy atelectasis on X-ray may be confused with pneumonitis on X-ray.
-In children with chronic or recurrent asthma, breathing and fitness exercise may assist the patient in aborting some attacks of asthma and improving muscular functions of the thoracic cage. Exerciseshould be encouraged rather than restricted, and exercise-induced bronchospasm can be

ameliorated by theophyllin 1-2 hours before exercise with or without disodium chromoglycate or salbutamol -Children with frequent overt asthma attacks as 1-2/week, and evidence of more or less constant pulmonary obstruction should be on constant pharmacological therapy. A daily regimen stimulating coughing and encouraging expectoration (postural drainage at least twice daily) may be helpful. Disodium chroraglycate 20mg 4 times daily by inhalation may be considered for chronic symptomatic asthma, alone or with other bronchodilator therapy.
The above treatment is for mild to moderate asthma.

STATUS ASTHMATICUS: (Severe acute asthma)

Then the patient continues to have a significant amount of respiratory distress Despite administration of sympathomimetic drugs and theophylline, status asthmatic is diagnosed. Thus, it is an increasingly severe asthma not responsive to drugs that are generally effective in treating an attack. Patient should be hospitalized, preferably to an intensive care unit. Analysis of arterial blood determination of p02, pC02, and pH is indicated. Well arterialized capillary blood suffices for suchestimations but arterial blood is preferable, especially if the patient had injections of epinephrine, which has a vasoconstriction effect on the peripheral vascular bed. Epinephrine (1:1000 sol,0.1-0.3 ml SC) is the drug of first choice. It can be repeated at 20-minute intervals for a total of 3 doses. If the Response is good but short-lived, a long-acting preparation, as Susphrine may be used. If the response is not good after 2nd or 3rd injection, especially in the face of epinephrine resistance, excessive use may aggravate asthma. Lack of therapeutic response to 2-3 injections of epinephrine may confirm presence of status asthmaticus. Epinephrine fastness (relative or apparently complete lack of responsiveness to epinephrine, may be due to hypoxemia and acidosis, bronchial obstruction with thick mucus plugs, pneumothorax, or simply severe asthma. Epinephrine sensitivity may improve after initiating other measures. Give 5% dextrose with 0.2%saline IV at the first sign of resistance to epinephrine or with poor fluid Intake, vomiting, dehydration. Dehydration is frequent present in the asthmatic child due to inadequate fluid intake, greatly increased insensible water loss due to tachypnea and the diuretic effect of theophylline. Adequate fluid intake must be maintained. Deficit therapy and

maintenance therapy is given but the patient should not be overhydrated. If steroids are being- used, potassium should be added to IV fluids (10-20 raEq/1 of IV fluids). Follow urine specificities as a guide. Patients in status have invariably hypoxemia and oxygen is indicated, evenwhen pCO2 is elevated. Hypoxemia in them is mainly due to ventilation/ perfusion imbalance.
In the presence of hypercarbia, oxygen should be given continuously and not intermittently. It can begiven by mask or nasal prongs (not by tent) at a flow rate of 2-4 liters/min. Others may aggravate asthma by its irritant effect on the airways leading to cough and worsening of the wheezing, the patient in the dense fog is also not observable, and water does not reach small airways, therefore tent (mist tent) should not be used.

If theophylline has not been used in previous 4-8hours 5mg/kg/dose can be given over a 10-20 min period and repeated 4-6 hourly. or given as a constant infusion beginning with a loading dose of 4-6mg/kg over 15 minutes and then 0.6-1 mg/kg/hour.

-Early during an asthmatic paroxysm, the patient usually hyperventilates and blows off C02with a resultant low PaC02. As the severity of the episode increases, patient becomes fatigued, and contributes to an increasing PaC02(therefore a normal or increased PaCO" in asthma indicates Respiratory failure).. If gas and pH analysis indicate presence of Respiratory failure (p02 less than 50mm, pC02 more than 50m»), an anesthetist is called and preparations for respiratory support made.

,

Correction of acidosis (pH 7.3 or below) with sodium carbonate is attempted. Sodium bicarbonate 1-3 mEq/kg should be given every 4-6 hourly. With tachypnea increased work of breathing and hypoxemia, metabolic acidosis may occur due to lactic acidosis, which may be compensated by a respiratory alkalosis due to hyperventilation. The appropriate bicarbonate doseis calculated: mEq of HC03 needed=Negative base excessx0.3xBW(kg)
Arterial or venous pH should be redetermined 5-10 min later, and further correction of acidosis, using bicarbonate considered if needed. In respiratory failure (without determining pH)
,2mEq/kg BW can be given initially.

Isoproterenol (1:200) or other adrenergic aerosols every 2-4 hourly may be given followed bypostural drainage if tolerated.

-If the patient is receiving corticosteroids already, the dose should be increased, temporarily. Hydrocortisone(100mg), prednisolone(20mg), dexamethasone(4mg) or methylprednisolone (20mg) is given 4 hourly around, the clock IV(=2mg/kg of prednisolone or its equivalent).Once thesymptoms are ameliorated, dose should be reduced as rapidly as possible. If patient dees not need corticosteroids, these are stopped abruptly rather than tapered; it is. feasible to stop corticosteroidsif patient has not taken high dose more than 48 hours). Jf prednisolone is to be used, oral prednisolone,1- 2mg/kg/d in one or two doses may be used followed ÏV use, and once status subsides, a switch onto alternate day regimen is made.

Antibiotics are given if indicated.

Chloral hydrate is the safest drug for sedation if needed (15mg/kg rectally) Narcotics and barbiturates depress the Respiratory center; tranquilizers may do the same in the presence of severehypoxemia. . Excessive use of epinephrine or adrenergic aerosols tend to thicken the secretions, deplete the glycogen stores, and increase apprehension.
-In Respiratory failure unresponsive to above therapy, IV isoproterenol therapy or assisted ventilation isgiven. 2 arterial determinations of pCO_2 above 45mmHg over a 15-30 minute period will call forinsertion of an indwelling arterial catheter, and if arterial pCO_2 remains above 45mm steadily, continuous isoproterenol infusion may give (to children, and not adolescents or adults)because of increased risk of cardiac arrythmias and should be given only in ICUs where continuous cardiac and BP monitoring facilities are available. An additional IV line for isoproterenol. the infusion is started at a rate of 0.1micg/kg/min and increased by this amount every 10-15 min until there is clinical improvement or until the heart rate approaches 200 beats/min. If arrythmias develop, rate of infusion is decreased. If Response is favorable, the patient isweaned very slowly from the infusion, decreasing the rate of infusion over a period of 30-36 hours.Rebound bronchospasm may occur if decreased too rapidly. –
If Despite isoproterenol infusion arterial pC02 remains high, endotracheal intubation is done andassisted ventilation given. When the patient is improved, and can take fluids orally, oral fluids should be given in the form of fruitjuices, but not fluids containing caffeine and chocolate. Give no milk or iced drinks. Adrenergic aerosols given every 3-6 hours followed by postural drainage for 20 minutes is applicable at this age, oral theophylline orally, and if corticosteroids have been started withdraw after 72 hours or taper gradually and discontinue as soon as possible.

PROGNOSIS

In majority of children, asthma can be brought under control and patient symptom free for long periods; the majority of children have less symptoms of asthma in their teens, and some lose any symptomatology for whole life(less than 30%).Others live with their asthma(about30%)die of asthma. Even with best management, some have chronic and disabling pulmonary andcardiopulmonary disability. Continuous night cough, breathlessness, and wheezing provoked by exercises or stress are usually indicative of serious disease than occasional spontaneous brief attacks due to recognizable allergens with symptom free periods in between. Infective asthma that begins early in life, are having a better prognosis allergy-induced asthma.

THE NEPHROTIC SYNMOME

Nephrotic syndrome results from increased permeability of the glomerular base- membraneto protein, and is characterized by general edema, hypoproteinemia, with serum albumin levels less than 2g% ,hyperlipidemia with serum cholesterol levels above 220 mg%, and excessive proteinuria, 2g/m2/d or more, the essential feature is marked proteinuria.

Proteinuria is from increased glomerular filtration of protein owing to increased permeability of the gl basement membrane. Plasma proteins of low mol wt (albumin, immunoglobulins, G, and transferrin)are excreted more easily than proteins of large mol wts(lipoproteins). Therefore, the relative clearance of the various plasma proteins thus vary with inverse relation to their size or mol wt (selectivity of proteinuria). Decrease in serum levels of albumin, lgG, and transferrin, is primarily due to excessive proteinuria, but increased protein catabolism is also involved. There is a reduction in total serum pleins, but a paradoxical increase in the concentration of some proteins of larger mol wt, especially of alpha-2 globulins(plasma lipoproteins are in this fraction) Plasma calciumconcentration mgc be low since 1/2 of plasma calcium is bound to albumin; the amount of ionized calcium remains normal.

Edema is a dominant symptom, but its presence or absence depends on fluid casait intake, etc, but is mainly due to excessive proteinuria. Many factors are involved in the causation of edema: reduction in plasma colloid osmotic pressure consequent to the decreased conc of serum albumin, which is responsible for redistribution of extracellular water, with an increase in the interstitial compartment relative to that in intravascular compartment marked reduction in urinary excretion of sodium due to an increase in tubula reabsorption of Na. A reduction in

intravascular volume resulting from, a shift of fluid to the extravascular space is the primestimulus for renin secretion, and secondary to renin hypersecretion, urinary excretion of aldosrone is also increased. Decreased plasma colloid osmotic pressure caused by the lowplasma albumin concentration has a direct effect on tubular reabsorption of sodium- reduction of plasma colloid osmotic pressure and retention of all ingested sodium are notsufficient for that much edema, for which retention of water should occur. For each 140 mEq of sodium ingested and not excreted one litre of water must be retained. Normal tonicity is maintained through the secretion of ADH which leads to reabsorption of water in the distal tubues and collecting ducts and the elaboration of a hypertonic or concentrated urine. If sodium intake is. markedly reduced, there is no need to restrict water intake (since the ability to excrete water is not impaired.. In some the water retention stretches to the point of becoming markedly hyponatremic, eye when their sodium intake is null this may be due to inappropriate continued release of ADH Despite plasma hypotonicity$_r$ in response to contraction,of intravascular volume, 'there are other causes also, for water retention.

Most of the lipid fractions normally found in plasma are elevated. There is a variable inverse relation between the degree of hyperlipidemia and the reduction in plasma albumin. Lipoproteinsare high mol wt proteins wrt album A decrease in plasma lipase activity is also found as a contributor to hyper lipidemia.

IDIOPATHIC NEPHROTIC SYHDBOME

Again there is proteinuria, hypoproteinemia, hyperlipidemia and edema, _the characteristic featurebeing responsiveness to corticosteroid therapy and characteristic histopathologic findings: the absence of significant glomerular lesions on light microscopy, absence of deposition of glomerular immune globulin, or complement, and fusion of epithelial foot processes without other significant Gl lesions on EM.

INCIDENCE:

Under 16 years of age, the incidence is 2/100,000(1 and 2.8:100,000 Respiratory white and nonwhites). Itusually occurs between 2-7 years of age,75% vases occur below 7 years,50% between 1-5 years, and peak incidence is between 2-3 years.. It is rare in first. 6 months, and uncommon in first year. 60% cases are males. Idiopathic nephrotic syndrome (INS) accounts for 80-90% cases of nephrotic syndrome in children.

ETIOLOGY.

Etiology is unknown, but hormonal causes and associated dysfunction of Tlymphocytes.

PATHOLOGY:

Light microscopy shows no changes except occasional areas of presence of the mesangial matrix, which become pronounced as the duration of proteinuria increases. EM showsfusion of epithelial foot processes of the gl. epithelial cells (podocytes), considered to be a nonspecific result of protein, If cessation of proteinuria is not achieved, some patients may develop progressive sclerosis of the glomeruli Prominence of mesangial matrix is due to mesangial protein trapping. Some metabolic, biochemical, or physicochemical disturbance in the gl. basement membrane leads to increased permeability to protein probability.

CLINICAL FEATURES:

Patients are usually in the preschool age (less than 5 years) at the time of first episode. Often following aflulike syndrome, the child is noted to have per orbital swelling and even-Anasarea perhaps oliguria. Increasing edema over several weeks is the usual presentation. There may be a h/o transient edema in preceding months Edema is the most conspicuous symptom; the onset of edema is usually insidious, at first periodical and then becoming increasingly extensive, and there is later generalized anasarca, including ascites and pleural effusion. The edema fluid accumulates first in dependent sites; after a night 's sleeps the face, lids, or sacral region nay be edematous, whereas during the day, swelling of the legs and abdomen is more prominent. An antecedent Respiratory infection is common and may precipitate a relapse. Other vague features are lethargy, anorexia, abdominal pain etc. A weight gain of 15-20% is common and is due to accumulation of edema fluid. The volume of urine is usually decreased, and concentrated urine may look to be dark. BP is usually normal, or slightly decreased; but in some cases, it may be increased because of hyperreninemia leading to excess production of angiotensin. There is an increased susceptibility to bacterial infection (partly due to decreased level of plasma gamuaclobulin). peritonitis or septicemia due to pneumococcus or coliforms and cellulitis are condoner infections. Venous or arterial thrombosis and thromboembolism are co- other infrequent complications and are accentuated by hypercoagulability and steroid therapy.

Shock is another infrequent Complication and is due to rapid diuresis induced by aggressive diuretic therapy in a patient with volume contraction. Liver enlargement, veins and the abdominal wall are associated with the edema. Diarrhea is frequent during episodes of edema (because of fluid infiltration in the intestinal wall). Respiratory difficulty (dyspnea) may result massive ascites (in some cases, needing abdominal paracentesis) or pleural effusions with massive edema. Due to the impressive swelling and weight gain, patient may show signs of intravascular volume depletion, and may even present in shock. Diarrhea is frequent during episodes of edema.

EVALUATION AND DIAGNOSIS:

- A h7o nephritis or infection must be sought.
- A careful assessment should be made including wt, BP, site and extent of edema, and cardiacstatus.
- 24-hour urine for protein estimation: Proteinuria may precede fluid retention by days or even weeks. Proteinuria more than 2g/m2/d is the main feature of the active phase; there may be aloss of 50 mg to 5g or more daily.
- Reduction in total serum protein, with albumin fraction reduced to less than 20% (hypoproteinemia mainly with hypoalbuminemia), elevation of alpha-2 and beta globulins, and gamma globulins are depressed (albumin reduced, globulin increased: A/G ratio reversed). Thereis hyperlipidemia. IgM may be raised, and IgG decreased.
- Urine sediment is usually normally rarely containing RBC, though oval fat bodies (tubular cellscontaining lipid) and hyaline casts are seen. Microscopic hematuria is rarely found, and its presence should raise suspicion of other glomeruli r diseases especially focal necrosis.
- Azotemia may occur (with raised urea and keratinize) being due to intravascular volume depletion rather than functional derangement of the kidneys. Usually, renal function tests are normal. (when present, azotemia is prerenal)
- Urinary protein electrophoresis shows high selectively of proteins (those of smaller molweights cleared more easily

and lost in urine).

- There is no anemia; hematocrit and Hemoglobin may be raised from hemoconcentration.
- VBC count is normal or mildly elevated to 10-12 thousand/cgm. ESR is raised -If the child iswell hydrated and hypervolemia is not significant, the patients GFR is normal.
- Serum level of beta-1c globulin is normal serum complement and its B, 1C component arenormal (if low, another disease is to be sought).
- Glomerular morphology 's shows fusion of foot processes of visceral epithelium, -Serumsodium is normal or often decreased (130-135 mEq/1).

All the features of disease need not be present especially early in relapse A combination of clinical features with proteinuria in excess of 1-2g/m2/d confirms the diagnosis, Fusion of foot processes of the visceral epithelium of gl basement membrane is found in any protein uric state, Presence of gross hematuria, a low C3, unselective proteinuria, an age of presentation between 2 months or after 10 years, a failure to respond to steroids, elevated blood urea, əlauated PP cast a doubt on diagnosis of idiopathic nephrotic syndrome, and renal biopsy should be done.

DIFFERENTIAL DIAGNOSIS:

This includes all glomerulopathies which lead to nephrotic syndrome, 20% cases of nephrotic syndrome, there is focal, proliferative, membranous disease, which may be primary, or secondary to anaphylactic purpura, SLE, sickle cell anemia, cyanotic heart disease, tuberculosis, malaria,syphilis, diabetes mellitus, multiple myeloma, amyloidosis, renal vein thrombosis or drug toxicity, (mercurial, penicillin nine, tolbutaride, bismuth, heavy metals, tridine) etc. -Idiopathic membranous glomerulopathy may present with identical features, only the age of onset is more than 10 years, and Response to corticosteroids poor. Proteinuria is selective less selective, renal biopsy shows thickening of 21. base membrane, deposits of IgG with or without beta-1c globulin. -Mebranoproliferative (hypocomplementenic)

glomerulonephritis is, distinguished by adepressed conc of serum beta-1c globulin, hematuria, proteinuria, azotemia, and hypertension.
Renal biopsy shows glorierular lobulation and meningeal proliferation. (onset is frequently beyond 10 years of age. - Rapidly progressive glomerulonephritis is manifested by nephritis as wellnephrotic features, but serum complement levels are normal. It is an idiopathic proliferative glomerulonephritis with epithelial crescent formation. - Membranous glomerulopathy is associated with SLE, malaria or syphilis, and distinguished by specific features. - Glomerulonephritis of anaphylactic purpura, a proliferative lesion primarily involved mesangiumwith or without crescent formation nephritic component is common. Toxic (drug or toxic induced) nephrotic syndrome (secondary to triwethadone therapy, ingestion of mercury, exposure Co poison oak, or to a beesting. Clinically and pathologically may be indistinguishable from INS; diagnosis being made only by n/o ingestion of the drug or toxin. -focal sclerosing glomerilopatnyis similar 10 INS at the onset, but less responsive to therapy and has a poorer prognosis. There is more microscopic nematurta, and renal biopsy is typical. - Acute poststrepiococcal nephritis may occasionally clinically present as the nephritis syndrome. - Nephrotic syndrome in infancy is a group of many disorders.

TREATMENT

-Goal in treatment is reduction of urinary protein to a normal quantity. steroids are ine drugs oi choice and as soon as the diagnosis is made, cortic steroids should be given the least expensive isprednisone, 2mg/kg/d, or 60mg/m2/d of prednisone, exceed 80mg/d. li is given in 3-4 doses. drug is continued: until the urine is proteinase for 3-46 days, or if urine fails to welcome protein free, for 4-8 weeks. If lor 10 days on prednisone, urine remains protein-free IOF 10 days, it is tapered to discontinuance OI 3-4 days. In more than 90% pus, protein excretion returns to normalwithin 4 weeks (mean response time 2 weeks). Lack of response (continued proteinuria) within weeks suggests steroid resistance and their chances of responding to prolonged treatment.

These are also less effective in steroid resistant cases but are more effective in frequently relapsing cases. Cyclophosphamide, dose is 1-2.5mg/kg/d given for 6 Weeks to O months. Prednisone should be given on alternate day therapy until. administration of cyclophosphamide.Side effects include sterility, hemorrhagic cystitis, and alopecia, especially with longer courses (shortercourses have more relapses). Besides this, nitrogen mustard, netjotrixate, b-tniogluanine, azathioprine, and chlorambucil can be used (all should be used under guidance of a children's nephrologist). Chlorambucil is slow-acting and less toxic than cyclophosphamide (dose is 0.1mg/kg/d weeks, then 0.2ng/kg/d for 6 weeks; prednisone given with it tapering it following the combined should be followed weekly and if leukopenia occurs, it is mild and transient, and resolves when the drug is stopped.

Spontaneous remission may occur, especially if the episode was precipitated by an intercurrent infection or illness. Also, there is a chance of latent bacterial infections spreading or reactivatingunder cover of corticosteroids (especially TB, and unrecognized UTI). Therefore, many advise that it is better to wait for 1-2 week(s) for spontaneous remission to avoid unnecessary use of corticosteroids. Others advise that corticosteroids be used as soon as diagnosis is made severe edema, and ascites lead to discomfort, anorexia, inability to move out, and skin nay breakdown and become infected. These are used with prednisone since use ci a diuretic alone can be hazardous in the presence of a low serum albumin since these can aggravate an already existing contraction of the circulating blood volume. Diuretics may be used alone in the following circumstances: a combination of oral hydrochlorothiazide(75mg/02/d) and triamterene(300mg /ma/d) in 3 divided doses for 4-7 days in patients who have problems with recurrent edega; Oral or parenteral furosemide, 1-3mg/kg/d if an immediate Response is needed(to mobilize edema fluid and alleviate symptoms from ascites, to help control infections, while the patient is edematous, and to alleviate the aggravation of edema, which can occur when steroids are first begun. There is a danger of contraction OI vascular volume, electrolyte disturbances, and shock with intensive diuretic therapy in nephrotic child, there extreme caution and hospitalization is needed, When diuresis is ineffective, or is pulse rate increases, or it bp drops, or goes up precipitously, diuretic should be used with albumin only or discontinued. When accumulation of edema fluid is severe, or diuretics alone fail, and generalized anasarra is results in acute distress ed. When accumulation of edema fluid is severe, or diuretics alone sail, and generalized anasarcais results in acute distress or when severe intravascular depletion occurs, salt-poor albumin is given (1g/kg IV slowly given over 1 hour period, and if needed 12 hourly). It is followed by IV furosemide(1mg/kg). Diuretics are more useful when used immediately after expansion of the intravascular volume by infusion of salt poor albumin; too rapid administration of salt poor albumin may cause pulmonary edema and CCF.

Diet should be normal for age; tendency to retention of salt in the nephrotic state is accentuatedby steroid therapy, dietary da salt is restricted to 1g =17 mq/d) if there is edema and proteinuria. If salt is restricted, fluid restriction occurs itself (and should be restriction only if there progressive accumulation of edema Despite sodium restriction or if there is an impaired ability to excrete a normal intake of water.) A clear level of dilution of fluids is shown a serum level 01 130mEq/1 or less. Activity is not restricted and is allowed as the patient tolerates it; the child can go to school but contact with sick children should be avoided. Enforced bed rest contributes more to patients wellbeing special care should be taken to avoid infection of the peritoneal cavity, and fluid and protein depletion. Patients have a great susceptibility to infection, andpreviously pneumococcal peritonitis accounted for many deaths during acute infection occurs with bacteria, prognosis is guarded; presence of ascites mask symptoms Ol peritonitis Prognosis: 90-958 01 children snow an initial Response lo corticosteroids (80% snow complete Response);1/OI inose responding nave no subsequent disease activity; 1/2 relapse infrequently, and 1/2 frequently, and even may become steroid resistant. Initial response suggests later prognosis. Relapses are more common during first 1 yr (but can occur up to 1 years later); a patient regission lasuing for years is almost always permanent while as failure to respond or early relapse usually heralds a prolonged series of relapses free for 5 years, ne has 92 chances 01 Weing cured, 11 one relapse occurs, Subsequentcourse cannot be predicted, and number of relapses persedonc affect ultimate prognosis. Criteria predictive of the course OI disease include age at Onset, presence or absence of hematuria, and hypertension, Response co steroid clear level of dilution of wody flows is shown a serum level of 130mEq/1 or less. Activity is not restricted and is allowed as the patient tolerates the child can go to school but contact with sick children should be avoided. Enforced bed rest contributes more to patients wellbeing the virtubig. Thechild should we taugni LO by dipstick. -special care should be taken to avoid infection of the peritoneal cavity, and fluid and protein depletion. Pts. have a great susceptibility to infection, angpreviously pneumococcal peritonitis accounted for many deaths during acute oneself injection occurs with gm -ve bacteria, le prognosis is guarded, presence of ascites masks the usually.

CLINICAL FEATURES IN AIR-LEAK

Any type of air leak can be asymptomatic. But when it is symptomatic, the onset is usually acute,and extensive pneumothorax will present with PAIN, CYANOSIS, AND DYSPNEA Tension pneumothorax presents with rapid onset of marked respiratory distress , particularly in newborns,in which it may be associated with significant hypotension. There may be physical evidence of impaired venous return and shift of the cardiac Impulse and trachea towards the normal side. In infancy both symptoms and signs a may be difficult to recognize. If the pneumothorax is moderate in extent, there may be little displacement of the intrathoracic organs and few or no symptoms. Even in severe cases there may le few. Physical findings except for cyanosis and dyspnea or tachypnea. "The percussion note over the involved area is tympani tic Breath sounds are feeble or absent on the affected area in both newborn as well as children. Larynx, trachea, andheart may be shifted towards the normal side the breath sounds may have an amphoric quality If there is an open fistula. from air-bearing tissues into the pleural cavity. When fluid is present, there is a sharp delimited area of time tympany above a level of flatness to percussion. It is important to determine whether the pneumothorax is an open. (tension pneumothorax) or a closed one. The presence of emphatic heeathing or of gurgling sounds synchronous with Respiratory rations when fluid is present with in the pleural cavity is suggestive of an: open fistula. confirzatory evidence is provided when the pneumothorax fille rapidly artery aspiration of It Another means to determine whether the fistula is open in examination of the aspirated air for its. Oxygen content. If a fistula is present, the oxygen content of the air in pheunot borax remains constant. If there are 10 connections with the bronchial tree, the oxygen content is low, since it is: rapidly absorbed The older child is likely to experience sudden sharp chest pain, and there may be hyper resonance on percussion of the involved area. With pneumothorax- pericardium, there may be muffled heart sounds and severe circulatory insufficiency, most infrequently causing death by cardiac tamponed. In most cases am isolated pneumomediastinum causes no symptoms other than mild repotto tachypnea Rarely severe tension pneumomediastinum may develop, causing symptoms like those of the tension pneumothorax X-

RAY establishes the diagnosis. Both AP and Lateral voews should be taken.

The definitive diagnosis of any type of air Leak is given by X-ray. Cross-table lateral and lateraldecubitus x-rays within the upon affected side up, are best for demonstrate pneumothorax.
Occasionally the extra pulmonary intrathorax air may not shift with changes in body position because of loculation within the pleural space of localization of the air beneath the visceral pleura. Pneumomediastinum appears as a radiolucent line following the contour of the mediastinum. Pneumo pericardium is best distinguished from the pneumomediastinum by the factthat the radiolucent line is continuous along the diaphragmatic cardiac border. Pulmonary interstitial emphysema appears on X-ray as a collection of small linear, reticular, or cystic radiolucency that tend to be wider in the more peripheral lung tissue. Particularly in the newborninfant increased trans illumination of the involved hemi thorax using a high-intensity light sourcemay strongly suggest space or localization of the air beneath the visceral pleura. Pneumomeg Lasuruum appears as a radiolucent line following the contour of the mediastinum. Pneumopericardium is beat distinguished from the pneumomediastinum by the factthat the radiolucent line is continuous along the diaphragmatic cardiac border. Pulmonary interstitial emphysema appears on X-ray as a collection of small linear, reticular, or cystic radiolucency that tend to be wider in the more peripheral 1ung tissue. Particularly in the newborn infant increased trans illumination of the involved hem thorax using a high-intensity light source may strongly suggest the presence of tension pneumothorax. The air in the pleural cavity may cause collapse of the underlying lung and shift of the mediastina structures to the opposite side.

DIFFERENTIAL DIAGNOSIS

Pneumothorax must be distinguished from localized or generalized emphysema, extensive emphysematous bleb, large pulmonary cavities, or other cystic formations, diaphragmatic hernia,and gaseous distension of the stomach. Most of the times a simple X-ray will solve the issue. Occasionally it is difficult to distinguish it from diaphragmatic hernia, lung cysts, localized lung hyperinflation (pulmonary interstitial emphysema, lobarvemphysema) or artifact due to overlyingskin folds or clothing. A small amount of bar um may be needed in cases of diaphragmatic herniathat a portion of the GIT is in the thoracic cavity. Treatment In mild cases, oxygen may be needed for relief of dyspnea. When there is no fistula between the air-bearing tissue and the pneumothorax, the air is usually absorbed within a week or 50, and no treatment is necessary unless there are symptoms of excessive pressure, in which case the air should be aspirated.

Tension pneumothorax in a newborn or young infant requires immediate emergency needle aspiration and of the pleural air followed by chest tube insertion and underwater closed system drainage for several days. Needle aspiration should be performed using a needle orc catheter ofappropriate size for the patient (20 to 22 gauge in newborn infants) inserting it into the 2nd intercostal space in the midclavicular line. If the bronchopleural fistula is large, -ve pressure in the tube may be necessary. If the tension pneumothorax is not relieved by this means surgical closure of the fistula should be considered. Pneumopericardium requires emergency treatment consisting of aspirating the pericardial ugh a needle introduced in the subxiphoid or left parasternal position. A drain age tube should be placed in the pericardial sac if there is repeatedaccumulation of pericardial air.

Pneumomediastinum rarely requires aspiration.

The air in the mediastinum is usually lobulated into multiple cysts and therefore cannot be effectively removed by needle or mediastina tube. There is no proven way to remove the abnormal air in the pulmonary interstitial emphysema other than stopping it reaccumulating. Any patient with an air leak who needs resuscitation or assorted ventilation should be treated by the lowest possible inflate pressures. Small pneumothorax (less than 20% of the hemi thorax) in stable patients of any age can be treated with bed rest. In some cases, Spontaneous resorption of pleural air can be hastened by having the patient breathe 100% oxygen. But this is not appropriate in newborn infants because of the risk of retrolental fibropl sia. Conservative therapywhile awaiting spontaneous resorption is more often indicated in older ots. A chest tube may be indicated for patients with chronic sma pneumothorax to cause some pleural reaction to seal the air leak, Surgical procedures are occasionally needed for a persistent air leak as a broncholeural fistula. Significant respiratory distress is always an indication for cest tube drainage of the pleural space (thoracotomy).

HYDROTHORAX

In Hydrothorax, the fluid is no inflammatory in origin, and has a lower specific gravity (less than1015) than that of a serofiibrinous exudate it contains Less protein and fewer cells, which are mesothelium rather than Leukocytic, and is usually associated with an accumulation of fluid in other parts of the body a peritoneal cavity and the subcutaneous tissues. Hydrothorax Is most often associated with cardiac or renal disease, although occasionally it may be a manifestation of severe nutritional edema, and rarely from venous obstruction by neoplasms, enlarged Lymph nodes or adhesions. Hydrothorax is bilateral in renal disease, nutritional edema: and may be in myocardia disease (but in the last case may be limited to the right side or may be more on the right than on the left side). Physical findings are those of serofibrin us pleurisy, but the shifting of dullness is more rapid with changes of positic, the treagent is that of primary disorder; if pressuresymptoms appear, aspiration may be needed.

NEMOTHORAX

Accumulation of whole blood in the pleural cavity is most caused by surgical. or accidental trauma, but extensive bleeding into the P.I cavity may be caused by erosion of a bloodvessel by an inflammatory process as TB, and empyema, or occasionally may result from blood dyscrasias, coagulation defeat, tumors. of lung, and pleura, it may be iatrogenic, associated withsubclavian vein annulation, Bleeding may be rapid or slow. Rupture of an aneurysm is not likely during childhood. Symptoms are related to blood 1066. or compression of pulmonary parenchyma by pleural accumulation of blood. When a hem thorax occurs in association with a pneumothorax, as in cases of trauma, it is called hem pneumothorax. The diagnosis of hemothorax can only be made by thoracentesis. There is a significant risk a hemo-empyema. In many cases of uncomplicated hemothorax, thoracotomy tube draining may not be necessary since blood is absorbed must be determined since the treatment depends on the cause. Surgical intervention may be needed to control active bleeding and transfusion is necessary where the lossof blood is excessive.

CHYLOTHORAX

Chylothorax is accumulation of chyle in the pleural cavity, which is usually due to accidental or surgical trauma to the thoracic duct. When the chyle escapes from the duct into the pleural cavity, Sometimes escape of chyle may occur apparently without rupture because of the pressure of enlarged lymph node or neoplasms:(when the spreading cancer eats away the duct or enlarged node obstructs the duct). In the newborn chylothorax may be congenital or secondary birth trauma. There may be a 2–10-day latent period between the injury to the thoracic duct and the appearance of chyle in the thoracic cavity. Thrombosis of the duct, or of the subclavian vein and congenital anomalies of the duct system has been reported as causes. Chylothorax is usually on the left side and is only rarely bilateral. It is a rare disease at all the symptoms are dependent onthe amount of fluid, and symptoms and signs are those of fluid in the pleural cavity. X-ray also issimilar to pleural effusion. There is no associated pain, but tachypnea and dyspnea occur with large accumulations. A white eerily or milky fluid obtained at thoracentesis justifies diagnosis the chylous fluid is a milky fluid containing fat, protein, and other constituents of chyle. In newborn infants who have not been fed the fluid may be clear. and grossly like pleural effusion. Chylothorax must be differentiated from the accumulation of fatty material is a chronicpleural effusion. A pseudostyles milky fluid has been seen in cases of serous effusion in whichthe fatty material is assumed to be due tom the degenerative changes within the fluid

It has been suggested that this type of fluid can be distinguished from one con training chime by:shaking it with alkalis or ether, the fluid containing chyle tends to become clear. Chylothorax canbe differentiated from the accumulation of fatty material in a chronic pleural effusion by demonstrating the appearance of a fat-soluble dye ingested by the pt. into the pleural fluid.

Spontaneous closure of the defect in the thoracic duct Occurs in about 1/2 cases in infants less than 1 year of age. Repeated aspirations may be needed to relieve respiratory distress . And other symptoms of pressure. Continuous removal of repeated accumulations of chyle can be the cause of significant depletions of the patients proteins and lymphocytes. The aspirated chyle has been injected without any untoward reactions. Since in 1/2 cases spontaneous closure occurs, with recovery, therefore every case should be treated conservatively for about 4-6 weeks. conservative therapy consists of repeated continuous chest tube drainage, first discontinuing all oral feedings, then reinstituting

feedings with MCT fats the die should be low in fat and rich in protein, and hyper alimentation may be used to avoid significant protein malnutrition. Low fat intake of fat is associated with a decrease production of chyle. The high protein diet intake is needed for
108s of protein in the chyle. The total calorie intake must also be above the required intake, fat soluble vitamins intake should be much. If 4-6 weeks of conservative therapy are not successfulin decreasing or stopping the accumulation of chyle, ligation of the duct is attempted or closureof the site of the leak; but this surgery is often unsuccessful.

MEDIASTINAL MASSES

Most mediastina masses are asymptomatic and discovered during routine chest x-rays, but pressure symptoms may occur respiratory symptoms are more common in children than in adults,and result from pressure on the airways, with cough, incomplete airway obstruction with wheezing or air trapping, complete obstruction or atelectasis, Pressure on the left recurrent laryngeal nerve may cause hoarseness of the voice due to left. V.C paralysis. Pressure on the esophagus can lead to dysphagia.

Dilatation of the neck vessels may occur because of SVC obstruction. Physical findings are rare except in very large masses. Most types of the mediastina tum ours tend to be localized to a specific mediastina compartment and enhance the accuracy of diagnosis, but some are either intrapulmonary but appear to be in the mediastinum, or some are seen the in different or several compartments. An enlarged thymus is the commonest mediastina mass in the children. Mediastinal lymph nodes may be enlarged in benign or malignant disease. Benign cystsare usually abnormalities of the emphrologic development. X-ray is mostly diagnostic, butt ECG, echocardiogram, thoracic ultrasound, fungal and mycobacterial skin, urinary catecholamine, peripheral lymph node biopsy, and mediastinoscopy treatment depends on the type of the mass, but surgery is required for diagnosis or treatment.

INFANTILE(Congenital) Labar emphysema

It is progressive over distension of the lung tissue, usually a single lobe, producing respiratory distress within the first 6 months of life, especially during the first 2 weeks. The left upper Labe and the right middle lobe are most affected. There is usually no identifiable cause, butin some cases localized bronchial cartilage deficiency causing a ball-valve obstruction has been

reported. Sometimes the airway obstructionist present at birth, and early chest X-ray way show alocalize delayed clearance of the fetal, lung fluid (increased opacity) from the affected area.

During the first week of the life this is replaced by air and there is gradual development of increasing hyperinflation of the affected lung. Respiratory distress classically increases within the first days or weeks of life, with tachypnea, retractions, chest asymmetry intermittent cyanosis,expiratory wheezing, and localized decreased air entry. Other causes of the similar clinical hectare are bronchogenic cysts, or musicales, an errant or large pulmonary arteries (especially. those associated with large L-R shunts), mucous plugs, FB, andiredund and bronchial mucosa. Chest X-ray shows localized hyperinflation of the lung tissue with compression adjacent lung and mediastina shift towards the contralateral hemithorax with manuntien honor inflation there maybe anterior herniation of the abnormal lung done for ant aberrant or enlarged vessels Differentialdiagnosis in addition to above mentioned cases including lung cysts, pneumatoceles, localized pulmonary interstitial emphysema diaphragmatic hernia and localized pneumothorax.

Lobectomy is the treatment in cases with significant respiratorysymptoms if symptoms cannot be relieved by any other method. Postoperatively many patients will have persistence of recurrent coughand wheezing episodes and 10% will develop hyperinflation of another lube in future.

CYSTIC ADENOMATOID MALFORMATION

This rare congenital anomaly of the lung is a multicyclic mass of pulmonary tis sue containing disordered, polypoid proliferation of respiratory epithelium and bronchiolar structures that may or may not communicate with normal airways. The cysts are lined by cuboidal or columnar epithelium. The affected infants are born prematurely, and usually begin to experience respiratory distress at birth or within the first weeks of life. The cystic mass, which may occur inany lobe, produces symptoms of tachypnea, cyanosis, and retractions by enlargement, with secondary compression of the normal lung tissue. Chest X-ray shows an intrapulmonary mass thatmay be radio dense or radiolucent with sharp irregular borders. There is oft ten a shift of the mediastinum as the abnormal area becomes hyper inflated. With symptomatic infant, and the abnormality being localized to one lobe or lung, surgical resection is indicated to avoid further compression of the normal lung.

PULMONARY CYSTS

Congenital pulmonary cysts may be congenital or acquired, associated with the trachea or main bronchus (extrapulmonary) or with the smaller airways or alveoli (intrepid monary) and may be symptomatic or asymptomatic. The differential diagnosis of lung cysts includes congenital cysts,cystic adenomatoid malformations, pneumatic cells, lung abscess, pulmonary sequestration, lobulated pyopneumothorax, infantile Isobar emphysema, diaphragmatic hernia, FB aspiration, a variety of mediastina masses, and localized pulmonary interstitial emphysema. Distinguishing congenital from acquired cysts (post-infectious) is important since in the congenital ones, surgery is indicated, and in the post-infectious ones, contraindicated. True congenital cysts are very rare, and the true congenital pulmonary cysts are bronchogenic is cysts and congenital cystic adenomatoid malformations.

BRONCHOGENIC CYSTS

These characteristically occur adjacent to the airway near the tracheal bifurcation. Those at the carina are usually the most serious, causing obstructive respiratory symptoms, often from birth, dueto tracheobronchial compression. Hilar cysts attached to one of the main or lo bar bronchi are more common in older children and are usually asymptomatic. There is no relationship between thesize of the cysts and the degree of the resultant respiratory distress . Cysts are thin-walled and contain clear mucous fluid. The contents of the cyst may become infected, or the airway compression by the cyst may cause the distal lung parenchyma to become hyperinflated, and attelectasaisi are infected. Cysts adjacent to the esophagus may cause dysphagia. Occasionally an infected cyst may develop a communication with a bronchus, resulting in hemoptysis, purulent sputum, and associated fever. Chest X-ray may demonstrate the cyst, obstructer, emphysema, atelectasis, mediastina shift, or in young newborn, an opacified. Hemithorax due to delayed clearance of fetal Lung fluid. Esophagoscopy may show the presence of the cyst if it is not apparent on Palin x-ray. Sometimes the cyst in often positioned between theesophagus and the trachea. Occasionally a fluid. Level may be evident in a cyst, indicating communication with the tracheobronchial tree. Treatment is by surgical resection, and vigorous pulmonary physiotherapy. Acquired pulmonary cysts include pneumatoceles and lung, abscesses.

PIERRE ROBIN SYNDROME

A congenital malformation is characterized by a triad of micrognathia glossator sis with pseudomacroglossia., and left palate or high arched palate.

Posterior displacement of time attachment of the senioglos and Ųs muscle to the hypoplastic mandible prevents the normal anchorage of the tongue under the influence gravity; the tongue assumes a returned position, obstructing the pharynx post alveolar cleft of the hard and soft palates is a common feature, while as in other cases the palate is high arched. The tongue isof normal size, the floor of mouth is foreshortened, and the buccal cavity reduced in size. The lack of space further contributes to the glossoptosis. The obstruction of the air passages especially of inspiration, requires treatment in order a to avoid suffocation. These children present as emergency during the neonatal period because of the infringement of the airway by the tongue. The main objective of the treatment is to prevent asphyxia until the mandible becomes enlarged enough to accommodate the tongue. The infant should be placed in prone position or so that the tongue falls forward to relive respiratory obstruction. In other cases, this isnot. Sufficient, and temporary suturing time ventral surface of the tongue to the lower lip, tracheotomy or a or pharyngeal airway are used. Feeding also requires great care, Normally growth of the mandible will progress so that an essentially normal profile is achieved with 4-6 years.

Diaphragmatic hernia can be congenital or acquired (the latter being usually traumatic). Congenital variety may be due to a defect in the poster lateral port ion of the diaphragm (foramen of Bochdalek), and in 5% cases, to a defect in the retrosternal area(foramenof Morgagni)..Diaphragmatic hernia represents the failure of division of the thoracic and abdominal cavities at the 8th to 10th weeks. of fetal life. Herniation occurs most often in the poster lateral segments of the diaphragm, and more often on the left than the right side. The defect represents the failure of the pleuroperitoneal canal to close completely during the embryonic development (foramen of Bochdalek). The defect in the anterior portion of diaphragm in the retrosternal area (Morgagni) represents failure of the fusion of the two anlagen of diaphragm with elements of the pericardium. All degrees of protrusion of the abdominal viscera through the diaphragmatic openings into the thoracic cavity may occur. The extent of herniation will deter mine the severity and timing of the fewer than 2% cases are secondary to retrosternal defect in poster lateral variety more than 80% cases involve the left diaphragm. In the retrosternal defect, there may be herniation of the intestine, into the pericardial sac or conversely ectopic cordis with displacement of the heart into the peritoneal cavity. Umbilical defects are commonly associated with herniation through the foramen of Morgagni. In Bochdalek lesion usually the entire gastrointestinal tract is present in the left chest. In severe cases of the stomach and large part ofthe intestine, and in rare cases, spleen, liver, and even kidney displace the heart and lungs. There may be associated incomplete rotation of the cecum, umbilical defects, and duodenal constricting bands. The lungs on the affected side are compressed and often hypo plastic. Hypoplasia of the oppo and site lung has also been seen.

CLINICAL FEATURES

Symptoms of mild to severe respiratory distress and cyanosis are usually present from the birth. Congenital herniation of the abdominal contents into the thoracic cavity may be responsible for serious embarrassment of respiratory, and usually constitutes a medical-surgical emergency in the immediate neonatal period, but infrequently there is no or little respiratoryembarrassment, and the hernia may not be detected until later in infancy or childhood, when the finding of a largediaphragmatic hernia with air-filled coils on X-ray is incidentally found on X-ray chest. Severe respiratory distress including dyspnea and cyanosis, is usually present from birth. If symptoms are not present at birth, they may appear at any time during the neonatal period or later, these include vomiting, severe colicky pain, 6 discomfort, after eating, constipation and dyspnea. Signsand symptoms of acute intestinal obstruction when the condition is detected on chest x-ray. The physical examination varies considerably, depending on the degree of displacement of abdominal contents into the thoracic cavity.

With extensive displacement: in the newborn, the abdomen. is, small and scaphoid, the infant being cyanotic and in as obvious retractions. If the respiratoryembarrassment is not relieved., shock and rapidly progressive hypoxia Occurs, and severe metabolic and respiratoryacidosis can occur in contrast, id mildly affected patients there may be no or only minimal respiratory distress , and no digestive disturbances. The percussion notes on the part of the thorax containing the stomach and intestines. may be moretympanic or duller than usual breath sounds are absent in the affected hemi thorax. Occasionally spends of the intestinal peristaltic movements can be heard over the chest, but this is an unreliablefinding. More dependable is the absence of the point of maximal impulse of the heart (displacement of the point of maximal impulse) Presence of the point of maximal impulse of the heart in a newborn with respiratory distress indicates either extra pulmonary air as pneumothorax or mediastinum, or diaphragmatic hernia. Further differentiation is made clinically by the presence or absence of abdominal distension favors pneumothorax or pneumomediastinum, and scaphoid abdomen a diaphragmatic hernia. Fatal cases (30%) have circulatory problems secondary to mediastina shift, giving rise to stretching and kinking of the great vessels. Pulmonary infections, prematurity, cardiac anomalies, malrotation, are usual causes of death, but the most frequent cause of death in them is pulmonary insufficiency. The long on the affected side is compressed and hypo plastic with decreased number offs of airways and prudery arteries throughout. and1 though. hypo perfusion, and a pre-emphysematous state can be. identified, hypo plastic Lungs remain asymptomatic at least until late in children X-RAY establishes the diagnosis, usually without the aid of contrast medium, or by injecting air into the stomach. Characteristically, in theneonatal period there are fluid and air-filled loops of intestine in the chest simulating cysts. The Mediastinum is displayed towards the unaffected side, usually the right occasion in cases of cystic adenomatoid malformations of the lung or congenital lober emphysema, use of contrast medium is necessary that shows presence of stomach/intestine in the abdominal cavity.

TREATMENT

Diaphragmatic hernia is a surgical emergency, and resuscitation of the newborn is mandatory prior to undertaking reduction of the hernia' and closure of the diaphragmatic defect. As soon as the diagnosis is made, the infant must be positioned with his head and thorax higher than the abdomen and feet to facilitate the downward displacement of the abdominal organs. Nasogasyric intubation with intermittent suction will decrease the entrapment of air and fluid within the herniatedviscera and lessen the degree of the Berniated- ventilator compromise. Intravenous fluids are given. Positive pressure ventilation should be administered cautiously through an endotracheal tube since pneumothorax may result due to uneven distribution of the intrapulmonary pressures in lungs affected by compression atelectasis or pulmonary hypoplasia. Arterial blood gas determination, including pH should be obtained preoperatively and metabolic and respiratoryacidosis should be corrected with appropriate IV doses of NaHCO3.Via a subcostal lesion, the gastrointestinal contents are brought into the celomic cavity, and after the reduction of the hernia,the defect is closed. The abdominal cavity should be stretched, or the creation of an incisional hernia should be performed. The postoperative course is extremely demanding and associated with high mortality Survival of this lesion is no greater than 50% when the diagnosis is made within the first 18 hours of life. Re-expansion of the hypo plastic ipsilateral lung may take several days. No attempatient shouldbe made to forcefully inflate the lung as this invariably causes a pneumothorax. There is a greater incidence of pneumothorax on the contralateral side, and the role of the PDA in return of fetal circulation is extremely critical for this lesion.

EVAPORATION OF DIAPHRAGM

There is an abnormal elevation of one or both leaves of the diaphragm, with an upward displacement of the abdominal contents into an out pouching or saclike structures of the diaphragm resulting from a weakness or absence of the diaphragmatic musculature without an abnormal opening. It may be due to congenital maldevelopment of normal diaphragmatic muscular or tendinous structures or acquired abnormality of the phrenic nerve. In congenital eventuation, the diaphragmatic abnormality may be complete or only localized, and is characterized by inadequate or absent masculinization, leaving only a translucent membrane separating the thoracic and abdominal cavities. Many different processes may interfere with phrenic nerve conduction, thereby causing diaphragmatic paralysis or Levant ration. Some causes of phrenic nerve dysfunction are neuritis (infectious, toxic, an allergic) compression of the nerve roots at the level of the cervical spine, CNS disease. Or peripheral phrenic nerve damage due to surgical or other trauma, pressure, or inflammation. Phrenic nerve palsy in the newborn is usually the result of birth trauma, particularly after breech or forceps delivery in such cases phrenic nerve palsy is, associated with ipsilateral Erbs palsy. Phrenic nerve palsy may also be due to surgical trauma, especially during correction of the congenital heart defects. Both congenital and acquired event rations are more common on the left than on the right. Symptoms are due to decreased intrathoracic v lumen (decreased functional residua l capacity) and of inefficient ventilation due to paradoxical movement of the abnormal diaphragm with associated mediastina mobility. Typical clinical findings are tachypnea, cyanosis, sternal retraction, asymmetric chest movements, and sub costal retractions. There may be decreased breath sounds and dullness to percuss ion at the base of the affected lung. Recurrent fevers may result from the bronchopneumonia due to ineffective cough and persistent atelectasis. Most patients with event rationhas no or minimal symptoms after the first 1-2 years., but in the neonatal period and infancy, the above symptoms are more common, and may be associate with recurrent respiratory infections, poor feeding, and EFT. Regular AP and lateral chest X-ray and fluoroscopy establish the diagnosis-complete or partial elevation of the abnormal diaphragm will be evident on regular X-ray chest. The amount of paradoxical diaphragmatic movements and mediastina shift is best evaluated by fluoroscopy. In some cases of congenital eventuation, there may be no paradoxical movement of the diaphragm because of the presence of some muscles in all parts of the diaphragm. Occasionally it may be difficult to distinguish between a partial eventration and a low thoracic mass. Injection of a small amount of nonirritating fluid or air into the peritoneal cavity will help outline the diaphragm. Asymptomatic-eventration needs no treatment. For patients with significant disability, prolonged increased oxygen or ventilator requirement, recurrent lower respiratory tract infections, feeding problems, ETT need diaphragmatic plication. Those with the acquired lesions, such as birth trauma or surgical injury, improve significantly over the first month; and if there is no improvement over 2-4 weeks, plication is indicated. Vigorous chest physiotherapy is administered to all patients with less than-normal diaphragmatic function.

Spontaneous recovery should be awaited before going for surgery in cases of mild lesions. Clinically, COF is the failure of the heart to meet the circulatory and metabolic needs of the body. It is a clinical syndrome in which the heart fails to supply an output sufficient to meet the metabolic requirements of the tissues. The heart is either unable to maintain cardiac output at therequired level or is unable to dispose of adequately the venous return or, more often, a combination of the two. The result is elevated venous and capillary pressure and effort dyspnea, which indicates that the cardiac output can 't be adequately raised to meet the demands of effort. A low cardiac output by stimulating the renin-angiotensin mechanism causes an increased secretion of aldosterone resulting in salt and water retention and an increase in blood volume. Elevated venousand capillary pressures and increased blood volume are responsible for hepatic congestion and transudation of fluid in the subcutaneous tissue.

ETIOLOGY

-CHD, usually with large left-to-right shunts or obstructive lesions of the left or right ventricle. -Acquired disease of the heart, including myocarditis, acute or chronic RHD, and infective endocarditis.
-Arrhythmias including paroxysmal atrial tachycardia, atrial fibrillation, or flutter, or completeheart block
-Iatrogenic causes include damage to the heat at surgery (ventriculostomy), fluid overload, ordoxobian therapy
-Non cardiac causes such as thyrotoxicosis, systemic arteriovenous fistulas, anemia 's, acute or chronic lung disease, glycogen storage disease, or connective tissue or neuromuscular disorders. By far the commonest cause of COF in childhood is CHD in infancy. Cardiac causes include CHD(producing volume overload, obstruction, myocardial impairment), congenital vascular disease (coarctation of the aorta, peripheral arteriovenous shunt), acquired myocardial

disease (myocarditis), arrhythmias, rheumatic fever(rare), Cardiovascular causes are potentially the same in child, but rheumatic fever plays a more important role in children. Non cardiovascular causes may be acidosis, respiratorydisease, CNS disease, anemia, sepsis, or hypoglycemia; these become less important with increasing age especially., acidosis, and hypoglycemia.

CLINICAL FEATURES

These fall into 3 categories.

1. Signs of impaired myocardial function include growth failure, sweating, cardiac enlargementgallop rhythm, alterations in peripheral pulses including pulsus paradoxes and pulsus alternans.
2. Signs of pulmonary congestion include tachypnea, dyspnea with effort, cough, rales wheezing and cyanosis.
3. Signs of systemic venous congestion include hepatomegaly, neck vein distension andperipheral edema
4. In the older child, the signs and symptom of COF are like those in adults, Fatigue, effortintolerance, anorexia, abdominal pain, and cough are frequent, in adaption to breathlessness at rest, the systemic venous pressure is elevated as gauged by clinical assessment of the jugular venous pressure, the liver is enlarged and tender, and edema may be present.

Orthopedic and rales (basal rales) are commonly present, and edema usually occurs in the dependent portions of the body. An older children may prefer to lie in a flat position, which may cause generalized anasarca. Cardiomegaly is invariably present. Auscultator findings are those produced by the basic lesions, but gallop rhythm is common. The 3 cardinal signs of COF are cardiomegaly, tachypnea(right) and hepatomegaly(right). Cardiomegaly represents a homeostatic (compensatory) mechanism thatmaintains the adequate cardiac output by enlarging the capacity of the pump. Up to a point the enlarged heart can deliver a greater stroke volume output, but limits are soon reached (Starlings law of the heart). One should be very cautious about diagnosing COF in absence of cardiomegaly (One exception is total anomalous venous return below the diaphragm, which will for a short time be characterized by other signs of COF without an enlarge heart). Cardiomegaly without other signs of COF may be taken as early or compensated heart failure. Tachypnea is a cardinal signs of left sided heart failure, and it may be present for a short time before hepatomegaly occurs.

Pure left or right sided failure does not commonly exist independently for long. Hepatomegaly isthe cardinal sign of right sided heart failure. The liver is capable of trapping relatively large amounts of edema fluid in the infant that would be more evident as peripheral edema in the olderchild and adult. It is therefore common in the infant in moderately severe heart failure to have anenlarged liver with no perennial or even presacral or facial edema. Peripheral edema is found in infants only in the most severe cases of CCF. Additional features of COF are feeding difficulties,dyspnea, restlessness, easy fatigability, weak pulses, pallor, rales, peripheral edema, weight gain from fluid accumulation, tachycardia, sweating, pneumonia, orthopnea, and growth failure.

During infancy, the presence of COF may be more difficult to determine Symptoms. are dominated by tachypnea, feeding difficulties, poor weight gain, excessive perspiration, irritability, weak cry, and noisy, labored respiratory with costal and subcostal retractions. Flaringof the alae nasi and sternal retractions are frequent. Signs of pulmonary congestion and those ofbronchospasm are indistinguishable. Pneumonitis with or without collapse of part of the lung is common. Dyspnea and hepatomegaly and cardiomegaly are always present. DITEpronounced tachycardia, gallop rhythm can be recognized frequently The other auscultatory signed are those of the basic cardiac lesion. A sudden increase in weight that decreases after diuretic therapy is common. Owing to the shortness of the neck, estimates of jugular venous pressure in infant may be difficult (also difficulty of securing a relaxed state), but should be attempted. Edema in infants with COF is frequently not detectable clinically, but when present may be generalized involving the eyelids as well as the sacrum, legs, and feet.

Right sided failure is identified by the presence of tachycardia, tachypnea, hepatomegaly, cardiomegaly; the presence of all the 4 features is present to establish the diagnosis. Visible signsof water retention and engorged neck veins are not always seen in infants and children.

The left sided failure in infants and children is recognized by the presence of dyspnea on exertion, or orthopnea, wheezing, or chronic hacking cough, tachycardia, and cardiomegaly all being manifestations of pulmonary venous hypertension. The classic picture of COF in childrenis one of the Right sided or combined R and L sided failure; isolated left failure is rare.

In the neonate, the COF may be from many causes; PDA in premature infants is the most common cause of COF in the neonate period. Other causes of failure are hypo plastic left heartsyndrome, complex CHD, myocarditis, A-V fistulas in the brain and liver, and idiopathic paroxysmal tachycardia. Common signs of COF in neonate are tachycardia, tachypnea, hepatomegaly, cardiomegaly, and diaphoresis. The diagnostic procedures used in these cases are arterial blood gas analysis, chest x-rays, ECG,echocardiography, radionuclide angiography and cardiac catheterization.

MANAGEMENT IN CCF

The underlying cause of cardiac failure must be removed if possible or alluvia ted if the cause isa congenital cardiovascular anomaly, medical treatment must precede surgical treatment, and should be extended to postoperative period. For some diseases as hyperthyroidism, hypothyroidism, anemia and beriberi, specific therapy is available, but in most cease only general measures can be adapted.

Bed rest in a comfortable position is essential; some patients prefer to lie flat, but for most breathing is easier in the semi reclining position. Even babies feel more comfortable in a propped-up position, and sometimes it may be all that is needed to quite an irritable infant. The compensated and mildly distressed patient requires rest only, whereas the severely distressed and anxious patient requires sedation to produce complete relaxation;0.1 mg/kg of morphine is used, which is sedative as well as analgesic and is useful for acute pulmonary edema also but should be given only with good airway control. Other drugs used for sedating a fretful, anxious, agitatedchild with or irritable infant may be codeine, barbiturates, chloral hydrate. Morphine is given sc in the patient with left and right failure with wheezing in the chest indicating cardiac asthma.

Oxygen, administered by any method will relieve dyspnea and will raise the systemic PaO2 in patients with CCF, overcoming the capillary alveolar block of pulmonary edema and alleviating the hypoxemic contribution to CCF. Oxygen will not make a patient with cyanotic heart disease pink. If the baby is very uncomfortable in the 02 tent or only dry oxygen through a nasal catheter can begiven, then one should not force the issue. Cool moist oxygen via a tent, mask or nasal prongs isideal A sitting or s3mirecumbent position may be achieved in infants using a cardiac chair.

Diet It is generally held that a low sodium diet is efficacious in the treatment of cardiac edema and paroxysmal cardiac dyspnea. The oral intake of sodium is reduced to 0.5g/d; patients receives a high calorie, low volume, low sodium diet, while as. The diet is made more palatable by adding a salt substitute. Formulas are available with specially reduced sodium content for infants, but many hold that there is no place for sodium restricted- free formulas in the treatment of

COF in infants, since some such formulas have a sodium content equivalent to that in human milk, and half that of cow 's milk. Most cases of the low-salt COF are mostly due to overly vigorous Balt restriction and vigorous diuretic therapy. Salt foods as potato chips and bacon should be avoided, but ordinary cooking with normal amount of salt is allowed. Since the patient may be undernourished due to chronic poorly compensated heart failure, food should be made palatable to be it attractive to the child. Salt restriction is therefore necessary is infants.

Fluids are moderately restricted to 50-90 mg/kg/d. If salt is restricted, stringent fluid restriction may not be necessary. But in general; IV fluid should low in salt or salt free. Diuretics are used ifdigitalis alone is not adequate in achieving satisfactory compensation. These relieve edema and pulmonary congestion of heart failure. Usually for rapid inpatient diuresis, furosemide is used while as for maintenance therapy thiazide or furosemide may be given with spironolactone.
Effective ness of a diuretic is dependent on renal perfusion, and electrolyte and acid base balance. Diuretics may cause profound changes in electrolyte composition, and frequent electrolyte evaluations must be made. In the presence of shock or acute renal failure, they will have little effect; Potassium depletion especially. in the digitalized patient is dangerous and may be lethal. Itis better not to use them routinely and should be reserved for emergency cases that don 't respondsto digitalis, sodium restriction and bed rest only.

Mercurial diuretics are not used now. (can be given only parentally, toxicity is very low, absolutecontraindications being azotemia and advanced liver disease Dose in neonate 0.1-0.25 ml, and after first month,0.2-0.5 ml).

Furosemide and ethacrynic acid, both are extremely potent

diuretics. They differ structurally but have similar diuretic effects. Because of the massive diuresis they produce, they should be used rarely in the previously untreated child unless careful observation of electrolytes. especially. serum K and blood volume is possible Both inhibit reabsorption in the ascending loop of Henley of sodium, thereby increasing renal excretion of Na and Cl and an accompanying volume of water. These interfere with sodium transport and diluting mechanism, also a redistribution of blood intothe venous pool precedes. The diuresis of furosemide. Both can be given orally as well as parentally with parenteral therapy, the onset of action is rapid, 5 min (furosemide) to 15 min (Ethacrynic acid), but is short-lived, lasting for 2-3 hours only. The usual parenteral, IV or IM, is 1 mg /kg, though in resistant cases up to 3mg/kg have been used. A single dose daily should be given, and not repeated more than once a day Furosemide is more convenient since it can be given both IV and IM, while as ethacrynic acid must be used IV only. It is important to measure serum electrolytes during therapy since hypokalemia or hypochloremia alkalosis can be inducedwith these drugs. Since induced hypokalemia exaggerates the digitalis toxicity, supplementation with K is advisable. The efficacy of therapy is judged by measuring the urinary volume and by comparison of daily body weights. When a constant weight is reached it should be maintained. A decrease in venous ails toxicity, supplementation with K is advisable. The efficacy of therapy is judged by measuring the urinary volume and by comparison of daily body weights, when a constant weight is reached it should be maintained. A decrease in venous pressure and hepatic size with improvement of dyspnea and signs of edema parallels the diagnosed - diuresis. Once cardiac failure is compensated, these can be given orally-both are well absorbed orally. Given orally action starts within 30min (ethacrynic acid) to 60(furosemide), reaching a peak in 1-2 hours.,but lasting for 6-8 hours. Usual oral dose is again 1mg/kg once or twice daily. But in exceptional circumstances, 2-3 mg/kg may be used. Both are potent and clinical toxicity will be manifested by hypovolemic or hypokalemia. Both competitively inhibit urate secretion in the PCT causing hyperuricemia, and in susceptible persons gout Transient and even permanent deafness has been reported especially. with ethacrynic acid, possibly due to electrolyte changes in the end lymph, They candehydrate the pt. Both are bound to plasma proteins and mostly excreted via the kidney.

Thiazide is moderately potent diuretics. Since they can be given orally, they are mostly used for long-term management of COF in infants and children. They inhibit resorption of Na and cl in the ascending loop of Henle, and thus facilitate sodium excretion and an accompanied water excretion. They are rapidly absorbed from the gut begin to have diuretic effect within 1 the peak of effect reached at 4 hours and duration of action of chlorothiazide is for 6-12 hours and that of hydrochlorothiazide 12 hours or more. They are excreted by kidney with some subsequent resorption. The dose is 20-40mg/kg/d for chlorothiazide, while as it is 2-5 mg/kg/d for hydrochlorothiazide for these are given with spironolactone daily. They are contraindicated in anuria or progressive renal insufficiency. Potassium depletion occurs with long term use especially withchlorothiazide (therefore potassium should be given with chlorothiazide), they should not be given for pro longed periods, except when used spironolactone. Serum electrolytes should be monitored routinely. Alternate day therapy intake of food high in potassium, administration of liquid K, or addition of K-sparing diuretic as pironolactone or triamterene may protect against K-depletion. However, periodic measurements of serum K are essential especially early in therapy.

Allergic reactions especially after hydrochlorothiazide as thrombocytopenia, leukopenia or vacuities arerarely seen. Hyperglycemia and aggravation of preexisting diabetes mellitus or hyperuricemia may occur.

Spironolactone is a weak diuretic by itself but may be useful

as an addition to the other diuretic drugs, both because of its different site of action and its potassium sparing action. It is useful supplementary diuretic in patients with resistant peripheral edema. It is structurally like but antagonist to aldosterone and is competitive inhibitor of the mineralocorticoids that normally stimulates Na absorption and K excretion in the DCT. It blocks the aldosterone exchange of K for Na. It is absorbed orally, but diuretic effect may not be manifested for 2-3 days and may persistfor 2-3 days after cessation of therapy. The dose is 1-3 mg/kg orally in 2 divided doses.
Spironolactone is contraindicated in renal insufficiency; the major complication is hyperkalemia,resulting from inhibition of K-secretions with normal or increased K intake. Therefore, serum K must be monitored carefully. In chronic toxicity studies it has been found to be oncogenic. Acetazolamide, a carbonic anhydrase inhibitor, starts acting within 1 hr and can last up to 24 hours; its dose is 5mg/kg/d. Itmay cause drowsiness anesthesia.

Digitalis is the keystone of the treatment in CCF. It should be used in all forms of cardiac failure. The most satisfactory Response is obtained in failure due to rheumatic heart disease, paroxysmal tachycardia, and myocardial diseases. In general, patients with primary left ventricular failure responds better than those with primary right ventricular failure. The Response of the patients with COF from cyanotic congenital heart disease is unpredictable since hypoxia, acidosis, and hypoglycemia may complicate the picture. It improves cardiac function by increasing myocardial contractibility, which in turn increases cardiac output by reducing venous pressure, relieving venous congestion, and slowing the heart rate, increasing the diastolic phase of the cardiac cycle, during which coronary arteries are perfused. The major effect sought in improvement is that in myocardial performance (inotropic effect), by which the force of contraction is increased, thereby increasing the stroke volume. Many preparations are there; digitalis and digoxin are mostly used for slow digitalization and maintenance, while lanatoside C is for rapid digitalization. The dose of digitalis and the rapidity of administration depend on the weight of the pt, the severity of CCF, the type of preparation, and, later on, the Response of the pt. Digoxin is a universally used drug in pediatric practice since it is available in liquid form and can be used orally as well as parentally, in emergencies as well as in chronic situations; it can be given IV, IM, or orally as per the clinical urgency. The elixir contains 0.05mg/ml and tablet 0.2 5mg. The maximum effect occurs within 4 hours of administration, 70-90% of the drug is absorbed orally, the half-life is 2-3 days, and about 1/3 of the drug is excreted daily, which implies that a steady state will be achieved if this small amount is replaced. For routine digitalization, 1/4 of the DD is given 6 hourlies for 4 doses. For rapid digitalization, ż of the DD is given IV or IM and then repeated in 4-6 hours. For very rapid digitalization, full DD is given iv with very close monitoring.

For maintenance, 1/3-1/4 of the DD is given in 2 equally divided doses, morning, and evening. The total DD dose is for newborn and premature, 0.03-0.05mg/kg, with an MD of 1/5-1/10 of DD for infants beyond the neonatal period, 0.006-0.08mg, MD being 1/3-1/5 of DD(if the parenteral route is involved, DD is 0.04-0.06mg, and parenteral MD will be 1/5-1/10DD) for children beyond 2 years, DD is 0.04-0.06mg, daily MD being 1/3-1/5 of this. If a parenteral route is involved, 0.02.-0.0478,). Some estimate it on the body area, for neonates and premature, 0.75mg/sq meter of the body surface, and 1.5mgfor older infants and children. (Total DD should not exceed 2.5mg in the pediatric age group). MD is started 12 hours after the last. DD. (Lanatoside C is used for rapid iv digitalization and should be reserved for emergencies only. It begins to act within 3-15 minutes after administration, and the maximum effect is reached within 1 hr; it is excreted within 24-36 hours. (DD is 0.325-0.75mg/sqm). Neonates (full-term or premature) have distinct intolerance for digitalis preparations. Digitalization should be controlled by repeated physical examinations supplemented by ECG (In some infants, the only dependable guide to toxicity is ECG evidence of arrhythmia). The maximum effective dose is close to the toxic dose. But to get maximum effect maximum tolerable dose should be given on an individual basis without causing signs and symptoms of toxicity. IN outpatient, digitalization is affected by giving MD in 2 divided morning and evening doses, and in less than a week, adequate digitalization is obtained. Digitalization is effective if dyspnea, cough is lessened, there is a sense of bitterness and better appetite (symptoms), there is slowing of the heart and respeciallyirate t towards more physiological levels, venous pressure and liver size is decreased, ECG signs are shortening, systole, depression of ST segment, with T Wave inversion, and lengthening of the PR interval. Mechanisms of action: Inotropic effect -interferes with the ATPase involved in the Na pump that removes. Na from the myocardial cell. The accumulation of Na at the inner surface of the cell membrane allows for an increased influx of calcium into the filament, thus potentiating myocardial contractibility. Antiarrhythmic affect cholinergic effects of digitalis slow the sinus rate prolong the AV node refractory time and slow AV conduction. Additionally, digitalis results in hyperpolarization of atrial conducting cells and decrease the slope of phase 4 depolarization, thus slowing or suppressing atrial ectopic impulse formation Digitalization prolongs the PR interval, shortens the QT intervals, and decreases the ST segment.

DIGITALIS TOXICITY:

Early symptoms are nausea and vomiting, anorexia, diarrhea, and abdominal pain. Occasional vomiting and spitting are quite common in healthy infants also and I presence of

vomiting and nausea overall clinical picture helps.
*Any rhythm disturbance should alert to the possibility of digitalis. Toxicity, and should be taken to be due to digitalis unless proved otherwise. Occasionalextra systoles are seen often in severe cases of CCF, but presence of multiple extra systoles, pulses big minus, coupled beat sand various degrees of AV block is usually due to digitalis toxicity. In children supraventricular and in adolescent ventricular arrhythmia is common. The arrhythmias include a trial and ventricular extra systole, paroxysmal atrial tachycardia, with block, atrial flutter or fibrillation, bundle branch block, ventricular tachycardia, and intra-arterialblock.
*Slowing of heart rate below 100 in infants, below 80 in young children and below 80 in olderchildren is often taken as a guide to reducing the dosage of digoxin.
*ECG signs of toxicity will be prolonged PR interval, second degree heart block with, changing PR interval (Wenckebach phenomenon), coupled beats, rarely paroxysmal atrial tachycardia withblock; sinus node depression and AV conduction disturbances are due to vagal actions.
*Age specific serum levels suggestive of toxicity during maintenance therapy a newborn more than 4ng/ml, up to 1 yr over 3ng/ml, after 1 yr, over 2 ng/ml. Neurological and visual disturbances are rare in children. Predisposing factors that lead to toxicity should include electrolyte disturbances especially hypokalemia caused by administration of potent diuresis, alkalosis,hypoxia, and renal suppression, especially during the postoperative period. An adequate Intake shouldbe maintained in the form of fruits as oranges and bananas or K salts in a palatable form. Digitalis poisoning is an acute emergency that must be treated without delay. Stomach should be emptied, and then attention can be paid to maintaining an adequate cardiac rate and output, and to controlling arrhythmia.. A useful basic solution is 10% dextrose in water, to which3 mEq of KCl/kg/d and 20mnitis of regular insulin/1000 ml. Administration of KCl may correct digitalis induced arrhythmia} but is contraindicated in

presence of high grade AV block. To thissolution may be added isoproterenol (0.1 microgram/kg/min.) titrated to maintain adequate heartrate and output in the face of complete heart block. Phenytoin 300-600mg/d) has been used as a specific antiarrhythmic drug specific for digitalis induced. It is given IV beginning with 1mg/kg followed by doubling doses every 5-10 minutes to a maximum total dose of 5mg/kg. Electrolytesare checked. Lidocaine or propranolol is also used as antiarrhythmic. If medical treatment fails, temporary trans venous pacemaker may be needed for high grade AV block. Cardioversion is used as a last resort since it may exacerbate rather than halt and occasionally induces ventricularfibrillation. Infusion of isoproterenol or more recently dopamine (5-10 microgram/kg/min) may be used in those who fail to respond to other methods. Their use is not without risks and may be helpful in carefully selected patients preliminary to emergency surgery. Thus, in the treatment of COF the steps in management include, general treatment increasing efficiency of the heart by digoxin or isoproterenol etc., reducing work of the heart by bed rest, diet, restriction of fluids and diuretics and fir ally afterload reduction. Corticosteroids produce water retention but are Sometimes used in patients whose diuretic resistant cardiac failure is due to inflammation disease e.g., rheumatic carditis. Cardiac failure that is resistant to therapy or breakdown of Response to previously successful management may be due to infection (as reactivation of Rh fever superimposed sub-acute bacterial endocarditis or intercurrent pulmonary or urinary tract infection), electrolyte imbalance (hypokalemia, hypochloremia alkalosis hypernatremia), development of arrhythmia as atrial fibrillation with rapid ventricular Response , or pulmonary embolism (rare in children). In renal disease in children, decreased excretion of digitalis may occur, the fore MD is calculated as = % of digoxin excreted (replaced).

KERATINIZE CLEARANCE

In neonates, the treatment is again diverted to decreasing workload of the heart. Digoxin is againthe mainstay of the treatment, but recent work suggests that digoxin may be of little help to the very immature preterm infant with COF secondary to PDS. Other measures are diuretics, fluid restriction, use of a low solute formula or breast milk, maintenance of the neutral thermal environment, decreasing the work of the feeding by giving gavage rather than the nipple, maintenance of adequate oxygenation of the myocardium is sought by maintaining in
Cardio tonic drugs as digitalis and isoproterenol are the cornerstone of the treatment. Dopaminehas been used in the newborn for the treatment of severe hypotension. It has also been used to reverse the hypotensive effect of tolazoline when it is used for the treatment of persistent fetal circulation.

EMERGENCY TREATMENT

The acute emergencies of COF are usually related to fluid retention with pulmonary edema and low cardiac output. These include -morphine used for acute palm edema., 0.1mg/kg iv or sc. - diuretics, furosemide or ethacrynic acid may be given iv as an initial dosage of 1 mg/kg to produce a rapid diuresis. -positive pressure breathing pulmonary edema may sometimes be managed by intubation or mask with bag breathing or a respirator to raise the alveolar pressure above pulmonary capillary pressure. -peritoneal dialysis; there are 3 specific instances where peritoneal dialysis 1 with a hypertonic solution may be indicated'; when fluid retention, especially pulmonary edema, is life-threatening, and furosemide diuresis fails in low-salt COF when both the fluid retention and the electrolyte imbalance require correction in t the early postop care of an infant who may have an element of transient renal failure with both fluid retention and hyperkalemia Hypertonic peritoneal dialysis within minutes draws fluid into the peritoneal cavitywhere it is subject to immediate removal, while simultaneously correcting the electrolyte imbalance whether it is sodium-Hoch or potassium-high or both. - Afterload reduction: It is used in patients without intracardiac shunts, who fail to respond to digitalis and diuresis. It is a new form of therapy for pump-failure by reduction in systemic vascular resistance with an intravenous vasodilator. The procedure has been mostly used in postop patients with reduced cardiac output and peripheral vasoconstriction. Vasodilators drugs by reducing ventricular filling pressure and decreasing peripheral resistance may improve cardiac output. It is used only in a setting where central venous pressure, arterial pressure, cardiac output etc. can be monitored.

Sodium nitroprusside (0.5-1 mEq/kg iv) has b been used. If the drug is measured used for anextended period, thiocyanate level should be measured. For chronic treatment isosorbide denigrate (0.25-1mg/4-8 hourly or hydralazine 0.75-3mg/kg/d have been used.

In seriously ill small infants, it is not sometimes possible to rule out the presence of concurrentchest infection and therefore broad-spectrum antibiotics or penicillin-streptomycin should be used from the very beginning.

Part III: MYOCARDIAL DISEASES

Myocarditis(inflammation of ventricular myocardium.) may be due to infection, mesenchyme diseases, endocrine disorders, metabolic and nutritional diseases, neuromuscular diseases, blood diseases, tumors, hypertension, and congenital anomalies: The status of myocardium is the factor which most affects the prognosis of cardiac disease; ditecongenital cardiac malformations, 1€ acquired valvular disease, or arrhythmias if the myocardium is able to provide satisfactory circulation of blood, the child will be able to maintain adequate nutrition, growth and activity.
Inflammations of ventricular myocardium of nonthematic origin may be -which occurs during generalized infection as that occurs as a part of diphtheria and enteric fever, and in cases of viral infections, as mumps, measles. Small box and infectious mononucleosis... Here myocarditis is a complication of the primary infection Myocarditis complicating measles.
Chickenpox and mumps are rare. In poliomyelitis, hypertension is not uncommon but cardiac failure is rare. Terminal pulmonary failure may occur ECG abnormalities are not common. Severe myocarditis has been identified with coxsackie virus. B. Circulatory involvement in bacterial diseases is manifest by as peripheral circulatory collapse or toxic myocarditis. Toxic myocarditis as evidenced by tachycardia, gallop rhythm, and cardiac enlargement may complicate pneumonia, bacterial endocarditis, and septicemia. Lesions in the myocardium. Haveoccurred in association with histoplasmosis, coccidioidomycosis, toxoplasmosis, and trichiniasis. But in these conditions cardiac Lesion rarely produces clinical symptoms. Actinomycosis may involve the pericardium and myocardium by direct contiguity as from a pulmonary: ovary abscess. Hydrated cysts of the pericardium may be found on routine X-ray chest, producing symptoms only when it ruptures. Schistosomiasis may produce pulmonary

hypertension and corPulmonarynale Cruz: trypanosomiasis may produce acute or sub-acute myocarditis and sudden death. -Which occurs as an offshoot of the noninfectious disease process, as beriberi. In patients with malnutrition the deficiencies are often multiple. -The most important group is where myocarditis dominates the clinical picture, and there is no other recognizable disease, as myocarditis in neonate and infection due to various strains of CoxsackieB virus.

CLINICAL FEATURES OF MYOCARDITID

Essential features of myocarditis are -presence of muffled heart sounds and tachycardia out of proportion to fever, gallop: rhythm (which is an exaggeration of the normally audible. 3rd heart sound d), absence of any significant murmur, conduction defects recognized as rhythm disturbances clinically; evidence of cardiomegaly, due to ventricular dilatation recognized clinically or radio logically ECG is very valuable in diagnosis and may show one or more of lackof ventricular hypertrophy, presence of conduction defects, low voltage complexes use, and ST Twave changes.

Symptoms of early heart failure from acute myocarditis, in the infant or child can be very subtleand are likely to be easily overlooked until obvious signs of heart failure develop. Myocardial diseases are characterized generally by cardiac enlargement; murmurs may or maynot be present, ECG changes including left ventricular hypertrophy, ST depression, and T Wave: inversion.

MYOCARDITIS IN NEWBORN INFANCY

Presumed to be passed trans placentally. The mother may be having coryza, sneezing and malaise shortly before delivery. The virus may be recovered by virus cultures from nasopharynx, and rectal swabs, CSF, umbilical cord stump, or by tissue culture at biopsy. However, Coxsackie disease is a generalized infection, myocardium bears: the main brunt of the infection. Clinical picture of myocarditis is severe same as in other groups, the pericardium may occasionally be involved, and maybe I associated with peripheral effusion. Many series of fatal myocarditis in the neonate due to coxsackie have been reported; ininfants this is the principal cause of myocarditis and epidemics have been reported from various parts of the world.

MYOCARDITIS IN BERIBERI

In infant 's enlargement of the heart and liver is found as part of the general picture of the acute infantile beriberi. In older child, the symptoms are all related to heart and often the clinical picture of acute cardiac failure develops within a few days. There may be anasarca with edema invarious parts of the body the child becomes drowsy, dyspnea and walks with a very slow waddling or stamping gait. In the first stage of the rapidly developing edema, there is low diastolic and normal systolic pressure. The cardiac output increases and the circular
edematous with hypertrophic regenerations of myocardium. The systolic pressured drops, the pulse becomes feeble, the lungs are congested, and death results quickly, with symptoms of leftventricular failure.

Even with suspicion, treatment should be started immediately. B1,100mg.im daily for the first few days, followed by 50mg, im, daily for a fortnight. In a fulminant case, the use of B1 may notbe quick enough, since the return to normal lactic-pyruvic acid metabolism takes time, and vasopressor drugs as nor-adrenaline and partisan or pituitary may be lifesaving. Other supportive therapy as oxygen, low salt diet, and digitalis is useful.

DIPHTHERITIC MYOCARDITIS

All types of diphtheria including cutaneous form can lead to this complication. Diphtheria toxinmay lead to peripheral circulatory failure or as toxic myocarditis. Toxic myocarditis is characterized by the development of arrhythmia in the form of partial or complete heart block, bundle branch block or extra systoles. Late findings include development of CCT, which may occur during convalesce and is associated with cardiac enlargement and gallop rhythm In- addition The onset of heart failure may be suggested by pallor, breathlessness, precordial oppression and vomiting. In addition to arrhythmia there may be sinus tachycardia, and ECG showing depression of ST segment, or I wave inversion is most leads is suggestive of myocarditis. Otherwise, the pit may present with peripheral circulatory failure occurring within first 2 weeks of the disease, associated with thread pulse, cold clammy pale skin, and hypotension. Such early collapse has very bad prognosis. The toxin may cause degeneration and necrosis of the myocardium. The fibers lose their striation and present a swollen granular appearance. The lesions are patchy, and only short segments of individual muscle fibers, may be affected. Cardiac complications occur in the first or 2nd week, and immediate prognosis is grave, about 50% dying. Treatment includes strict bed rest until all signs of myocarditis have disappeared. Digitalis is reserved for patients with frank CCF. Prednisone or prednisolone 40 mg/d in 4 doses with luminal, may save some children, especially with frank CCF. Patients are treated as cardiogenic shock when in peripheral circulatory failure.

TYPHOID FEVER

Toxic myocarditis may be inferred if there is ECG evidence of T wave inversion in most leads.This sign may be transient and by itself is not clinically significant. Both cardiac failure and peripheral circulatory failure are rare.

Acute Glomerulonephritis

Myocardial involvement is evidenced by CCF, cardiac enlargement, gallop rhythm, an apical systolic murmur, and ECG abnormalities. Cardiac failure is evidenced by dyspnea, and pulmonary congestion, which are soon followed by increased venous pressure and hepatomegaly. Cardiac failure contributes to edema in acute nephrite while as hypervolemia contributes to cardiac failure. In this patients X-ray evidence of pulmonary edema is common. The ECG is frequently normal, but there may be Twar inversion, prolonged electrical systole, or signs of left ventricular hypertrophy. In addition to usual treatment of AGN digitalization is indicated in cardiac failure. The Response is good, and digitalis can be discontinued after a weekor two Endocrinal disorders Hyperthyroidism produces tachycardia, vasodilatation, wide pulse pressure, cardiac enlargement, and rarely atrial fibrillation. Cretinism seldom produces gross cardi: involvement, but ECG shows bradycardia, low voltage of all complexes (especially of PandT Waves), left axis deviation, and prolonged electrical systole. These signs disappear within a month of adequate thyroid therapy.

NEUROMUSCULAR DISEASES

In most patients of Frederic 's ataxia, cardiac symptoms are masked by the basic disease, but in some heart failure, effort intolerance, and chest pain have been presenting symptoms, due to myocardial disease which affects chiefly the left ventricle and results in congestive or obstructive cardiomyopathy ECG shows generalized T Wave inversion or signs of left ventricular hypertrophy. Arrhythmias atrial tachycardia, or fibrillation, or extra systoles X-ray chest shows. varying degree of cardiomyopathy (cardiomegaly, left ventricular prominence and pulmonary congestion). In progressive muscular dystrophy, 50% of children have myocardial involvement to the similarity of the striated muscle. Cardiac symptoms are not common, but ECG may show tachycardia, abnormal P wave, short PR interval, and abnormal QandT waves. Minimal evidence ofright or left ventricular hypertrophy may also occur and some patients have CCF.

BLOOD DISEASES

In infants and children, anemia is the most common blood disease associated with cardiac involvement, as in leukemia, hemolytic anemia, severe iron deficiency and hemorrhage. Though cardiac output increases when the Hemoglobin is below 76%, in infants, cardiac enlargement with or without COF occurs only with an extreme reduction in Hemoglobin to 3-4.8 or less. The heart rate is rapid, the pulse pressure sis widened, and the venous pressure is increased. An apical or left sternal border systolic murmur is usual, diastolic murmurs may occur in the same areas, and gallop rhythm is common. The ECG changes include depressed ST segments and flat T waves.Occasionally minimal signs and symptoms are present when extreme states: of anemia have developed gradually Treatment is directed towards the cause of I anemia: if blood transfusionsare needed in the presence of cardiac failure or cardiomegaly, small volumes, 4-5ml/kg of packed cells are preferred. Venous pressure measurements during transfusion can be used as guides to the rate of and volume of transfusion.

ENDOCARDIAL FIBROELASTOSIS

This is a common type of primary myocardial disease in which there is depiction and proliferation of fibroblastic tissue in the endocardium and sute endocardium. Etiology is uncertain, but it is a congenital anomaly; there are many theories: intrauterine infection with mumps or coxsackievirus: Inflammation before or after birth, mal development, and inadequate blood supply to the endocardium; others. Believe that it is due to primary changes in myocardium which results in cardiac dilatation, subjecting the endocardium to greater stretch, which initiates fibroblastic proliferation in the endocardium there is some dispute whether the disease is primary or secondary to cardiac dilatation produced by cardiomyopathy. The disease occurs sporadically and is seen in siblings. Pathology. There is a marked milky (white opaque) fibro elastic thickening of the endocardium, especially of the left side of the heart, the subendocardial layers of the left ventricle, and usually the left atrium; the process may spread to involve the valves especially mitral and aortic. Fibro elastic(sclerotic)layer obscures the trabeculation of the inner surfaces of the cardiac chamber. The myocardial fibers themselves are fibrotic and disorganizedthere is associated hyper vascularization.

Serial sections indicate that myocarditis is also present. Left ventricle shows the most marked changes. Other birth CVS anomalies may be present. Microscopy of the lesion shows that there is fibro elastic thickening of the endocardium which follows the course of the trabecular sinusoids and may result in subendocardial degeneration of necrosis of muscle with vacillation ofmuscle fibers. The involved valves, show a myxomatous proliferation of cells with an increase in collagenous elements.

CLINICAL PICTURE

Most are normal at birth, growth and development at-birth being normal for some months after birth, but most of them develop irritability anorexia, tachypnea, pallor, increased sweating, and other signs of left sided heart failure (dyspnea, easy fatigability, feeding difficulties, and eventually right and left failure. The classical signs of heart failure are present majority of the children are small and undernourished; there

is cardiomegaly, with the point of maximum impulse displaced laterally and downwards. The first and the 2nd heart sounds are normal, but wide splitting of 2nd sound may be heard. A loud 3rd hearts sound may be heard. A systolic murmur of mitral insufficiency may be heard. About 1/4 of the patients have a grade I or II blowing systolic murmur down the left sternal border, but murmurs are not significant. During episodes of COF (precipitated by reinfections often), the infant is acutely ill with dyspnea, cough; cyanosismay be found in the terminal phase or shows associated congenital heart defects. The JVP is raised, the liver is greatly enlarged, edema of the limbs, sacral area or face may be present. Rules and the rhonchi are due to pulmonary infection and congestion. The enlarged heart is of an indistinctive contour. There are 3 groups of pts; 1-young infants, usually less than 6 months, whoare in apparent health until, precipitated suddenly by a Respiratory infection, the child present with sudden onset of CCF. If Response to therapy for COF is not good, prognosis is poor.2-Infants with similar symptoms but of milder degree and with periods of re mission, but within the first 2 years they may manifest dyspnea, refusal of feeding, FIT, and recurrent pulmonary infections.
There are repeated episodes of COF which in some may be controlled by digitalis, and diuretics.3-A miscellaneous group in whom valvular lesions or associated congenital cvs defects are predominant. Most of the cases belong to group 1 and 2.

X-RAY:

Chest X-ray shows generalized cardiac enlargement with or without associated with pulmonary venous, congestion. All chambers of heart are involved. The enlarged heart is of an indistinctive contour There may be signs of intercurrent pulmonary inflation TCG is usually abnormal but not pathognomonic. Dominance of left ventricle shown by tall R waves and inversion of Twaves over the ventricular surface with inversion of the T waves in the standardlead's depression of ST segment, I These ECG changes are also seen in primary myocardial disease, gargoylism, glycogen storage diseases of the heart, aberrant origin of the left coronaryartery from the pulmonary artery and medial necrosis of or calcinosis of the coronary arteries.Cardiac catheterization reveals the absence of L to R shunts, and in addition it shows high ventricular(left) end-diastolic pressure and elevated pulmonary wedge, and left atrial pressure,and may show raised pulmonary pressure. Angiocardiography confirms the diminished myocardial contractility, the enlarged left atrium, and left ventricle if mitral insufficiency develops, this will be defined by left ventricular angiocardiography.

TREATMENT

Early and vigorous, treatment of cardiac failure is essential. There should be adequate and prolonged digitalis therapy, with continuous furosemide and Spironolactone. If the Response is not good, the dose of both digitalis and diuretic should be increased till there is Response or toxicity. Antibiotics are given for associated Respiratory infection. The prognosis is most favorable in infants 6 months to 3 years of age who respond promptly to the treatment Surviving patients remain well but may have residual signs of cardiomyopathy. In others all the abnormal signs vanish, when it is difficult to say whether it was myocarditis or end fibro elastic The mortality rate is 25-30%, others, becoming cured or chronic. Some cases improve clinically initially, but then develops recurrent bouts of heart failure. Complete recovery in such patients is very infrequent and most eventually die with intractable CCF.

GLYCOGEN STORAGE DISEASES OF THE HEART

The type that primarily involves heart is. Pompes disease

(type II glycogenesis) In this there is a complete absence of 1,4-glucosidase activity at pH 4, this enzyme-acid maltase-is necessary forthe hydrolysis of the outer branches of glycogen, and its absence results in marked deposition of glycogen within the myocardium. It is a rare autosomal disease... Affected infants are usually normal at birth, but onset usually begins by the 6th month, with marked cardiac enlargement, very large tongue causing feeding problem, and marked generalized muscular weakness; the liver is not enlarged unless there is CCF-these children have a h/o retardation of growth and development, feeding problems, poor weight gain and then CCF.

Physical examination reveals the generalized muscular weakness, a large tongue, cardiomegaly, nosignificant murmur, and evidence of CCF. Chest X-ray shows marked cardiomegaly with or without pulmonary venous congestion ECG shows left ventricular hypertrophy and ST depression and T Wave inversion over the left precordial leads Echocardiography shows extremely thick ventricular wall structures. These patients usually die within the first year of life;death may be sudden or progressive due to progressive CCF.

CORONARY DISEASE IN CHILDREN

The etiology of the disease, which is rare, is in the origin of coronary arteries. In most cases there is anomalous origin of the left coronary artery from pulmonary artery while as only one right coronary artery arises from the aorta while as the left coronary artery arises from the base of the pulmonary artery. Variable number of anastomotic channels between the 2 coronary arteries determines the clinical course and basis for the two types, infantile and adult Type. After arising from the wrong vessel, it assumes a normal distribution (In the neonatal period, while the pulmonary arterial pressure is high, blood is supplied to the left ventricle from the pulmonary artery. Therefore, the patient is normal during the neonatal period, but by the 2 months of age pulmonary arterial pressure starts to decrease towards normal. This results in a marked decrease of flow to the left coronary artery, which leads to infraction of heart. If the patient survives, collateral channels start developing that join the peripheral branches of the right with the branches of the left coronary artery. Since the flow previously was from the pulmonary artery to myocardium through the left coronary, now flow. Occurs from the right coronary artery through the collaterals to the left coronary artery and then into the pulmonary artery. In essence an arteriovenous fistula is formedthat further removes blood from the myocardium, which results in further myocardial infarction and fibrosis. Since the myocardium is deprived even of that blood which it got from the normal right coronary artery, symptoms of coronary insufficiency, angina and myocardial infarction occur. Therefore, the symptoms are not related to the perfusion of myocardium by the deoxygenated blood but due to the AV fistula reducing blood perfusion of the left myocardium, from reversal of flow, the left ventricle becomes dilated and hypertrophied, with patchy fibrosis, and microscopic deposition of calcium. Complicating mitral incompetence is frequent, due to papillary muscle infection. Localized aneurysms may develop the left ventricle.

CLINICAL FEATURES

Most patients are normal at birth, and most symptoms appear within the first 6 months of life (Usually in the first yr = infantile type), present with tachypnea, dyspnea, wheezing, cough, feeding difficulties (all pointing to a respiratorypathology), signs and symptoms of CCF, frequently associated with or precipitated by respiratory infections Characteristic features are episodes of colicky pain resembling angina attacks, which occur during feeding and last a few minutes. These are associated with recurrent attacks of discomfort, restlessness, irritability, sweating, dyspnea, and pallor, with or without mild cyanosis, all interpreted to be due to angina pectoris. Growth and development are normal for a few months, but proper history from the pedant's parents shows that there have been intermittent episodes of severe abdominal pain, pallor, and sweating especially during or after feeding. Physically patient is well-nourished and well-developed, shows evidence of COF only when death is imminent, has weak pulses, theheart is enlarged but not continually active, gallop: rhythm is present initially, there are no murmurs, butlater nonspecific murmurs as ejection murmur, or regurgitate murmurs may be heard precordial holosystolic murmurs of mitral insufficiency regurgitant, later becomes evident. There is tachypnea and tachycardia. Wheezing is present. Evidence of left heart failure may be there. X-ray shows gross cardiomegaly and features of pulmonary venous congestion (Large left atrium and ventricle with passive pulmonary congestion). ECG resembles the anterior myocardial infarction adults. A QR Cor QS pattern over the left precordial leads Q waves appearing in leads I and aVL, T wave inversions in the lead I and aVL T Wave inversions in leads V4- 7(precordial leads), deep, wide Q waves in the lead I aVL, V4-6, elevated ST segments (QR pattern followed but inverted T waves are in the lead I and aVL, and deep Q waves in V4,5,6 are diagnosticof anterolateral myocardial infarction. Cardiac catheterization may indicate the presence of AV shunts (but frequently the shunt is so small that it is detected only by hydrogen electrode catheteronly). Catheterization may show an elevated left ventricular end diastolic and left atrial pressure. The pulmonary artery and pulmonary wedge pressures are elevated. Diagnosis is confirmed by angiocardiography of the ascending aorta obtained after selective angiogram obtained after the aortic root injection which shows the right coronary artery, with no evidence of a left coronary artery arising at its natural place. A huge right coronary artery fills directly from the aorta, the collaterals may be visualized, when the die goes from right to left artery. Contrast the dye may be seen flowing into the pulmonary artery under cineangiocardiogra) by (aortography) With immediate o pacification of the large and tortuous right col nary artery after filling of the intracoronary anastomoses, the left coronary artery, and the pulmonary artery are in turn: pacified Selective pulmonary arteriography may pacify the anomalous left coronary artery.

Selective left ventriculography reveals a dilated left ventricle which empties poor. In most cases, death from heart failure occurs within 6 months of li. and the only exceptional patient that survives has an unusually abundant intracoronary anastomosis. The variable prognosis depends onthe severity of heart failure and the extent of the myocardial infarction. Symptomatic treatment- untreated pa are at risk of sudden death usually dying between 3-5 months. A few are symptom during infancy. Most of the survivors are asymptomatic during childhood but may die suddenly during adulthood or may get myocardial infarction (adult type).

TREATMENT

Seriously ill infants with retrograde drainage of left coronary art blood into the pulmonary arteryhave been treated with ligation of the left co: nary artery to prevent runoff of blood from the coronary circuit and to incite se myocardial perfusion via collaterals. Some have done vigorous digitalis and diuretic therapy to postpone the surgery beyond infancy, at which time the anomalous left coronary artery is detached from the pulmonary artery and reattached to the ascending aorta to establish arterial perfusion. It is usually done aft. 4 years.

DIFFERENTIAL DIAGNOSIS

- Similar clinical picture is presented by endocardia fibro elastic in both conditions, the signs, symptoms, and X-ray findings are the same. The main differences between the two are Anomalous origin, Endo fibroelastosis Age: 90% of patients are less than 1 year Rare after 2 years: when first seen, ECG: Most have evidence of anterior mycoses; only occasional patient has radial infarction, only a few have. Myocardial infarction, while as LHV, all cases have LHV. Aorta gram Only the right coronary artery is seen. Coronary arteries arise for the root of the aorta normally. Treatment; Surgical Med supportive Prognosis; Good after surgical ligation of left Poor coronary artery.

- 2 Pompes disease has all the clinical features, severe muscle weakness and macro glossitis. Family history and ECG show no evidence of anterior myocardial
- Infarction.

- Infants with pericardial effusion
- Other conditions leading to gross cardiomegaly, including myocarditis clinical course isshorter, ECG may have inverted I waves on the left precordium, but there is no pattern of anterior infarction or LHV. In cases where the signs of myocardial infarction are present, selective aortography rules out the diagnosis.

- Other causes of myocardial infarction or ischemia in ECG are inflammation, myocarditis, embolism from endocardia vegetation, RH carditis, SLE; metabolic as hypercholesteremia, states asfamilial hyperlipoproteinemia, myxedema, mucopolysac acidosis as Hurlers or homocystinuria degenerative conditions, as coronary atherosclerosis as seen in progeria and coronary calcinosis

.

GARGOYLISM:

In this disease, the lesions in the heart resemble those in the connective tissue elsewhere in the body. The most pronounced lesions are found in the valves and coronary arteries, but abnormalities may be seen in pericardium and aorta The heart is much enlarged with ECG changes of LHV-LVH. Cardiac murmurs are due to incompetence and stenosis of the mitral valves and aortic valves (Tricuspid and pulmonary valve may be involved). Coronary artery disease may result in angina which may lead to death. Many children die before 10 years of heartfailure and pulmonary infection.

CALCINOSIS OF HEART CORONARIES:

A rare disease where coronaries are tortuous and calcareous and the ventricle the left, ishypertrophied, cardiac failure ensues suddenly, and death occurs during infancy.

MUCOCUTANEOUS SYNDROME:

(Mucocutaneous lymph node syndrome);1/3 of patients have arteritis of an aneurysm, thrombosis, occlusion, infarction, and coronary artery symptoms and signs are as that of any acute febrile illness,but the coronary disease resembles polyarthritis nodosa in infants. Aspirin is given in high doses during the acuillness, with continued low doses of the same if coronary involvement is shown b ECG, X-ray chest, mode, and 2-dimensional echocardiography to watch for (3-5mg/kg/d). Coronary angiography is recommended for all.

CARDIOMYOPATHY:

Cardiomyopathy is the hypertrophy of either ventricle of unknown origin, which maybemassive and familial. The left ventricle is more frequently involved than the right.

OBSTRUCTIVE CARDIOMYOPATHY

Outflow of blood from the left ventricle is obstructed by muscular hypertrophy, producing symptoms and signs which may closely: simulate aortic stenosis. Right ventral

obstruction is less frequent and simulates the pulmonary obstruction. In other signs mimic those of mitral insufficiency when left ventricle outflow obstruction, a systolic pressure gradient is demonstrablebetween the left vent and aorta. Rapid ejection from the left ventricle occurs in early systole, but with further contraction, obstruction develops to the outflow of blood. The severity of obstruction depends on the force of the left ventricle contract and on the volume of the left vent cavity. Thus, a post-extra systolic beat does not result in the normally expected increase in arterial pressure.
Factors that red left vent systolic volume intensify the gradient (Valsalva maneuver, inotropic agents including digitalis, and administration of nitroglycerin and isoproterenol). The complianceof the hypertrophied ventricle is poor. Many children are asymptomatic except for murmurs.

Others have weakness, effort dyspnea, fatigue, palpitations, angina pectoris, dizziness, and syncope. The pulse is brisk because of the early systolic ejection of blood from the ventricle. The heart is enlarged with a prominent left ventricular lift and double apical impulse. The first and second heart sounds are normal, but the paradoxical splitting of the 2nd sound may be heard with alarge gradient (Systolic ejection click is rare, which differentiates it from valvular aortic stenosis), A 4th sound may be heard, but 3rd sound is nor heads commonly. Murmur is systolic ejection medium intensity and heard maximally at the left sternal edge and apex. ECG shows LVH, with or without ST depression and T-wave inversion. The Wolff-Parkinson-White syndrome or other intraventricular conduction defects are seen X-ray shows cardiomegaly with the prominence of the left ventricle and sometimes the right ventricle; ascending aorta and aortic know are usually normal. The echocardiogram shows asymmetrical VSD hypertrophy and systolic anterior motion of the anterior of the leaflet of the mitral valve. The diagnosis of left ventriculography show encroachment of the left ventricular cavity by the hypertrophied muscle, especially the interventricular septum. Prognosis is unpredictable, especially in the asymptomatic pt, but sudden death from dysrhythmia or sudden intensification of the gradient Digitalis and nitroglycerin bothintensifies the obstruction, should be used with caution propranolol is used successfully. Some use incision and resection of the left vent outflow tract.

NON-OBSTRUCTIVE CARDIOMYOPATHY

This is more common in children. The enlarged heart shows diffuse hypertrophy (of the vent septum) and disorganization of the alignment of the muscle bundles. The symptoms are those ofchronic CCF, sometimes with angina pectoris and palpitation. Physically there is cardiac enlargement, non-pacific systolic murmurs, and gallop rhythm, but apical murmurs of gross miti incompetence may be present. Chronic COF may result in tricuspid incompetence for right vent dilatation. ECG shows LVH. X-ray confirms the generalized cardiomegaly with left ventricularprominence and pulmonary congestion. Treatment is that of heart failure; the prognosis is poor.

RESTRICTIVE CARDIOMYOPATHY

Occasionally restrictive cardiomyopathy leads to poor ventricular compliance, so diastolic filling of the heart is compromised. This results in a clinical picture resembling constrictive pericarditis. In its overt form, it results in dyspnea, edema, ascites, hepatomegaly, increased JVP,and pulmonary congestion. There is cardiomegaly with nonspecific murmurs. ECG shows prominent P Waves, frequently normal QRS voltage, Sl segment de pression, and Twa inversion.Ray shows cardiomegaly with poor cardiac pulsations, and Prognosis is poor, and treatment is directedto edema with diuretics.

MYOCARDITIS

In the vast majority of cases, the cause of myocarditis remains obscure; Coxsacle B virus is the commonest agent, followed but coxsackie A, rubella, mumps, herpes, ad virus, cytomegalovirus, and many other viral agents are implicated. Clinical picture Clinically it may present as sudden onset of COF in a newborn, who has been in relatively good health 12-24 previously; as, an overwhelming viremia and tissue invasion of multiple organ systems includingthe heart In the older child, cardiac findings develop gradually; there is h/o an URI or GE within the month prior to the development of cardiac findings is a more insidious form and maybe a late post infectious or autoimmune component. Recovery from infection is followed by gradual and progressive development of early fatigability, dyspnea on exertion and malaise.
In the newborn infant, the signs and symptoms are usually apparent. The skin is pale and gray;peripheral cyanosis may be present. Pulses are rapid, weak, and thread. Edema of the face and limbs may be present. Cardiomegaly is present, and the left and right cardiac impulses (ventricular)are weak. Heart sounds are poor, muffled, and distant; 3rd and 4th sounds are common resulting in gallop rhythm Murmurs are usually absent, though tricuspid or mitral insufficiency murmur may be heard. Both lung bases elicit crepitation; the liver is enlarged andtender, and JVP is raised. In the older child group, the signs of COF are not as apparent as in the newborn. X-ray shows generalized cardiomegaly, all four chambers of the heart enlarged, with pulmonary venous congestion, and commonly pneumonitis is present ECG classically shows evidence of low voltage of the QRS throughout all frontal and precordial lead şand depression of STsegment and inversion of T Waves in leads I III and aVF and in the left precordial leads. During the acute malignant stage. There may be arrhythmias or AV or IV conduction defects withthe recovery phase of the malignant form or in

the benign form, there is the presence of LVH asevidenced by high voltage QRS.

TREATMENT:

All patients with clinical findings of myocarditis should be started immediately on digitalis since inflamed myocardium is overly sensitive to digitalis. Only two-thirds of the usual dose is used. During teinitial phase of recovery, frequent ECGs should be taken, and if serious arrhythmias or other evidence of digitalis intoxication develops, the drug should be stopped and not reinstituted until all evidence of digitalis. Toxicity has appeared-disappeared. Diuretics should be administered with caution since they may potentiate digital toxicity - use of corticosteroids ismore beneficial in the treatment of the more benign post-infectious, autoimmune cases, and if patient deteriorates, diteant congestive measures, corticosteroids are used. The prognosis depends on the age donset, the Response to therapy, and the presence or absence of recurrences. If the patient is less than 6months of age or more than 3 yr responds poorly to therapy, and manifests multiple recurrencesof CCF, the prognosis is poor. Many patients recovers clinically but have persistent cardiomegaly.
In some cases of subclinical cases - myocarditis in childhood is the pathophysiologic basis for someof the idiopathic myocardiopathy seen in later life.

RHEUMATIC CARDITIS

Group A beta-hemolytic streptococcal infection of the Respiratory tract is the essential environmental trigger that acts on predisposed individuals, producing the first attack of rheumatic fever. After a child has an attack, the risk of recurrences following subsequent inadequately treated streptococcal infections is 50%, at least for 5 years. Thus, the mere fact that a child has had rh fever once increases the risk of further attacks by 150 times. Therefore, penicillin prophylaxis isso important. The clinical presentation of an attack tends to repeat itself in subsequent attacks; therefore, a patient with severe carditis on the first attack is subject to a similar course if there is another episode of rh fever. Rh fever is a disease of multifactorial inheritance. There is a hereditary predisposition and an environmental trigger. However, the patient is predisposed and vulnerable to the presence of the streptococcal group. An infection is essential to produce rh fever.

Streptococci that are not from group A don 't cause beta-hemolysis and don 't infect the Respiratory tract are not associated with rh fever. The streptococci and the myocardium have antigens in common. The body in defending itself against streptococcal invasion raises antibodies against antigens of this organism, but the same antibodies are also capable of attacking similar antigens present in the individuals own heart (autoimmune reaction). The peak incidence is in children aged 5-15 years. Jones criteria: Major manifestations of carditis, polyarthritis, Sydenham's chorea, erythema, marginatum, Sc nodules. Minor manifestations Clinical Previous rheumatic fever or rh heart disease, polyarthralgia, fever; lab acute phase reactants, as elevated ESPECIALLY, CRP, leukocytosis; prolonged PR interval. Other supporting evidence of preceding streptococcal infection, such as increased titers of ASO or other streptococcal antibodies, throat culture for group A streptococci recent scarlet fever. Two major or one major and two minor criteria, supportingevidence of streptococcal infections, are sufficient for presumptive diagnosis. Clinical features of rh fever includes -Polyarthritis; two or more joints must be involved, and involvement of one jointis not sufficient; may be involved simultaneously or in a migratory fashion; the commonest jointsinvolved are ankles, knees, hips, wrists, elbows, and shoulders, with heat, redness, swelling, severe pain, and tenderness.

Subcutaneous nodules are usually seen only in severe cases, most commonly over the joints, scalp, and spinal column. They may be from a few mm to 2 cm in diameter, are not tender, and are freely movable under the skin.

Erythema marginatum usually occurs only in severe cases and consists of a macular erythematous rash with a circulate border appearing primarily on the trunk and limbs. The face isusually not involved Sydenham 's chorea is characterized by emotional instability and involuntary movements, which become progressively more severe, and are often followed by the development of ataxia and slurring of speech. Muscular weakness becomes apparent following the onset of involuntary movements. The individual attack of chorea is self-limiting, though it may last for up to 3 months. It may be one-sided only. Fever is typically low. Grade, but may reach 39-40. C. - Polyarthralgia of two or more joints without heat, swelling, and tenderness (pain on Isis a minor manifestation.

ECG changes include prolongation of PR interval; it does not qualify for active carditis.
Acute phase reactants include elevation of DESR; more specifically, CRP (C-reactive protein) is elevated; CRP is not affected by: CCF, and ESR also is not affected usually by it. Leukocytosisis the rule. There is a prior h/o acute rh fever or the presence of inactive rheumatic carditis. Except in cases of rh fever presenting solely as Sydenham's chorea or long-standing carditis, there should be clear supporting evidence of a streptococcal infection such as scarlet fever, a +ve throat culture for group A beta-hemolytic streptococci, increased ASO titers or other streptococcal antibody titers. ASO titire is significantly higher in rh fever than in uncomplicated streptococcal infection; Associated findings may include erythema multiform, abdominal back, and precordial pain, no traumatic epistaxis, vomiting, malaise, weight loss, and anemia.

RHEUMATIC CARDITIS:

Cardiac involvement in rh fever embodies pericarditis, myocarditis, and endocarditis. Rh endocarditis (where valves and endocardium are involved) is the most common type of endocarditis in children. Lesions begin as small verrucae composed of fibrin and blood cells along the borders of the valves. With recurrent attacks of rh fever, the valves become fibrotic andcontract. As the infection subsides, the verrucae tend to disappear and leave scar tissue with each infection, more small lesions form near the previous one, and the mural endocardium and chordate tendinae also become involved. The mitral valve is affected most often, and the aortic next, tricuspid, and pulmonary valves are less common.

ACTIVE CARDITIS

ACTIVE CARDITIS_is present in 50% of cases; it is heralded by any of the following -a significant new murmur that is clearly either of mitral insufficiency (with or without a transient topical murmur, i.e., apical diastolic Carey Coombs) or aortic insufficiency. Mitral insufficiency though commonly from rhfever, has many other causes in children. Either new or changing murmurs suggest carditis–
Pericarditis is manifested by a pericardial friction rub or evidence of pericardial effusion.

EVIDENCE OF CCF

Others are poor quality heart sounds with gallop or tic-tac rhythm, cardiomegaly, and tachycardia (uncommonly bradycardia). Rhotic pneumonia may occur with severe carditis rarely.In the absence of carditis, the average duration of rh activity is 89+ 27 days: when carditis is present the activity is persistent for an average of 124 + 6 8 days. The features that suggest that the RH fever has become inactive are the return of ESR and CRP to normal after discontinuing the anti-inflammatory treatment, the return of the sleeping pulse to normal, the rise of Hemoglobin to normal levels.

In some adolescent and preadolescent girls, the ESR does not return to normal when all other criteria for activity have disappeared, which in the face of clinical improvement, will not be important. Inactive rheumatic carditis will include mitral stenosis, mitral regurgitation, aortic incompetence, etc. There is a history of the fever and signs of heart disease, such as a murmurand cardiomegaly. The valvular lesions may be isolated or in combination. The more common lesions are mitral insufficiency and aortic insufficiency, while others are uncommon.

MITRAL INSUFFICIENCY

Mitral insufficiency is the most common valvular residual of acute RH carditis; it results from deformity of the valve cusps, contraction of the chordae tendon, and dilatation of the valve ring impeding the valve closure. There is usually, so me loss of the substance of the valve, and insufficiency prevents normal closure of the valve. Often there is associated MS because of thesclerosis of the base of the mitral ring and cups. During ventricular systole, blood regurgitates from the left ventricle to the left atrium, which may result in left trial enlargement which is sometimes aneurysmal. Due to the greater workload and filling pressure of the left ventricle, thatalso becomes enlarged. The increased left atrial pressure may be reflected through the pulmonary bed to the right side of the heart, producing enlargement of the right ventricle and atrium, with subsequent CCF. In most of the pts, the lesion is mild or moderate, is well tolerated, and The principal finding is the apical, blowing, pan systolic murmur, which well radiates to the left axilla and to the left sternal edge. This murmur appears exceedingly early in MI, depending on the severity of the damage, may disappear over the period of days or months or may persist for life. Occasionally the murmur may be short systolic or absent altogether. A diastolic murmur, dueto increased flow from he left atrium across the mitral valve, may be audible in the absence of MS (It is a soft, rumbling mid-diastolic murmur). The traditional long ejection or holosystolic murmur is best heard at the left lower sternal border and apex radiating to the left axilla.

Palpation of the heart reveals a hyperactive left vein impulse but no thrill. The first heart sound is normal and soft, 2nd sound is widely split (because of the shorter duration of the left vent systole), pulmonary Valvular closure is loud in the presence of complicating pulmonary hypertension, a 3rd 600 and is prominent (due to the large early diastolic filling of the left ventricle) If the lesion is mild, X-ray and ECG are normal, but with more severe lesions, ECG shows prominent P Waves(bi fid), signs of LVH, and sometimes associated with RVH. Prominent P waves are due to a large left atrium (P mitral). X-ray shows a prominent left atrium and left ventricle, thus cardiomegaly. The right side is enlarged only when the left side fails. When pulmonary hypertension of COF supervenes, the pulmonary artery segment and right heart chambers are also prominent. Signs of pulmonary venous pretension are also seen. Calcification of the mitral valve is rare in children, and Echocardiography shows an increased velocity of diastolic closure of the artery or mitral leaflet (greater than 120-180mm/sec) in moderate or severe regurgitation. If there is a rapid progression of the disease, and surgical treatment is needed, cardiAltanisation and left ventriculography are done. Cardiac catheterization.

Echocardiography shows an increased velocity of alaston2C closure mitral leaflet (greater than 170-180mm/sec) in moderate or severe regurgitation If there is a rapid progression of the disease and surgical treatment is needed, cardiac catheterization and left ventriculography are done. Cardiaccatheterization shows a pressure gradient across the mitral valve even in the absence of MS, and lei ventriculography opacities the left ventricle and left atrium. The degree of pacification is needed- used as a qualitative assessment of the severity c incompetence. Any patient with the murmur of MI should be followed up for many years. Though the fever I the most commonest cause of MI in children, it may be due to other causes, the most common being mitral dysfunction syndrome (characterized by a mild to late apical systolic murmur introduced by a click; echocardiographic finding of prolapse or redundancy of the mitral valve which characterizes mitral dysfunction, may also be found in acute rh fever and recently acquired RHD), others are myocarditis, endocardia fibroelastosis, anomalous left coronary artery, and congenital anomalies of the mitral valve(isolated or part of endocardia fusion. defects) The dominant symptoms are fatigue, poor weight gain, weakness, dyspnea on effort, and palpitations. During convalescence, milder cases often make a great improvement, while those with the far advanced cardiac disease suffer from the effects of rapid growth. If the RH infections recur, the valvular condition may become progressively worse.

COMPLICATIONS:

Severe MI can lead to cardiac failure; this may be precipitated by the progression of the RH fever, the onset of atrial fibrillations with the rapid ventricular Response , or Sabe. Pulmonary congestion is common, but frank left vent failure is unusual Right-sided heart failure may be accompanied by TI or PI. SABE may complicate the rheumatic mitral disease, especially when dominant incompetence is associated with moderate stenosis. Occasional atrial or extra vent systoles are well tolerated. First-degree heart block, due to initial infection or digital therapy, may persist for years. Atrialfibrillation is associated with a large hypertensive left atrium with MI.

TREATMENT

In the majority of patients with MI, prophylaxis against recurrences of Rh fever is all that is needed since the lesion is mild and well tolerated; if heart failure, arrhythmias, or SABE occurs it is managed. A minority who, diteadequate medical care, suffer from recurrent attacks of heart failure, extreme dyspnea with moderate activity, and progressive cardiomegaly with pulmonary hypertension. Most of them need valve replacement (Valvuloplasty, but some havegood results with annuloplasty. The prognosis is generally good.

MITRAL STENOSIS (MS)

MS is rare in childhood and occurs in 5% of patients with RHD, and structural stenosis is seen only 5-10 years after the first attack of the fever. Therefore, much more is is seenin adults than in children. It is rare in developed countries: but has been increasingly reported in the Middle East, India, and SEA. It is presumed that rhea tic fever runs a more malignant course in this part of the world. Others blame crowded ling conditions, poor nutritional status, and lack of adaptation of rhea tic fever prop axis programmers, which predisposes children and youngadults to the ravages of the fever. Mostly seen in patients who are in their teens but has been seen in cases as young as 10 years. Organic stenosis is nearly always rheumatic in origin, resulting from fibrosis of the mitral ring, commissural adhesions, and contracture of the valve leaflets chordae and papillary muscles. It may take more than 2 years of the lesion to become established fully, though the process may be accelerated in some children.MS is often associated with MI. MS of critical degree is considered to exist if the valve orifice is reduced to 25% or less of the expected norm. There is difficulty in left atrial emptying, which results in hypertrophy and increases pressure in this chamber, which in t turn leads to pulmonary venous hypertension, increased pulmonary vascular resistance, pulmonary arterial hypertension, which leads to right ventricularhypertrophy, and right atrial dilatation, which are followed by right ventricular failure (CCF).

Murmurs of the MS may be due to the legendary stenosis of the valve (structural due to a relative excess of flow as in large volumes of regurgitation, and those which are present during a cute valvulitis Carey Costenotic murmur, flow murmurs, and Carey Coombs murmur are short and heard in middiastol Established stenosis murmurs become progressively longer in duration, and they attain the classic crescendo, presystolic configuration. A low-frequency (low-pitched), long, rumbling, mid-diastolic murmur is the classic murmur with presystolic accentuation. (Apical presystolic murmur of crescendo type), it is accompanied by a loud first heart sound and an opening snap of the mitral valve (opening snap following the second heart sound). The murmur is best heard at the apex. Mitral diastolic murmur may be absent. In CCF, presystolic accentuation of the diastolic murmur disappears during atrial fibrillation. An apical systolic murmur may be heard even in the absence of mitral incompetence; in some, it is due to tricuspid incompetence. In the presence of pulmonary hypertension, pulmonary valvular closure is accentuated with prominent pulmonary sound. An early diastolic murmur may be due to associated aortic incompetence (pulmonary incompetence is not common). With mild disease, heart size is normal. The severe diastolic murmur may be due to associated aortic one competence; pulmonary incompetence is not common). With mild disease, heart size is normal; with severe disease, moderate cardiomegaly is seen but may be severe if atrial fibrillation and COF supervene. The apical impulse is brief and tapping; when pulmonary Vascular resistance is high, a parasternal right ventricular lift (heave) is felt. Pulses-pressure may be small. Exercise and turning the patient in the left lateral position may bring out the typical murmur. Symptoms correlate with the severity of the lesion. Patients with mild lesions is asymptomatic, but more severe cases have effort intolerance, dyspnea, orthopnea, paroxysmal nocturnal dyspnea, and overt pulmonary edema, and all these can be precipitated by uncontrolled tachycardia, atrial fibrillation, or pulmonary infections. COF is usually associated with moderate or severe pulmonary hypertension. Right ventricular dilatation may result in functional bicuspid incompetence, hepatomegaly, ascites, and edema. Hemoptysis may occur due to ruptured bronchial or pleurohilar veins and occasionally pulmonary infarction. Blood-streaked sputum occurs in episodes of pulmonary edema. Bacterial endocarditis and systemic emboli are uncommon in children with severe lesions. There is malar flush and cyanosis; in the presence of CCF, JVP is raised. Or it may be due to tricuspid valve disease or severe hypertension. An episode of pulmonary infarction may present as acute chest pail dyspnea, rusty sputum, hemoptysis, and fever. X-ray showing a triangular shadow, the appendages of which may promote the formation of clots. When some of these clots get detached systemic embolization occurs. If an embolus goes to the brain, it may lead to hemiplegia, and if the embolus travels down the descending aorta, then it may obstruct the blood supply to a limb or part of it. In juvenile MS, pulmonary hypertension develops rather early and may lead to COF and tricuspid regurgitation. Severe obstruction is present when the diastolic murmur is long, in the absence of MI, the time between the wave of ECG and the first heart sound (Q-1 interval is long, and the time between the aortic valve closure and the opening snap (2-03 interval) is short. X-RAY: Heart size is often normal but may be enlarged (mild to moderate cardiomegaly) with right ventricular and left atrial enlargement principally. Pulmonary one venous congestion is a prominent feature of tight MS. There may be a double shadow at the right border of the heart, suggesting the enlargement of the left atrium, which needs to be confirmed by swallowing the right anterior oblique or left anterior oblique view. Thus, X-ray shows varying degrees of absteustier-et- left atria enlargement, prominence of the pulmonary artery, prominence of right heart chambers, and normal or small aorta and left ventricle.

The lungs may show pulmonary venous congestion, and Kelley lines may become prominent. Severe obstruction is associated with a redistribution of pulmonary blood flow so that the apices of the lung show greater perfusion (reverse of normal). Serial films may show more pulmonary vascular obstruction markings at the apices with a prominence of the pulmonary veins. Septal lines at the costrophrenic angles are also prominent. ECG: Isolated cases of MS show right axis deviation (QRS axis in the frontal plane beyond +100), varying degrees of right vent hypertrophy (dominant waves in V4R and V1), and broad and notched P Waves (P mitral) in leads I and II, Sowing left ventricular atrial enlargement. In cases of longstanding obstruction and markedly enlarged left atrium, atrial fibrillation may set in, and on ECG, there are fibrillatory waves in V1 that indicate a huge enlargement of the right-left atrium. Echocardiography shows marked solving of the diastolic closure of the anterior mitral leaflet (less than 40mm/sec). Cardiac catheterization quantitates the diastolic gradient between the two chambers across the mitral valve, the degree of pulmonary hypertension, and the severity of the increase of pulmonary vascular resistance. There is a significant elevation of pulmonary artery wedge pressure in most cases of MS. Later, pulmonary artery pressure and the right ventricular pressure also rises. In severe cases, cardiac output is reduced and does not rise proportionately with an increase in heart rate during exercise.

TREATMENT:

Medical treatment consists of the management of cardiac failure, arrhythmias, and prophylaxis of the fever. Chest infections should be controlled. Indications of surgery are in patients in whom there are signs of recurrent pulmonary edema, high pulmonary resistance, or systemic emboli. Once the symptom presence of MI is established and there is evidence of significant left atrial enlargement and rt ventricular hypertrophy, if there has been no recurrence of the fever within the last few months, surgery should be offered. Since extreme valvular distortion and calculation is rare in children, closed mitral valvotomy is sufficient, but the prophylaxis should be continued for years after surgery. JMS is progressive, except in very mild cases, if the course is not interrupted by surgery.

AORTIC INSUFFICIENCY

In most cases, AI is due to RHD (may be congenital also), is the second most frequent of valves affected in polyvalvular or monovalvular disease. Aortic insufficiency usually occurs withmitral insufficiency. In chronic rh AL, sclerosis of the aortic valves resulys in distortion and retraction of cusps. Regurgitation of blood results in a volume overload with dilatation of and hypertrophy - tine 12+ antennal In order to compensate for the resulting low aortic devastation ofblood results in a volume overload with dilatation of and hypertrophy of the left ventricle. To compensate for the resulting low aortic diastolic pressure, the systolic pressure is raised Secondary mitral insufficiency may occur following progressive left ventricular dilatation. Left ventricular failure results in left atrial hypertension.COF may occur insidiously or be preceded bybouts of pulmonary edema. Symptoms: are unusual except in gross. AI. The large stroke volume and forceful left ventricular contractions may result in palpitations. Excessive sweating and heat intolerance are related to vasodilatation. Dyspnea on effort progresses to orthopnea and pulmonary edema. Angina pectoris may occur during heavy exertion. In adolescents with florid incompetence, nocturnal attacks of nightmares, sweating,

tachycardia, chest pain, and hypertension may occur. Children are usually asymptomatic. Owing to the reflux of blood through the aortic valve during diastole and associated vasodilatation, the radial pulses are
water-hammer in type, the carotid arteries show bounding Corrigan pulsations(increased and clearly visible pulsations with severe AI there may be capillary pulsations in lips and fingernails,an audible systolic shock over the peripheral arteries (Pistol shot),and systolic and diastolic murmurs over the femoral arteries if pressure is applied to the artery just distal to the stethoscope (Duroziez signs), the systolic pressure is raised and the diastolic lowered, therefore the wide pulse pressure. Heart is enlarged, there is a left ventricular apical heave (thrust), the sudden thrust of the left ventricle is both visible as well as palpable; the left chest is prominent. The thrill is absent unless there is an associated AS. Early The typical AI murmur is a soft, blowing, high-pitched, decrescendo,4-diastolic murmur, best heard in the 2nd and 3rd left space (heard over the upper and middle left sternal border with radiation to the apex and to the aortic area. It has a hollow fading quality of a whispered ping. Generally, the murmur is more easily audible in full expiration with the patient leaning forward, or it may become louder in the recumbent position. A short systolic ejection murmur, preceded by a click, is due to excess flow, and a large stroke volume may be heard. An apical presystolic murmur resembling that of mitral stenosis is heard sometimes (Austin flint murmur), which is due to interference with valvular function by the large regurgitant blood flow which deflects the aortic cusp of the mitral valve. X-ray shows enlargement and increased pulsation of the left ventricle and the aorta.

ECG may be normal, but in severe cases, it may show LVH and tall R waves, and deep Q waves in the left chest lead ST, and I wave; changes of left ventricular strain may be present. P Waves are prominent. Echocardiography shows diastolic

mitral valve flutter or Oscillation, having a frequency of 30-40 cycles/sec, which results from the regurgitation jet striking at anterior mitralleaflet. Cardiac catheterization is done only if surgery is intended for a progressive lesion.
Ascending aortography also is done to demonstrate the regurgitant flow across the aortic valve into the left ventricle. Mild and moderate lesions are well tolerated. Many adolescents with severe regurgitation are symptom free and tolerate advanced lesions well into the 3rd and 4th decade. Onset of CCF, recurrent episodes of pulmonary edema or development of angina pectoris are unfavorable signs. Treatment consists of prophylaxis against the recurrence of acuterh fever and occurrence of SABE, encouragement to lead an active and normal life. Valve replacement is done only when there is progressive deterioration from heart failure, pulmonary edemaor angina pectoris.

AORTIC STENOSIS

AS in children is almost always congenital, but in the disease may be associated with AI, anddominant as is never rheumatic in childhood.

TRICUSPID INSUFFICIENCT

TI is usually functional, being secondary to right vent dilatation resulting from severe left-sidedlesions. It leads to prominent pulsations of the jugular vein with a c-V wave, systolic pulsationsof the liver, and blowing systolic murmur in the 4th and 5th left space, which increases in intensity during inspiration. Concomitant signs of mitral or aortic valvular disease with or without atrial fibrillation are frequent when heart failureproduced by the left-sided lesions is treated, and signs of tricuspid incompetence disappear. Tricuspid involvement is rare. Acquired tricuspid stenosis is also rare and is usually associatedwith rh mitral or aortic valvular disease. The signs are increased JVP, with prominent a waves presystolic hepatic pulsation, and a rumbling diastolic murmur in the 4th and 5th space with severe lesions there is hepatomegaly, edema, and ascites.

PULMONARY VALVULAR DISEASE

Pulmonary insufficiency is usually due to functional causes rarely organic, secondary to pulmonaryhypertension or dilatation of the pulmonary artery. Occasionally it! Complicates severe MS (Graham Steel murmur). The murmurs are like those of AI, but the peripheral arterialsigns are absent. Pulmonary stenosis is usually congenital than rheumatic.

TREATMENT FOR ACTIVE DISEASE

Active disease: Absolute bed rest until there is no remaining clinical or lab evidence of inflammation (normal pulse rate, temperature, and ESR for two consecutive weeks). Gradual resumption of activity with vigil for recurrence of symptoms. Strict bed rest is needed for pte with arthritis and mild carditis without CCFPatients with severe carditis (CCF) should be kept in bed.The average duration of rh fever without carditis is 3 months (1 month + -), and with carditis 4 months (2months +-), thus in no case activity disappears before 2 months. Nutrition should be maintained and salt/fluid restricted if COF is present. The child can 't goes to school, during the period of rheumatic activity.

Anti-infective therapy: eradication and prevention of streptococcal disease is affected by penicillin (asoral, 125-250mg 6 hourly for 10 days, parenteral benzathine penicillin, 0.6-1.2 million units' single injection, or benzyl-procaine penicillin 400,000 units daily for 10 days. In patients sensitive to penicillin, erythromycin 250 mg orally four times a day may be given.
Anti-inflammatory drugs used are in the absence of carditis,

aspirin 100-120mg/kg/d for 4-6 weeks, it relieves fever and arthritis. The maximum dose that can be given is 58/d. For maximum benefit, the salicylate level of blood should remain about 25mg/100ul. The dosage is reduced to 50mg/kg/d in one week and maintained at this level for 1 month, or until the CRP is -Ve and ESR falls when aspirin can be discontinued, Aspirin is, discontinued after tapering off gradually to prevent recurrence from rebound phenomenon. - Steroids are used in more seriously ill patients with carditis. Thus, patients who are in mild COF are benefitted from digitalis may not be given corticosteroids since aspirin is slightly better in preventing residual valvular damage and rebound phenomena are more frequent in corticosteroid-treated pts, so with corticosteroids, the acute phase may even be prolonged. But the child with carditis and intractable or poorly compensated COF needs corticosteroids. Treatment is most effective when started early: prednisolone 2mg/kg/orally for 2 weeks, then in the third week reduced to 1mg/kg/d, when aspirin is begun(50mg/kg/d), prednisolone is stopped at the end of third week, and aspirin continued for 8 weeks or until the CRP is ve and ESR are falling.

CHRONIC DISEASE

For chronic disease, prevention is the most important step. The patient who has had rh fever has a greatly increased (150 times.) risk of developing rh fever following the next inadequately treated group A beta hemolytic streptococci infection. Intramuscular benzathine penicillin G, given for a lifetime, is the ideal protection. Oral regimes have demonstrably lower effectiveness, even in those who follow regular regimes. There is currently no age at which discontinuation is advocated. The different regimes used are

- 1-Benzathine penicillin G1.2 million units IM once a month.
- 2-Sulfadiazine, 500 mg orally daily as a single dose for patients under 60lb, 1g orally daily as a single dose for those

over 60 lb. Blood dyscrasias and less effectiveness in reducing streptococcal infections make it a less satisfactory second choice

- 3-Penicillin G, buffered, 250,000 units orally twice daily, parallels the sulfas in effectiveness and is much less than IM benzathine penicillin (5.5v/s 0.4 str infections/100 patient years).
- 4- Erythromycin, 250 mg orally daily BD, to those who are allergic to both penicillin and sulfas. COF may follow a single severe episode of acute rh carditis, but more commonly follows repeated episodes. Some children with severe valvular damage who cannot be managed effectively on medical treatment may be sent for valve replacement before the myocardial tissue is damaged irreversibly. The usual manifestationsof residual valvular damage in children are heart murmurs of mitral and aortic insufficiency without COF during pediatric years if repeated attacks are prevented. Asymptomatic patients needs no treatment. Symptomatic patients need restrict ion of activity especially with aortic lesion.

INFECTIVE ENDOCARDITIS

SUBACUTE BACTERIAL ENDOCARDITIS (infective endocarditis with preexisting cyst disease). This is the bacterial infection of the endocardial surface of the heart or the intimal surface of an arterial vessel (corrected segment of the aorta and duct arteriosus). It is a rare condition that occurs when an abnormality of the heart or great vessels exists. The infection is more insidious and protracted than the acute form (which may develop in a normal heart during septicemia. The organisms produce an ulcerative-vegetative process on the previously damaged site. The process may spread to the adjacent endocardium. Vegetations that are friable may break off and seed the circulation with small emboli (a characteristic feature of the disease). The vegetation in the SABE is usually smaller than those in the acute type. They may destroy the endocardia lining and underlying muscle and even perforate the valves or septa. When superimposed upon the acquired cardiac disease, this usually attacks the left rather than the right side of the heart. In congenitally deformed hearts, the bacterial invasion begins near or at the site of the defect. The difference between the acute and subacute forms lies in the infecting organism rather than the type of the basic defect. Thus, Strep viridian is a sub-acute infection, and staph aureus causes highly subacute infection. Cyanotic hearts, mostly Fallot's tetralogy, are at the highest risk, followed by aortic stenosis and VSD. Etiology The commonest causative organism is. Strep viridans: other infecting organisms are enterococci (group D streptococci), staphalbus or aurous, and fungi. Predisposing factors are not always clear, but strep viridians may follow oral or pharyngeal surgery, especially dental extractions. Though almost all patients gives h/o heart disease, h/o infection, or a surgical procedure such as tooth extraction or tonsillectomy is not always there. Enterococci enter the bloodstream after the instrumentation of the genitourinary or GIT tract. After an open-heart surgery, organisms that are usually nonpathogenic may cause SABE.

CLINICAL FEATURES:

The onset is insidious, and the symptoms are nonspecific as pyrexia, malaise, lassitude, pallor, anorexia, weight loss, arlutulgia, chills, and night sweats. There are signs of heart disease, and new murmurs may appear during the disease as mitral incompetence or aortic incompetence. Unexplained heart failure in a patient previously well controlled is an early sign. There is often a h/o surgical procedure or a h/o previous infection. The patient looks ill. Murmurs may change character. Petechiae are common and are usually located in oral mucosa, conjunctivae, and around the ankles and wrists. Splinter hemorrhages may be seen under the fingernails and toenails; occasionally, retinal hemorrhages are present.

Splenomegaly may be present; left upper quadrant pain may be produced by splenic infarction. Hepatomegaly may be noted. The older manifestations are Osler 's nodes (small tender palpable erythematous lesions in the pads of fingers and toes), Jane ways lesions (painless hemorrhagic nodules in the palm and soles rotting spots (hemorrhagic areas with a white center seen in the retina and clubbing of finger: all these are late findings and now rarely seen. Anemia (normochromic normocytic) as usual. Proteinuria is common, hematuria (microscopic) may be there, and Tachycardia and gallop rhythm may occur in severe cases. COF occurs, and hemiplegia may occur.

DIAGNOSIS:

The essentials of diagnosis are a preexisting organic heart murmur persistent fever, increasingsymptoms of heart disease ranging from easy fatigability to heart failure, changing murmurs, splenomegaly (70% cases), emboli phenomena (50% cases), laboratory findings of raised ESR, anemia, leukocytosis, albuminuria and hematuria, cardiomegaly on x-ray, and prolonged PR internal or T-wave changes on ECG, and +ve blood culture. Six blood cultures, three anaerobic and three aerobic, are taken over a period of 2-4 days. If these are -ve subsequent cultures can rarely be present.

PROGNOSIS

The course and prognosis depend on how early treatment is instituted with early treatment most children recover completely. The disease may rum a mild course for its first week (sometimes formonths) so that the diagnosis is made only after serious damage to valves has occurred. With inadequate therapy r recurrences are usual. The prognosis is better in patients in whom blood culture is positive. On the whole prognosis in treated case is good. Even though

bacteriologic cure of theinfectious process is achieved death may occur from COF secondary to severe valvular destruction. Intractable COF may occur weeks or months following bacteriological cure.
Embolization may occur following bacteriologic cure when the vegetation tears off from the involved area. Acute bacterial endocarditis progresses rapidly with destruction of tissue and earlydeath if therapy is not instituted. To prevent the disease, proper antibiotic cover should be given be fire any type of dental work as tooth extraction, cleaning, or operations within the oropharynxGIT and genitourinary tract. Continuous antibiotic prophylaxis is not recommended for congenital heart disease, as for RHD.

TREATMENT:

- In a patient with known heart disease, presence of an otherwise unexplained fever should alert for the possibility of infective endocarditis, blood culture should be taken, and antibiotic selected onthe culture sensitivity.
- Antibiotics can be started pending the culture report. Blood levels of the antibiotics exceed theminimal inhibiting concentration of antibiotics in the broth. Bacteriostatic agents are seldom successful in eradicating bacteria from cardiac vegetation. Therefore, bactericidal drugs should beused. Strep viridian's is always sensitive to penicillin. For this organism, IV penicillin (0.6-3 million units of penicillin Giv or im) four hourly for 2-6 weeks, plus sptropmyocin in the same way as above.
- For gram -ve bacteria, mostly a complication of open-heart surgery, it depends on the c7s of the organism. -Oral penicillin has been used, instead of parenteral, penicillin V, 600-750mg/4 hourly for 2-6 weeks. There was no case of inadequate absorption or GIT disturbances, such as vomiting, nausea, or diarrhea.

When giving penicillin, some prefer to give oral prednisolone first, and thena gradual buildup of penicillin dosage given at one-half hourly intervals as follows 1-10 units ID, 2-100 units: SCA#,3-1000 units SC,4-100,000 units in. If no reaction occurs, the usual schedule of penicillin therapy may be followed even if urticarial is observed during treatment. - Clinically suspected but bacteriologically unproved endocarditis; generally, it is assumed that the organism is sensitive to penicillin, given in doses of 10 million units daily for at least 4 weeks, + IM streptomycin. Clinical course guards the treatment, and when there is no Response , either doseof penicillin i is increased, probenecid added, or other antibiotics added

A condition clinically indistinguishable from bacterial endocarditis or en arteritis is seen in ventricular-cardio-vascular shunts for the treatment of hydrocephalus. The colonization of the bacteria usually occurs in the valve of the artificial shunt Management is like that of SABE, but the shunt has t to be removed and replaced with an uncontaminated substitute, for success. Patients of SABE should be observed for at least 4-6 months after completion of treatment,and blood cultures should be repeated at each follow up examination. Corrective surgery for congenital diseases can be done once the infection is controlled.

ACUTE OR MALIGNANT ENDOCARDITIS

Infective endocarditis without preexisting CV disease:

Acute endocarditis has been seen at all ages and may have been even acquired prenatally, thuspresent in neonates. The infection may occur suddenly in a healthy child or may complicate a heart disease that is rheumatic or congenital. The commonest infecting agent is Staph areus, but Gm -ve bacilli, enterococci, pneumococci, and fungi. Infection may occur during septicemia. The se patients have vegetation ‘s developing on the endocardium of valves, and cardiac chambers, more frequently on the left sidethan the right

Vegetation consist of bacteria in an exudate of fibrin and blood. Ulceration and theformation of friable granulation tissue occurs early; destruction of valves progresses rapidly resulting in acute incompetence of valves, usually the mitral or aortic. Cardiac performance is further impaired by extension of the infection into the myocardium. Parts of the vegetation 's or necrotic tissue may embolize to any part of the body, obstructing the blood flow and establishing secondary foci of infection.

Clinically the onset is explosive, with high fever, prostration, the patient is extremely ill with evidence of severe sepsis. Involvement of the heart becomes clinically manifest with the development of heart murmurs and cardiomegaly. Cardiomegaly may or may not be present. Involvement of the heart is only a part of a total systemic infection. Retinal hemorrhage, splenomegaly, or the loss of pulsation of a major artery may be detected. In many patients the cause of the infection is not clear, but in some there is a h/o recent furunculosis, osteomyelitis, or infectedpilonidal BEAUA cyst. Neutrophil is usual, albuminuria, microscopic hematuria, and pyuria are common. Blood cultures are usually +ve. Acute bacterial endocarditis is rare in childhood. Septicemboli may produce e paralysis of parts of the body and there may be abdominal pain, hematuria, and diarrhea Disease is usually due to a septic focus, elsewhere in the body caused byany organism. There is usually no underlying cardiac disease. The process is rapidly destructive. Mortality rate is high (about 50%), death occurring within a few days unless the treatment is started early. Cause of death is either toxicity from the infection or relentless progress of cardiac disease (latter occurring weeks or months after the infection is cured, owing th rupture or development of defects in the valves (usually mitral or aortic). Even if bacteriologic cure is affected residual cardiac damage is the rule, and COF and death may occur. Treatment consists of three blood cultures taken within 1-2 hours and treatment instituted taking the

organism as staph.
Therefore, large iv doses of methicillin, oxacillin, or nafcillin, should be used till culture reports come. The treatment should be continued for at least 4 weeks. If the organism is sensitive to penicillin, Penicillin G, 20-40 million units daily, should be used, and blood levels still increasedby giving bprobenecid. Supportive therapy, including blood therapy and Tv fluids is same as for other infections. COF is treated as usual. Emboli to major vessels, especially in the lower extremities, should be removed surgically in an emergency.

PERICARDITIS

Pericarditis is inflammation of pericardium (its visceral and parietal surfaces) Pericardium is only rarely affected as an isolated structure, usually its involvement is associated with more generalized processes. The commonest cause is rheumatic In children pericardial disease takes the form of acute pericarditis and in most cases, there is effusion of fluid into the pericardial cavity. The consequences of such effusion will depend on its amount, type, and speed of formation. Under certain circumstances serious compression of the heart occurs. The direct compression and the body's attempatients to correct it results in cardiac tamponed. Unless the pericardial fluid is evacuated, death occurs very rapidly. The effects on circulation depend on theamount of fluid, speed of accumulation, and myocardial efficiency; a small amount of fluid with normal myocardium is compatible with normal CVS dynamics. In comparison, the accumulation of large amounts of fluid in the pericardium with a normal myocardium may result in cardiac tamponade. Smaller amounts of fluid with a diseased myocardium may also result in cardiac tamponade, as in acute rheumatic fever. In long standing chronic constrictive pericarditis. also, cardiac compression. The physiologic abnormality in cardiac compression is inadequate diastolicfilling of the ventricles, which results in increased pressure in both atria and in the venous systems. The stroke volume is small and almost fixed. Cardiac output is maintained by tachycardia, and reflex vasoconstriction maintains the blood pressure.

ETIOLOGY

Rheumatic fever is the most common cause of pericarditis in pediatric age group. Pericarditis may be primary (rheumatic, viral, post cardiotomy, purulent, traumatic or tuberculosis), or an intercurrent manifestation of systemic disease (effusion resulting from CCF, or associated withuremia, Rheumatoid arthritis, SLE, polyarthritis nodosa, primary or secondary neoplastic disease, hemolytic disease as leukemia, Cooley 's anemia, and congenital hypo plastic anemia).
More common causes are rh fever, Rheumatoid arthritis, pyogenic or viral infection, uremia, neoplastic, and cardiac surgery (postpericardiotomy syndrome); less common are TB, collagen disorder, anemia (thalassemia), ulcerative colitis, Friedrich ataxia, and following owing radiation Pericarditis maybe acute or chronic; when acute the exudate may be serous, fibrinous, serofibrinous, purulent or hemorrhagic when chronic, pericarditis is always associated with fibro elastic proliferation, leading to pericardial thickening or pericardial sac obliteration with or without the constriction of theheart.

CLINICAL FEATURES:

Essentials of diagnosis in pericarditis are retrosternal pain made worse by deep inspiration, and decreased by leaning forward: fever, shortness of breath and grunting respiratorys; tachycardia, pericardial friction rub, hepatomegaly and raised JVP. The symptoms will chiefly depend on the cause of pericarditis. Pain is common but may not be present and varies in intensity location or distribution. Since the lower one-third of the pericardium is innervated by phrenic nerve, pain may be referred to the neck or shoulder. The pain is usually sharp and stabbing, located in the midchest and in the shoulder or neck, made worse by inspiration and coughing (especially when it is pericardial ang pleural), when it may be referred to the back. Otherwise, it may be a localized dull precordialache. The pain may be localized to left shoulder, neck, scapula, precordial region, it is exaggerated by deep inspiration, coughing, or lying down, but relieved by sitting up and leaning forward. Shortness of breath and grunting respiratory are common in all pts. Physical signs usually depend on the amount of fluid present. In the absence of significant accumulation of fluid, the pulses are normal and the level of the JVP is normal. A characteristic, friction rub maybe heard, it is superficial, high pitched (but may be of varying intensity has no definite r relation with heart sounds., may be only transiently heard, is heard usually over the heart (precordial area), but frequently over the lower left sternal border. It can be heard by both bell and diaphragm of the stetho and remains audible when the patient holds his breath. Friction rub may be heard even with large accumulation of fluid. The heart sounds are usually normal, and the heart isnot enlarged on percussion. At this stage, ECG may show Widespread ST-T changes. X-ray chest is not of help. When there is considerable accumulation of fluid, the precordium on inspection is hypo dynamic and very quiet. But on percussion heart is enlarged. Apical impulse is difficult to locate. With large accumulation of fluid, fluid may be detected by percussion, and shifting dullness, and by recognizing that the apical impulse is well within the border of cardiac dullness. Heart sounds are muffled and distant. The friction rub is usually absent but may be audible at the base. Since the venous pressure varies with the intracardiac pressure, if intracardiac pressure is raised, venous pressure also is raised, especially during inspiration. Thus, neck veins become distended, but there are no pulsations usually. Hepatomegaly, ascites, and edema may also be present. The pulse is normal and small in volume, or it is paradoxical the pulse becoming smaller or disappears during inspiration (This s sign can be confirmed by measuring the blood pressure during the phases of respiratory.) Systolic BP falls during inspiration, but diastolic pressure may be high. In the absence of cardiac tamponade, peripheral venous and arterial pulses are normal. A small rapid pulse is found in patients with a tense pericardium and a low cardiac output. Cardiac tamponade is characterized by distension of jugular veins, tachycardia, enlargement of the liver, peripheral edema, and pulses paradox (in which systolic BP falls by more than 10mm Hg during inspiration; it is an accentuation of a normal event only during the normal inspiration, systolic BP falls by not more than 5 mm Patient with tamponade is critically ill, anxious, has dyspnea and discomfort may be so severe that the patient prefers a sitting position with the head bent on his knees. An irritating cough may be present, caused by t the pulmonary congestion, or by pressure of the pericardium on the trachea. If t the patient is extremely ill and has evidence of pericarditis and effusion (other findings may not all be present), treatment for tamponade should be instituted. Patient may have all the signs and symptoms of right sided CCF. Effusion may result in pressure on the left main bronchus, with collapse of the left lung leading to percussion dullness and bronchial breathing at the left base (Ewarts sign); similar changes mayoccur with secondary pleural effusion. ECG changes: The findings very of acute pericarditis withor without effusion often show a decrease in amplitude of all the waves, especially of QRS complex.; Low voltage is commonly seen in patients with significant pericardial effusion (but the voltage may be normal): In the earlier cases, ST segment is elevated, T wave exaggerated and QRS low, but after the acute stage subsides, ST becomes depressed and T wave, rounded, flattened, diphasic, or inverted, and lower in voltage. Usually during the first week, ST is elevated, T upright; after first week, ST normal, T flattened after second week, T Wave gets inverted; the graph returns to normal when the pericarditis heals, but Twave inversion persists for weeks to months after recovery. In contrast to patients with myocardial infarction, there is no reciprocal relationship between the findings in lead I and lead III in the frontal plane and the right and left precordial leads.

X-RAY

These vary with the extent of fluid accumulation. In dry pericarditis, there are no abnormal findings with large accumulation, the cardiopericard radial shadow is enlarged, and the normal contours are Fluoroscopy shows absent or diminished marginal pulsations. The heart assumes a pear-shaped, globular, or bottle-shaped shadow, with blunting of the cardioparenic angles. Other features may be changes in the shape of the cardiac silhouette with changes in posture, divergent vascular shadows at the base, an acute right cardio phrenic angle, and rapid changes in the size of the cardio pericardial shadow. The X-ray changes may closely be simulated by acute cardiac dilatation. With cardiac tamponade, pulmonary fields are clear, in contrast to myocardial dilatation, where there is pulmonary congestion). Fluoroscopy shows the absence of cardiac pulsations of the cardiac borders, while as in myocarditis, pulsations, even if feeble, are present.
Pericardial calcification because of constrictive pericarditis is rare in children. Echocardiography confirms pericardial effusion-separation of the cardiac chambers from the pericardium by echo-free fluid is evident, and the amount of fluid can even be quantified in older child. Cardiac catheterization reveals an increased pulmonary capillary and right atrial pressure.

PERICARDIOCENTESIS:

If the purulent fluid is suspected, exploratory pericardiocentesis is indicated, and cultural sensitivity of the fluid is done. Usually, the culture is -ve in cases of pyopericardium, which is a sequela of septicemia; staph may sometimes be detected. Cardiac tamponade is a medical emergency, and if fidaccumulates rapidly and remains undetected, death occurs. If the cardiac output is not maintained during cardiac compression, patient goes into shock. The intrapericardial pressure must berelieved immediately, usually by pericardiocentesis. In milder cases, primary disease and cardiac failure should be addressed, in cardiac tamponade of any cause, the fluid should be removed in an emergency by needle insertion, but it best is to perform a wide set resection of the pericardium through a surgical insertion. In chronic cases, to prevent the accumulation of fluid or to relieve obstruction, pericardiectomy is needed. By percussion or X-ray, the location of the left cardiac borders the location of the left cardiac border is determined. The safest site for the introduction of need le is through the diaphragm head ward under the xiphoid cartilage. The other site is 1-2 cm within the area of cardiac dullness in the 4th or 5th space. The site is infiltrated with procaine then a needle is inserted. A relatively blunt needle (18-20 gauge) on a sterile 10 ml syringe is inserted as the needle passes the rough chest wall, aspiration is started, and as much fluid is withdrawn as possible with ease. Underlying conditions and cardiac failure are treated. If pus is too thick, or when there are fibrous bands of chronic adhesive pericarditis, surgery is indicated if treated early; development of restrictive pericarditis is rare.

RHEUMATIC PERICARDITIS:

When pericarditis occurs with acute fever, there is pericarditis (there is pericarditis, myocarditis, and endocarditis). Thus, heart murmurs are always present. Pericarditis is usually fibrinous or serofibrinous, usually there is no significant accumulation of fluid. The fever, dyspnea, pericardial pain heart is enlarged. Treatment is directed to the illness, the relief of pain, and if in rare instances tamponade occurs, pericardiocentesis occurs.

Pericarditis dramatically responds to cortical steroids, usually disappearing within 1 week of the treatment. Constrictive pericarditis never occurs following this disease, Rh pericarditis does not produce serious side effects, but there is usually extensive carditis and potentially poor long- term prognosis. Differential diagnosis is by echocardiography, from acute cardiac dilatation. It can be differentiated from other forms of dry pericarditis (as acute beniga pericarditis) significantsystolic or diastolic murmurs and other evidence of RHD.

VIRAL PERICARDITIS:

Acute viral or idiopathic pericarditis frequently follows an upper respiratory tract infection, andthere is usually a previous h/o a protracted Reinfections The average latent period is 12 days.
Viral pericarditis is rare in children ad and usually due to Coxsackie virus B-4, but influenza virus may be involved. The onset is acute with fever, pericardial pain, and friction rub. Effusionis straw-colored, of varying amounts, but cardiac compression is rare. Effusion lasts for severalweeks, and recurrences of pericardial effusion are quite common or even months or years after the initial episode. Although the disease is usually benign without benign without any aftereffects, multiple recurrences are noted in 20% cases, and constrictive pericarditis has been reported in this disease. Aspirin is all that is needed, but corticosteroid therapy may be considered in the severe patient or patients with multiple recurrences.

PURULENT PERICARDITIS

Produced by a variety of bacteria, such as H influenza, Stap aurous, strep and pneumococci, E. coli.This is always secondary to an infection somewhere else, though the primary site is not always apparent. Usually follows pneumonia. It is mostly seen in infants than older children.

Generalized septicemia or osteomyelitis may also cause septic pericarditis (metastatic lesion). The purulent exidate is of varying consistency, and a coagulated mass of fibrin and pusare common. The patients is acutely ill, with fever, pericardial pain, tachypnea; thus, the patients in addition to hating cardiac compression are very septic and have very high fever; the flu id collected is usually quite thick and filled with polymorphs. The heart is enlarged, murmurs are insignificant, friction rub may or may not be present. Culture is done and antibiotics given.
Though antibiotics sterilize the fluid, tamponade commonly develops, and evacuation of the pericardial sac is usually necessary since pericardiocentesis yields only small amounts of pusdue to consistency of the exudate and multiple locutions. Therefore, wide resection of the pericardium through a surgical incision performed in the theatre is most desirable. Drainage offluid and antibiotic gives excellent results, and the long-term prognosis is usually good.

CHRONIC PERICARDITIS

Chronic constrictive pericarditis rare in children usually the cause is unknown, but often the disease follows tuberculosis, occasionally septic or acute nonspecific pericarditis may lead to it. It is insidious in onset and may not be detected early, sometimes the chronic pericarditis remains small and does not need removal, but some cases slowly progress to develop constrictive pericarditis, when cardiac tamponade occurs, which must be differentiated from chr COF and restrictive cardiomyopathy. Atrial fibrillation may occur if the constriction is severe, pericardiotomy is needed. 2-Uremie-perieardi tiB-In SEA countries, constrictive pericarditis is not rare, but is missed easily the features are that of cardiac tamponade with hepatomegaly, ascites, engorged neck veins, in a patient once the diagnosis is suspected search for TB must be made elsewhere, and for calcifications in the pericardium on x-ray. 2-Uremic pericarditis, pericardial involvement in collagen diseases. SLE and Rheumatoid arthritis are quite rare inchildren. Pericarditis may occur at any stage of Rheumatoid arthritis and may precede the typical joint manifestations. Effusion is and friction rub is common. Pericarditis improves when the disease is stabilized. In the terminal stage of uremia, a friction rub may appear, or significant accumulation of pericardial fluid may occur. Echocardiography confirms the diagnosis. The fluid resolves with dialysis or after successful renal transplantation. 3-Tuberculous pericarditis is usually secondary to a lesion in the hilar nodes or in the lung. Effusion is common and followedby a fibrotic reaction which may result in constrictive pericarditis. The onset may be insidious orassociated with cough, dyspnea, fever, weight loss and night sweats. The diagnosis depends on finding of Tb elsewhere, or recovery of the organism from the sputum, gastric washings, or the pericardial fluid. The effusion clears more rapidly if corticosteroids are added to antil B therapy.

POSTOPERATIVE PERICARDITIS

Postoperative Pericarditis may follow any direct surgical procedure in the heart.

Friction rubs are common during the first 2 weeks after operation. Some patients may have thepostcardiotomy syndrome.

CYANOSIS:

The two major clues to the presence of heart disease in infants and children are COF and cyanosis. Since the presence of 4-58% reduced Hemoglobin is necessary for cyanosis, a patient with sufficient anemia may not appear blue, and if Hemoglobin is very high (polycythemia), patient can appear blue even withsufficient oxygen saturation. Cyanosis may be due to CNS diseases, blood disorders, heart disease or pulmonary disease. Absence of a heart murmur, an ECG showing the usual right ventrhypertrophy of the newborn, and a chest X-ray showing borderline heart size and vascularity could befound to be caused by heart, lung, blood, or CNS disease. A chest X-ray showing no evidence of pulmonary disease and a rise in arterial po2 from 35-38mm would be assesses which can provide strong evidence of cyanosis being of cardiac origin. In all the four major CVS diseases of children-CHD, RHD, atherosclerosis, and hypertension-there is a genetic component and an important environmental interaction (except for very small percentage of causes ofCHD, atherosclerosis, and hypertension that have a mend Elian or chromosomal basis).

Cardiac disease in children may be congenital or acquired. In the neonates and during infancy, most cardiac lesions are congenital anomalies. In later childhood acquired lesions are commonespecially RHD and myocarditis following infectious diseases. Degenerative diseases of the heart andthose due to metabolic disturbances are infrequent during childhood.

CONGENITAL HEART DISEASES

Congenital heart diseases are the most common category of congenital structural malformation and isseen in 1% of children (8-9/1000 live births). Severe disease is seen in 1:400 infants. More than 50% patients will be dead by the first birthday if not treated (accounts for 50% of the deaths caused by congenital defects in the first-year curative or palliative surgery is available for over 90% of the lesions. Most lesions are single lesions and don 't causes any difficulty during childhood. The more complex lesions often present with severe cardiac symptoms soon after birth. Of all the deaths attributable to CHD, one-third rd occur during the neonatal period, and an additional 1/3 before the age of 1 year The commonest lesion is VSD, followed by tetralogy of fallot and PDA, pulmonary stenosis, ASD, aortic stenosis, and transposition and coarctation of the aorta. The commonest cyanotic lesion is VSD, and the commonest cyanotic lesion is tetralogy.

ETIOLOGY:

All known causes, including German measles, account for only less than 2% of CHD. Therefore, CHD is preventable to a certain extent only. Forces causing the abnormal development of the heart should operate between 2-8 weeks of embryonic life, as the fetal heart is completely developed by the end of 8 weeks of fetal life. other associated anomalies of CHD may be mongolism, arachnodactyly, Turners syndrome and transposition of viscera. Three of CHD is of single mutant gene origin (usually as part of a syndrome such as Ulrich-Noonan syndrome; 5% are associatedwith chromosomal aberrations such as Downs syndrome, and others have multifactorial inheritance, where there is apolygenetic hereditary predisposition interacting with an environmental trigger as dextro-amphetamine, progestogen-estrogen compounds many drugs, virus, and other environmental teratogens. Among genetic factors are chromosomal factors, such as Turner's syndrome is associate with aortic coarctation or conditions resulting from single gene defect aamutation such as Ellis-Can Crevelds syndrome, single atrium, or atrial defects. Environmental factors include viral infections, such as rubella associated with peripheral pulmonary stenosis, drugs, oraggressive perinatal care of premature RDS requiring respiratory therapy associated with persistent PDA. The great majority of cases are explained by multi factorial genetic-environmental interaction. Maternal rubella is associated with PDA and pulmonary arterial branch stenosis especially. It does not require a hereditary predisposition to produce PDA and pulmonary artery branch stenosis, but for lesions like VSD, a family history is often found even when it occurs with maternal rubella. The special etiologic relationship of rubella with PDA and pulmonary artery branch stenosis may be related to the active proliferation of the virus in the vascular intima Coxsackie B has been implicated in the causation of endocardia fibroelastosis. The role of mump virus is not established, the presence of toxoplasma virus in the heart does not produce any functional cardiac disturbance; late manifestations of congenital syphilis may include sortitis andaneurysm. The implication of CMV and adenovirus is not definite yet.

The highest incidence of CHD has been seen with thalidomide syndrome. The off springs of mothers on anticonvulsant therapy also have a higher incidence of CHD cleft palate and cleft lip. The incidence of PDA is higher among populations living at high altitudes, and cardiac malformations (especially TGA and VSD) are more common in children of prediabetic mothers. Though the incidence of CHD in the general population is 8-9/1000, the incidence in siblings is 14- 22/1000. The empiric recurrence risks are about 4.4% on VSD,3.4 in PDA, 3.2 with ASD, 52.9%for pulmonary stenosis and 2.7 for tetralogy. Generally, only one of the two twins is affected. Associated non-cardiac malformations are common especially with VSD and double outlet right ventricle. These are uncommon with TGA and aortic stenosis. The more common-associated anomalies are cleft palate and renal anomalies. Scoliosis occurs more frequently with cyanotic CHD. The more common the lesion, the higher the recurrence risk. Most often, the diagnosis of CHD is made on history, physical findings, and X-ray and ECE. If doubt is there, cardiac catheterization, selective angiography, angiocardiography, and aortography are done to confirm.

CLASSIFICATION OF CHD

CHD is divided into cyanotic, a cyanotic and potentially cyanotic diseases. A cyanotic CHD: (inorder of frequency) with L-R shunt With R-I shunt VSD, PDA, ASD, persistent AV canal, Pulmonary stenosis, aortic stenosis, aeration-of-Serta partial anomalous coarctation of aorta, vascular ring, pulmonary venus return, aortic pulmonary endocardia 1'i

broclastosis, coromilly window. Artery abnormalities.
Cyanotic (R-L shunt) Tetralogy, TGA, common ventricle, hypo plastic left heart syndrome, total anomalous, pulmonary venous return, tricuspid atresia, pulmonary atresia, persistent truncus arteriosus, double outlet right ventricle, and Ebstein's anomaly of the tricuspid valve.
Potentially cyanotic disease is those which under certain adverse conditions manifest cyanosis,as with high pulmonary resistance, as VSD, PDA.
Persistent cyanosis in CHD is due to shunting of venous blood from the right to left side of the heart, so that it passes the- into the systemic circulation without being oxygenated in the lungs. By convention, patients with R-L shunts fall into the cyanotic category, whether they have readily recognizable cyanosis or not patients who do not have R-L shunts, even if they are cyanotic for other reasons as low cardiac output, are placed in the non-cyanotic group
Whatever brings 4-58 of unsatrtdHemoglobin to the capillary bed produces cyanosis. If 4-56 of unsaturated Hemoglobin is not present, asin CRD with anemia, cyanosis is not present.

PHYSIOLOGIC AND HEMODYNAMIC CONSIDERATIONS

The fetal circulation has two parallel circulations. Blood is oxygenated in the placenta and is returned to the heart via the umbilical veins and inferior vena cava. The inferior vena cava return is made up of oxygenated placental blood and deoxygenated blood from the lower body and represents 60-70% of the total venous return to the heart. A further 20-25% of the total venous return occurs through the superior vena cava. Of the IVC return, about one-third is directed across the patent foramen ovule into the left atrium, where it is joined by pulmonary venous blood and a small contribution from the SVC. This mixture of left atrial blood has a higher concentration of oxygen than SVC blood) is distributed to the coronary circulation, upper extremities, and head through the left ventricle. The total ventricular output is about 35% of the total venous return to the heart. The remainder of IVC blood, together with nearly all superior VC and coronary sinus: blood, is directed through the tricuspid valve into the right ventricle and pumped into the main pulmonary artery. Because the lungs are unexpanded and the pulmonary arteries are tortuous and kinked with extremely high resistance to blood flow, only a small quantity of blood can enter the pulmonary circulation; the res passes through the duct's arterioles into the descending aorta, where it is joined by a small stream of blood crossing the isthmus of the aorta from the arch. This blood, which has a lower oxygen saturation than blood leaving the left ventricle, is distributed to the lower body and to the placenta for oxygenation. The placental component makes up about 40% of the combined ventricular output during birth, and immediately afterward, the circulation undergoes dramatic changes. The pulmonary and systemic circulations, in parallel in the fetus, now become established in series. With the removal of the low-resistant placental bed by umbilical artery clamping, there is a marked increase in systemic resistance and a fall in vena cava blood return to the right atrium. Consequently, a slight fall in right atrial procedures and pressures occurs. At the same time, lung expands ion produces a dramatic fall in pulmonary vascular resistance and a marked increase in pulmonary blood flow. These changes result in an increased return of blood to the left atrium through the pulmonary veins and a rise in left atrial pressure. Since the left atrial pressure exceeds that in the right atrium, the valve of the foramen ovule is closed. This normally occurs within a few minutes of birth, but anatomic closure may take many months, and any abnormality resulting in a higher right atrial pressure will allow the reopening of the foramen ovule, permitting blood flow from the right to the left atrium. The ductus arteriosus has a thick muscle coat that constricts in a high 02 environment. With the establishment of breathing and a rise in the oxygen center of the blood, the ductus constricts and finally closes, separating the pulmonary and aortic circulations. Functional closure occurs within 10-15 hours of birth, but the ductus may remain probe-patent for up to 21 days. However, the ductus may remain open when disturbances of oxygenation are present, such as RDS.

The initial fall in pulmonary vascular resistance and increase in pulmonary blood flow is sudden and marked. A more gradual fall in pulmonary vascular resistance occurs over 6-8 weeks. Pulmonaryarterial and right ventricular pressure also falls, stabilizing at about 1/5 of the systemic pressure. After circulatory adjustments following birth occur, the right and the left sides of heart communicate only indirectly through the pulmonary capillary bed and through the systemic capillary bed. Since pressure enhances- is usually higher on the left side than on the right side of the heart, any abnormal communication results in blood flow from left to right and no cyanosis is present. When defect is large, equalization of pressure may on the two sides of the defect occurs, a flow across the defects then becomes dependent upon the resistance to sulci flow Cyanosis is visible when venous blood enters the left side of the circulation
from the right side and when the magnitude of the shunt is sufficient to cause a concentration of 5€ or more of reduced Hemoglobin/100ml in the arterial system or an oxygen saturation of below 80%. This may occur when, in addition to an abnormal communication or defect, the pressure on the right side of the heart is higher than on the left. Such increase in right heart pressure is due to obstruction of blood flow distal to the abnormal communication and may be of congenital originas stenosis of tricuspid or pulmonary valve or acquired as progressive pulmonary obstructive vascular disease.

Most patients with CHD is asymptomatic, some are blue or present in cardiac failure. Physical examination may reveal bulging of the precordium due to cardiac enlargement and a prominent apical impulse indicating an enlarged left ventricle. Peripheral pulses palpated simultaneously inthe arm and leg may establish the diagnosis of coruscation when the femoral pulses are not palpable or weaker those at the prist. The reverse situation may be indicative of hypo plastic leftheart syndrome. Bounding pulses usually suggest an aortic-pulmonary shunt or semilunar valvular insufficiency. Cyanosis should be sought by examining the mucous membranes, lips, and nail beds. Cyanosis of upper limbs only without cyanosis of the lower half of the body, or vice versa, is associated with some specific abnormalities. Clubbing of the nails usually accompanies moderate cyanosis that has been present for a long period of time. In the neonate, cyanosis of pulmonary disease is confused with that of cardiac disease. Crying usually increases the cyanosis of cardiac disease, while pulmonary cyanosis usually improves. Administration of 100% oxygen may improve the patient with cardiac disease, but the cyanosis of pulmonary disease usually disappears Arterial oxygen tension in an atmosphere of 100% oxygen in cardiac cyanosis will bebelow 100 mm but in pulmonary disease it will rise above 100 mm Hg. Cardiac cyanosis usuallyindicates severe disease in neonate. In older child with cyanosis is, functional deterioration may be monitored with hematocrit and hemoglobin determinations that will show a steady increase asR-L shunting increases and pulmonary blood flow falls.

Cardiac failure due to congenital heart disease is rarely seen after the age of 6 months. Its presence indicates a severe cardiac anomaly. The manifestation of cardiac failure in older child isthat in the adults. In infants, neck vein distension and peripheral edema are rarely observed manifestations in the pulmonary neonate are related to impairment of myocardia} function and congestion in the pulmonary and systemic venous systems. Impaired myocardial function is manifest in cardiac enlargement tachycardia above 160 beats. /min in infants and above 100/min in older child, gallop rhythm, and weak peripheral pulses associated with low blood pressure andcold extremities, and less frequently pulsus alterans and pulsus paradoxical. Growth failure is seen when the cardiac failure is chronic. Pulmonary venous congestion is manifest by tachypnea, shallow respirator, dyspnea retractions of the suprasternal notch and at the level of the diaphragm, wheezing and rales may be present. The hall mark of systemic venous congestion is hepatomegaly. Typical murmurs pinpoint the lesion. Murmurs may occur during any phase of the cardiac cycle and are graded from 1-4 depending on their intensity. Those of loud intensity are usually accompanied by a palpable thrill. Systolic murmurs may be ejection type (crescendo or decrescendo) or holosystolic. The ejection murmur may be benign or organic (depending on the quality and site of origin, and the age of the pt, and usually occurs shortly after the first heart sound. When innocent (occurring in 60% of children) they are low-pitched have a vibratory quality and are usually localized to the mid-parasternal area. These murmurs vary in intensity with changing position. Organic ejections murmurs may be due to stenosis lesions of semilunar valves, or shunt lesions at the atrial level. Holosystolic murmurs commence with the first heart sound, are heard throughout the systole, have a plateau type of configuration, and end with the second heart sound; these are always organic in origin. Diastolic murmurs are always of organic nature. These either indicate semilunar valve regurgitation, or when occurring later, may be associated with increased flow. ECG helps in estimating a trial enlargement and ventricular hypertrophy. The normal full-term neonate has a dominant right ventricle (since much of fetal circulation has been supported by right ventricle), therefore the ECG shows right axis deviation and right vent predominance. As the left ventricular takes over the support of the systemic circulation, the mean cardiac axis shifts to the left deviation from the expected normal pattern forage may suggest) a specific anomaly.

References:

1. Dr Benjamin Alli. Bureaucrats undermine Trump's COVID-19 plan, bolstering Joe Biden. RealClearHealth - Opinion, News, Analysis, Video and Polls. https://www.realclearhealth.com/articles/2020/03/25/bureaucrats_undermine_trumps_cov id-19_plan_bolstering_joe_biden 111002.html
2. Alli, B. (2019, May 8). Will Congress stand up for healthcare innovation? Patient Daily. https://patientdaily.com/stories/512482138-will-congress-stand-up-for-healthcare- innovation
3. Alli, B., and Contributor, O. (2019, April 15). 3 signs the PBMs are desperately in need ofreform. The Hill. https://thehill.com/opinion/healthcare/438943-3-signs-the-pbms-are- desperately-in-need-of-reform
4. American Academy of Neurology. (2019, April 30). Cannabis-based medicine may reduce seizures for children with difficult-to-Treat epilepsy. PR Newswire: press release distribution, targeting, monitoring, and marketing. https://www.prnewswire.com/news- releases/cannabis-based-medicine-may-reduce-seizures-for-children-with-difficult-to-treat-epilepsy-300841365.html
5. BENJAMIN ALLI. (2019, September 3). Surprise billing: A blight that needs to be fixedby doctors, not the government. Morning Consult. https://morningconsult.com/opinions/surprise-billing-blight-needs-fixed-by-doctors-not-government/
6. Benjamin A. Alli, (n.d.). National Center for Biotechnology Information. https://www.ncbi.nlm.nih.gov/pmc/articles/PMC2536916/pdf/jnma00009-0039.pdf
7. Billiamin A. Alli, (n.d.). National Center for Biotechnology Information. https://www.ncbi.nlm.nih.gov/pmc/articles/PMC2537146/pdf/jnma00017-0059.pdf
8. Dr. Benjamin Alli. (2020, March 27). Would a long-term

COVID-19 shutdown be detrimental to public health? Real Clear Health - Opinion, News, Analysis, Video andPolls. https://www.realclearhealth.com/articles/2020/03/27/would_a_long-term_covid-19_shutdown_be_detrimental_to_public_health_111006.html

9. Dr. Benjamin Alli. (n.d.). How Trump can save rural health care. American Thinker. https://www.americanthinker.com/articles/2020/02/how_trump_can_save_rural_health_c are.html

Conclusion

This book can provide a comprehensive overview of neonatal care, covering a wide range of topics related to the care and management of newborn infants. We have explored the anatomy and physiology of the neonatal period, the common medical conditions and disorders that affect newborns, and the various diagnostic and treatment options available to healthcare professionals.

As we have seen throughout the book, neonatal care requires a specialized set of skills and knowledge, as well as a high level of attentiveness and care. The care provided to newborn infants can have a profound impact on their health and development, both in the short and long term.

While this book provides a thorough overview of the current state of knowledge and practice related to neonatal care, there is still much to be learned and explored in this field. Further research is needed to better understand the underlying causes of neonatal conditions and disorders, to identify new and effective treatment options, and to improve the overall quality of care for newborn infants.

In the meantime, we encourage healthcare professionals to continue to stay up-to-date with the latest research and best practices related to neonatal care, and to work collaboratively to provide the highest level of care possible to the newborn infants under their care. By doing so, we can help to ensure that all newborns have the best possible start in life.

Appendix 1: Dubowtiz Scoring of Neurological Signs

Dubowtiz scoring of neurological signs for assessment of gestational age:Neur sign Grades 0 1 2 3 4 5

Posture 0= arms and legs extended

Popliteal angle; 0=180, 1=160, 2=130, 3=110, 4=90, 5=less than 90 degree. Heel to ear; 0=heel touches the head, and the degree of extension at the knee is 180

4=heel is far off from the head, and the knee extension is 90

Scarf sign: 0=elbow reaches opposite axillary line

1=elbow between midline and opposite axillary line2=elbow reaches midline,

3=elbow will not reach midline.

Head lag; 0=complete lag,

1=partial head control,

2=able to maintain the head in line with the body,

3=brings the head anterior to the body.

Ventral. Suspension 0= the child droops with loosely falling extremities,

4=head raised, limbs flexed, and spine straightened.

Physical maturity scoring.

Skin; 0=gelatinous red, transparent 1=smooth, pink, visible veins, 2=superficial peeling or rash, few veins,3=cracking, palereas, rare veins,

4=parchment, deep, cracking, no vessels,5=leathery, crackled, wrinkled.

Lanugo 0=none, 1=abundant, 2=thinning, 3=bald areas, 4=mostly baldPlantar creases; 0=no creases,

1=Faint red marks,

2=Interior transverse crease only3=Creases interior 2/3rds only 4=crease cover entire sole.

Breast; 0=barely perceptible,1=flat areola, no bud,

2=stippled areola, bud 1-2 mm.3=raised areola, bud 3-4 mm.

4=areola, bud 5-10 mm

Ear: 0=pinna flat, stays folded,

1=slightly curved pinna, soft, slow recoil,2=well curved, soft, ready recoil.

3= Formed and firm, instant recoil,4=thick cartilage, ear stiff,

Genitalia, male; 0=scrotum empty, no rugae,

2=testes descending, few rugae,3=testes down, good rugae,

4=testes pendulous, deep rugae,

Genitalia, female; 0=prominent clitoris and labia minor,,

2=both labia major and minor equally prominent3=labia major large, minor small.

4=Clitoris and labia minor completely covered.

Score:	5	10	15	20	25	30	35	40	45	50
Weeks:	26	28	30	32	34	36	38	40	42	44

Appendix II: FIRST DAY OF LIFE

Descriptive Analysis of Special Problems, needs and care of infants in tropical countries,List of contents

A) General principles of Newborn Evaluation and Care:

Delivery room care 1. Establishing respiratory,

2. Apgar scoring
3. Conservation of body temperature
4. Care of the skin and cord
5. Care of the eyes.Birth recovery period
c. Regular nursery care

B) Physical Examination of the Newborn Infant

a) General appearance
b) Skin
c) Head
d) Face
e) Nose, eyes,
f) Ears
g) Mouth, throat, neck
h) heart, and CVS
i) abdomen; Anus
j) Genitalia; Extremities
k) Neurological examination
l) Feeding
m) Chest and respiratory system

C) Special Care of the High-Risk Infant

D) Multiple Births (Twins)

E) Low Birth Weight and Prematurity

a. Low birth weight
b. preterm infants with no fetal growth retardation

c. assessment of Gestational Age
d. pathology in LBW infants
e. Problems of Prematurity

F Care of the Preterm and LBW Ordinary and Special

a) General
b) Conservation of body temperature
c) Care of the umbilical cord
d) Role of the special care baby units
e) Transport of the baby
f) Feeding the premature baby

G) Intrauterine Growth Retardation

H) Small for Gestational Age Care of SGA infant (LFD and SFD) prevention of hypoglycemia inSGA infant

I) Post-term infants

J) Large for Gestational Age

K) Placental Dysfunction Syndrome

L) Delivery room care of the High-Risk Infant

a) Respiratory distress and failure
b) Failure to initiate or sustain respiratory
c) Delivery room care of the high-risk infants

M) Hypovolemic Shock in the Neonates

N) Oedema in the neonate

c) Phrenic nerve palsy, Facial nerve palsy, liver rupture,

Fractured clavicle.

Respiratory distress in Neonates

a) Causes of respiratory distress in the neonates
b) Heart Failure in the Newborns

c) Congenital Atelectasis
d) Meconium Aspiration
e) Transient Tachypnea of the Newborn
f) Persistent fetal circulation
g) Bronchopulmonary Dysplasia
h) Pneumonia in the Neonate
i) Aspiration of foreign materials

j) Air leak in the neonates
k) Idiopathic Respiratory distress Syndrome (RDS)
Complications of the Intensive Care

l) Use of oxygen in the neonates
m) Wilson Mikity Syndrome
n) Fung Cysts
o) Pulmonary Hemorrhage
p) Congenital pulmonary lymphangiectasia
q) Chylothorax
r) Apnea in the neonates
s) Necrotizing Enter colitis
t) Cyanosis in the Neonates
u) Some disorders are the special problems of premature.
v) Anemia in the neonates (Full-term and Premature)
w) Blood in the vomitus or stool
Some other Symptoms in the neonates

Appendix III: Special Care for the High-Risk Infant.

Special Care for the HIGH-RISK INFANT

Criteria for admission to the special care neonatal unit; -

Oligohydramnios and polyhydramnios

Duration of labor prime more than 24 hours. Multigravida more than 12 hours. OrSecond stage of labor more than 2 hours.

Ruptured membranes of 24 or more hours.LGA and SGA infants.

Maternal fever or infection

Placentae prevail or abruption placenta

Any difficult delivery or Apgar score of 5 or less at 1 min after birthHigh or mid-forceps delivery

Primary cesarean section for a brief duration, same for the breech delivery

Birth weight of under 2300g or over 4000g

Infant requiring resuscitation.

Appendix IV: Causes of Neonatal Respiratory distress.

CAUSES OF NEONATAL RESPIRATORY DISTRESS

1. Mechanical causes: Choanal atresia, Tracheoesophageal fistula, tracheal stenosis, Laryngeal web, Laryngomalacia Diaphragmatic hernia
2. Congenital lobar emphysema, pneumothorax, pneumomediastinum, chylothorax,Phrenic nerve palsy 2
3. Metabolic causes: Cold stress,
1. Acidosis, hypoglycemia hyponatremia,Shock,
2. Thyroid storm,Anemia
3 Maternal medication
4. 3) Cardiovascular: Congenital heart disease
5. CNS diseases Intracranial hemorrhage, cerebral edema
6. Primary pulmonary: Aspiration of amniotic fluid, blood, meconium Pneumonia, bacterial orviral, intrauterine, or postnatal
7. Congenital hypoplastic lung or agenesis
8. Alveolar hemorrhage
9. Transient tachypnea of the newborn (wet lung)
10. RDS (Pulmonary immaturity)

SCORING SYSTEM FOR EVALUATING THE SEVERITY

OF RESPIRATORY DISTRESS

	Grade 0	Grade 1
Upper Chest	Synchronized	Lag on Respiratory
Lower Chest	No Respiratory	Just Respiratory
Xiphoid Retraction	None	Just Minimal
Nares Dilation	None	Minimal
Expiratory Grunting	None	Stopped

Made in the USA
Monee, IL
13 May 2025

17411787R00272